Eicosanoids in Inflammatory Conditions of the Lung, Skin and Joints

ADVANCES IN EICOSANOID RESEARCH

Series Editor Keith Hillier

Eicosanoids and Reproduction
Edited by Keith Hillier

Eicosanoids in the Gastrointestinal Tract
Edited by Keith Hillier

Eicosanoids in Inflammatory Conditions of the Lung, Skin and Joints
Edited by Martin Church and Clive Robinson

Eicosanoids in the Cardiovascular and Renal Systems
Edited by Perry Halushka and Dale Mais

ADVANCES IN EICOSANOID RESEARCH

Series Editor Keith Hillier

Eicosanoids in Inflammatory Conditions of the Lung, Skin and Joints

Edited by

Martin Church

and

Clive Robinson

Department of Clinical Pharmacology
Faculty of Medicine
University of Southampton
UK

WKAP ARCHIEF

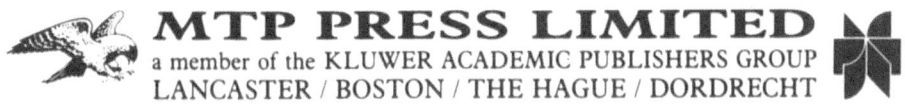

MTP PRESS LIMITED
a member of the KLUWER ACADEMIC PUBLISHERS GROUP
LANCASTER / BOSTON / THE HAGUE / DORDRECHT

Published in the UK and Europe by
MTP Press Limited
Falcon House
Lancaster, England

British Library Cataloguing in Publication Data

Eicosanoids in inflammatory conditions of the lung, skin and joints.
  1. Man. Inflammatory diseases. Role of eicosanoids
  I. Church, Martin, *1942–*   II. Robinson, Clive, *1958–*
  616'.0473

  ISBN-13:978-94-010-7070-6   e-ISBN-13:978-94-009-1283-0
  DOI: 10.1007/978-94-009-1283-0

Published in the USA by
MTP Press
A division of Kluwer Academic Publishers
101 Philip Drive
Norwell, MA 02061, USA

Library of Congress Cataloging in Publication Data

Eicosanoids in inflammatory conditions of the lung, skin, and joints.

  (Advances in eicosanoid research)
  Includes bibliographies and index.
  1. Inflammation — Pathophysiology. 2. Arachidonic acid — Derivatives — Physiological
effect. 3. Lungs — Pathophysiology. 4. Skin — Pathophysiology. 5. Joints —
Pathophysiology. I. Church, Martin, 1942–   .
II. Robinson, Clive, 1958–   . III. Series: Advances in eicosanoid research series. [DNLM:
1. Eicosanoic Acids — metabolism. 2. Inflammation — metabolism. QU 90 E343]
RB131.E45   1987   616'.0473   88-552
ISBN-13:978-94-010-7070-6

Copyright © 1988 MTP Press Limited
Softcover reprint of the hardcover 1st edition 1988

Typeset by Lasertext, Longford Trading Estate, Thomas Street, Stretford, Manchester M32 0JT

Contents

List of contributors

R. D. R. Camp
Institute of Dermatology
St. Thomas's Hospital
Lambeth Palace Road
London SE1 7EH
UK

M. K. Church
Clinical Pharmacology Group
University of Southampton
Southampton General Hospital
Southampton SO9 4XY
UK

O. Cromwell
Dept of Allergy/Clinical Immunology
Cardiothoracic Institute
76 Cale Street
London SW3 6NX
UK

F. M. Cunningham
Institute of Dermatology
St. Thomas's Hospital
Lambeth Palace Road
London SE1 7EH
UK

G. de Nucci
The William Harvey Research Institute
St. Bartholomew's Hospital Medical College
Charterhouse Square
London EC1M 6BQ
UK

B. J. Fitzsimmons
Medicinal Chemistry Department
Merck Frosst Canada Inc.
PO Box 1005, Pointe-Claire-Dorval
Quebec H9R 4P8
Canada

P. G. Hellewell
Department of Medicine and Pediatrics
National Jewish Center for Immunology and
    Respiratory Medicine
1400 Jackson Street
Denver, CO 80206
USA

B. Henderson
Pharmacology Department
Wellcome Research Laboratories
Langley Court, Beckenham
Kent BR3 3BS
UK

A. N. Payne
Department of Pharmacology
Wellcome Research Laboratories
Langley Court, Beckenham
Kent BR3 3BS
UK

E. R. Pettipher
Department of Pharmacology
Wellcome Research Laboratories
Langley Court, Beckenham
Kent BR3 3BS
UK

C. Robinson
Clinical Pharmacology Group
University of Southampton
Southampton General Hospital
Southampton SO9 4XY
UK

T. J. Rogers
Department of Microbiology and
    Immunology
Temple University School of Medicine
3400 N. Broad Street
Philadelphia, PA 19140
USA

J. Rokach
Research Administration
Merck Frosst Canada Inc.
PO Box 1005, Pointe-Claire-Dorval
Quebec H9R 4P8
Canada

T. J. Williams
Section of Vascular Biology
MRC Clinical Research Centre
Watford Road, Harrow
Middlesex HA1 3UJ
UK

Series Editor's Foreword

The original series, *Advances in Prostaglandin Research,* edited by Sultan M. M. Karim, was published by MTP Press in three volumes in 1975 and 1976. A glance at those books illustrates the progress that has been made since then. The thromboxanes were mentioned twice (first publication 1975) and prostacyclin not once (first publication 1976); leukotrienes were only on the horizon.

The amazing generation of research data in the last 10–15 years has given new, broad insights into many areas, including asthma, inflammation, renal, cardiovascular and gastrointestinal diseases and in reproduction, and has led in some instances to real clinical benefit.

This series, *Advances in Eicosanoid Research,* reflects the current understanding of prostaglandins, thromboxanes and leukotrienes. The aim is to provide an introductory background to each topic and the most up-to-date information available.

Although each book stands alone, the eicosanoids cut across many boundaries in their basic actions; selected chapters from each book in the series will provide illuminating and productive information for all readers which will advance their education and research.

In the production of this series, I must acknowledge with pleasure my collaboration with editors and authors and the patient endeavours of Dr Michael Brewis and the staff at MTP Press.

KEITH HILLIER
University of Southampton
England

*They are ill discoverers that think
there is no land, when they can see
nothing but sea*

Francis Bacon

Preface

Inflammation research continues to progress at an outstanding pace. In such a rapidly expanding subject it is difficult for specialists to keep abreast of current thinking and developments in disciplines which are outside their immediate sphere of interest but which may have a close bearing on their own research. In this volume we have sought to draw together a series of personal introductions and reviews on the likely roles of eicosanoids in inflammatory diseases of the lung, skin and joints. The book is not intended to be an introductory text on the biochemical mechanisms of eicosanoid biosynthesis, nor is it solely intended to be a treatise on the recent developments in particular spheres of eicosanoid research. Instead the book aims to bridge the gap between basic texts and the research literature, and we hope this will supply a valuable requirement of colleagues in other aspects of inflammation research.

We are indebted to all our colleagues who contributed a range of lively and informative chapters to this volume, and to Keith Hillier, the series editor, for his helpful suggestions. We would also like to thank Michael Brewis of MTP Press for his helpful and efficient guidance during the production process. Finally, we would have been lost without the most able and cheerful assistance of our secretary, Dianne Wilson.

MARTIN CHURCH
CLIVE ROBINSON
Southampton, October 1987

1
The Cellular and Molecular Basis of Eicosanoid Generation

M. K. CHURCH

Activation of eukaryotic cells almost invariably stimulates the cleavage of phospholipids and the resultant metabolism of the liberated fatty acids into biologically active intracellular and intercellular chemical messengers. Of these, the eicosanoids, or, more particularly, those products derived from arachidonic and closely related eicosapolyenoic acids, are the best characterized. Following its cleavage from the *sn*-2 position of membrane-associated phospholipids by phospholipase A$_2$, arachidonic acid undergoes either of two routes of metabolism to form cyclo-oxygenase or lipoxygenase products which have a plethora of biological functions. The possibility that these products, which include prostanoids and leukotrienes, are intimately related with the pathogenesis of inflammatory and allergic diseases has fascinated scientists and clinicians alike since long before their chemical characterization.

WHAT IS INFLAMMATION?

Inflammation is characterized clinically by redness, heat, swelling, tenderness and loss of function. At a cellular level it is characterized by tissue damage associated with a local accumulation of inflammatory leukocytes, including neutrophils, eosinophils, macrophages, lymphocytes and platelets. An adequate inflammatory response is an essential defence mechanism against invasion of the body with foreign insults, such as bacterial infections, parasites etc. However, some inflammatory reactions appear to be inappropriate and are the cause of considerable morbidity and, sometimes, mortality. Examples of such inflammatory reactions are asthma in the lung, urticaria in the skin and arthritis in the joints.

Clearly, inflammatory responses may differ in their nature largely depending on the stimulus for their initiation. As this chapter is not a treatise on inflammation, I have chosen inflammation subsequent to allergen provocation

1

in allergic asthma to illustrate some of the cellular events which occur. The most obvious event which follows allergen inhalation is an immediate bronchoconstriction. This is mediated by the action of bronchoconstrictor and vasoactive mediators released as a consequence of the activation of mast cells in the bronchial lumen and associated with the bronchial epithelium. These mediators, which are summarized in Table 1.1, include preformed granule-associated histamine and newly generated eicosanoids. Besides causing bronchoconstriction, mast cell mediators may also initiate the accumulation of inflammatory leukocytes which are associated with the late asthmatic reaction occurring 6–8 hours after provocation, and bronchial hyper-reactivity. Mast cell-derived histamine, leukotrienes, chemotactic factors and platelet activating factor (PAF-acether) all have chemokinetic and chemotactic potential for inflammatory leukocytes. The actions of mast cell mediators are augmented by the IgE-dependent release of leukotrienes and PAF-acether from resident and accumulating macrophages, eosinophils and platelets. The first event observed under the microscope is leukocyte margination or adherence of

Table 1.1 Preformed and newly generated mediators of human mast cells

Class	Mediator	Function
Amine	Histamine	H_1- and H_2-receptor stimulation, smooth muscle contraction, vasodilation, increased capillary permeability
Neutral protease	Tryptase	Cleavage of C_3 and C_{3a}, fibronogen and fibronectin
	Chymase (connective tissue mast cells only)	Cleavage of Type IV collagen, glucagon, neurotensin, fibronectin and heparin
	Carboxypeptidase	Acts together with tryptase and chymase
Acid hydrolases	β-Hexosaminidase	Cleavage of β-linked hexosamine from glycoproteins and complex carbohydrates
	β-Glucuronidase	Cleavage of glucuronic acid from complex carbohydrates
	β-D-Galactosidase	Cleavage of galactose from complex carbohydrates
	Arylsulphatase	Hydrolyses aromatic sulphate esters
Reducing enzymes	Superoxide dismutase	Converts O_2^- to H_2O_2
	Peroxidase	Converts H_2O_2 to H_2O
Chemotactic factors	ECF-A	Eosinophil chemotaxis, chemostasis and activation
	NCF-A	Neutrophil chemotaxis, chemostasis and activation
Proteoglycans	Heparin	Anti-coagulant, anti-complementary
Prostaglandins	PGD_2	Bronchoconstrictor, vasodilator, weak chemotactic agent for neutrophils and eosinophils
Leukotrienes	LTC_4 (LTD_4)	Bronchoconstrictor, vasodilator, weak chemotactic agent for neutrophils and eosinophils

2

leukocytes to the capillary walls. This is followed by extravasation of leukocytes which then migrate towards the source of the stimulus which, in asthma, is the bronchial epithelium and lumen. That this cell accumulation is organized rather than random is exemplified by a guinea pig model of asthma[1]. Examination of lung sections and cells recovered by broncho-alveolar lavage (BAL) has shown an influx of neutrophils which is demonstrable 2–6 h after provocation and reaches a maximum at 17–24 h. By 72 h, neutrophil numbers have returned to prechallenge levels. Eosinophil accumulation is, however, slower and more persistent. By 6 h after challenge, eosinophils may be seen tracking through the bronchial smooth muscle towards the lumen but few are recoverable by BAL. By 17 h, large numbers of eosinophils are seen beneath and between the bronchial epithelial cells, and by 72 h, they represent the dominant cell recoverable by BAL. The persistence of a lung eosinophilia in human asthma is well documented histologically.

To understand the mechanisms underlying the accumulation and activation of inflammatory cells and the effects of these inflammatory cells on the local environment in which they accumulate, we must understand the nature of the intercellular communication which mediates these events. This book will consider the role of eicosanoids as chemical mediators of inflammation.

PRODUCTION OF EICOSANOIDS

Eicosanoids derive primarily from arachidonic acid contained in phospholipids and, possibly to a lesser extent, in neutral lipids and cholesterol esters. It is possible that arachidonic acid may also be derived from cytoplasmic lipid bodies in mast cells and macrophages[2]. A necessary prerequisite for the majority of eicosanoid biosynthesis is the liberation of free arachidonic acid from membrane phospholipids (Figure 1.1). This event, which is thought to be the major rate-limiting step, presents arachidonic acid at the correct time and place for further metabolism. The major enzyme(s) for arachidonic acid liberation from membrane phospholipids[3] is the membrane-associated phospholipase A_2. The activity of this enzyme may be inhibited by lipocortin, a 30 000 dalton protein whose generation is induced by corticosteroids[4-6]. Generation of eicosanoids from mast cells is not, however, inhibited by corticosteroids. One possible explanation for this is that the majority of mast cell arachidonic acid is not generated by phospholipase A_2 but by diglyceride lipase cleavage of diacylglycerol generated from membrane phospholipid by the phospholipase C-like action of polyphosphoinoisitol phosphodiesterase[7-9]. Phospholipase C enzymes are not susceptible to inhibition by lipomodulin[4].

CYCLO-OXYGENASE PRODUCTS

Oxidation of arachidonic acid by the prostaglandin synthase enzyme complex results in the production of prostaglandins (PG) and thromboxane (Tx). In all tissues so far studied, arachidonic acid is oxidized initially by cyclo-oxygenase[10]

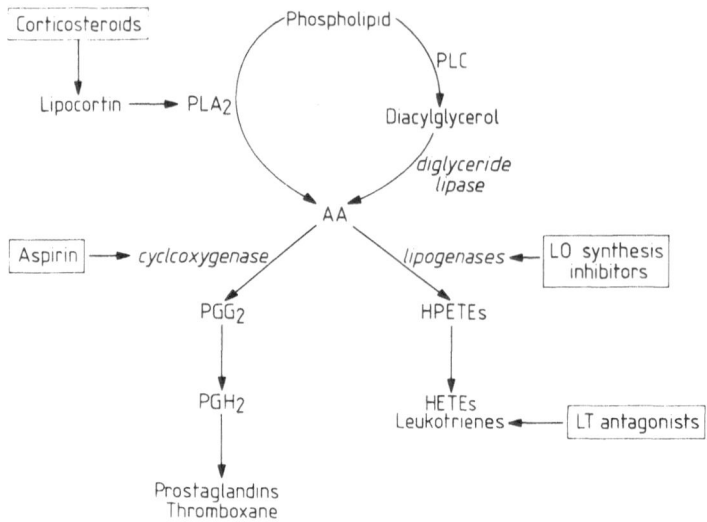

Figure 1.1 Generation of eicosanoids from arachidonic acid indicating the site of action of synthesis inhibitors and antagonists

to the 15-hydroperoxy endoperoxide PGG_2. Classically, PGG_2 is converted by a peroxidase to the endoperoxide PGH_2[11] which is subsequently metabolized by prostaglandins and thromboxanes by a series of cell- and species-specific enzymes whose activation may also be stimulus specific[12]. Formation of the PGH_2 intermediate is not, however, mandatory in the synthesis of some prostaglandins, e.g. PGE_2 which may be formed by the direct action of endoperoxide isomerase on PGG_2 and subsequent peroxidase-dependent metabolism of 15-hydroperoxy-PGE_2[13].

The spectrum of cyclo-oxygenase products which lung tissue is capable of generating include PGE_2[14-16], $PGF_{2\alpha}$[14-16], PGI_2[17,18], PGD_2[18-20] and TxA_2[18,21]. A qualitatively similar spectrum of prostanoids is generated by the skin[22-24].

This simple list of prostanoids does not take into account the many variables which have complicated research into prostaglandin generation, such as species, age, sex, immunological status and stimulus which provoked their synthesis. Species variation may be exemplified by the observation that TxA_2 is the major prostanoid produced by antigenic challenge of sensitized guinea-pig lung, accounting for more than 70% of total prostanoid biosynthesis[25]. In contrast, TxA_2 comprises only a small proportion of prostanoid release from human lung tissue[18,26] and is produced in negligible amounts from rat or rabbit lung[26,27]. Age may affect prostanoid generation, particularly around the time of birth. The ability of neonatal rabbit tissues to generate PGE_2 falls markedly at birth and recovers rapidly afterwards[28]. This transient fall in PGE_2 production may well be associated with the closure of the ductus arteriosus which is inhibited[29] by PGE_1, PGE_2 and PGI_2. Sex may also cause variations, particularly in the female where the oestrus cycle influences PG production[30]. It has even been suggested that exogenous arachidonic acid produces greater

PG generation from lungs of male rats compared with females[31].

Sensitization of animals is known to affect the ratio between PGI_2 and TxA_2 synthesis by guinea-pig lungs. Infusion of arachidonic acid into the lungs of unsensitized guinea pigs results in the release of PGI_2 as the predominant prostanoid. Following sensitization, the release of PGI_2 falls, whilst that of TxA_2 rises. After repeated challenge of animals with antigen, TxA_2 contributes more than 80% of the total prostanoid generation following infusion with arachidonic acid[21]. Berti et al.[32] have suggested that this change may result from the conversion of histamine H_2-receptors, which stimulate PGI_2 production, to H_1-receptors which, at least in the guinea pig, are associated with TxA_2 generation. Stimulation of histamine H_1-receptors has also been associated with prostanoid generation from human lung fragments[33] but not from cell dispersed from lung by enzymatic digestions[20]. That prostanoid generation is not secondary to bronchial smooth muscle contraction per se is suggested by the experiments of Hardy and colleagues[34].

LIPOXYGENASE PRODUCTS

Slow-reacting substance of anaphylaxis (SRS-A) was originally described by Kellaway and Trethewie[35] as a product of the immediate hypersensitivity reaction in guinea-pig lung which contracted smooth muscle more slowly than did histamine. The realization that the effects of SRS-A were not blocked by H_1-antagonists[36], which are of little use in the treatment of asthma[37], led to the hypothesis that this substance may be an important chemical mediator of asthma. However, it was not until 1979 that SRS-A yielded the secret of its chemical composition[38]. Until then, all that was known was that it was a polar sulphur-containing lipid of molecular weight around 500 daltons which could not be volatilized for structural analysis[39]. The experiments of Jakschik et al.[40] revealed that small quantities of radiolabel were present in SRS-A generated from rat basophil leukaemia cells which had previously been incubated with radiolabelled arachidonic acid and the recognition of dihydroxyeicosatetraenoic acids as a novel series of lipid products released from human neutrophils[41] paved the way for the identification of SRS-A released from murine mastocytoma cells by calcium ionophore A23187 as 5(S)-hydroxy-6(R)-S-glutathionyl-7(E),9(E),11(Z),14(Z)-eicosatetraenoic acid for which the group name leukotrienes was proposed[42]. The structure of LTC_4 was confirmed by total synthesis and comparison of the biological properties of the natural and synthetic products[43]. At about the same time, independent experiments employing mass spectrometry identified the covalent structure of LTD_4 as a product released following the challenge of guinea-pig lung[44]. Subsequent studies[45-47] have demonstrated SRS-A to be composed of LTC_4, LTD_4 and LTE_4.

The initial step in the production of leukotrienes and related products is the oxidation of arachidonic acid by one of a series of lipoxygenase enzymes. These enzymes require a penta-1,4-cis-diene in their substrates. Three such pairings are present in arachidonic acid, C5–C9, C8–C12 and C11–C15

5

(Figure 1.2). Single lipoxygenase reactions, catalysed by 5-, 12- and 15-lipoxygenase enzymes respectively, results in the formation of 6 possible hydroperoxyeicosatetraenoic acid (HPETE) products which rapidly undergo one of several different further transformations. A simple reduction yields the monohydroxyeicosatetraenoic acids (HETEs), of which 5-, 8-, 9-, 11-, 12- and 15-HETE have been identified. Further reaction of HPETEs, followed by reduction of their hydroperoxy groups, yields the di-HETEs of which 8,15-diHETE is the most common. A further transformation undergone by HPETEs is the formation of an epoxide derivative (e.g. LTA$_4$) which allows the formation of a variety of di-HETEs by non-enzymatic nucleophilic attack, specific di-HETEs by enzyme-catalysed reactions, e.g. to form LTB$_4$[48], or sulphidopeptide leukotrienes (LTs). Furthermore, 15-HPETE may also undergo transformation into tetraene tri-HETE derivatives of arachidonic acid known as the lipoxins of which lipoxin A ($5(S),6(R),15(S)$-trihydroxy-7,9,13(E)-11(Z)-eicosatetraenoic acid) and lipoxin B ($5,14,15(S)$-trihydroxy-6,8,10,12-eicosatetraenoic acid) have been identified[59-51].

The lipoxygenase products which have attracted most attention to date in the investigation of allergic and inflammatory diseases are the sulphidopeptide leukotrienes obtained from the 5-lipoxygenation of arachidonic acid. Following its generation by 5-lipoxygenase, 5-HPETE undergoes an elimination reaction to form the 5,6-epoxide, LTA$_4$, a reaction also catalysed by 5-lipoxygenase enzyme[52,53] (Figure 1.2). Under the influence of leukotriene C$_4$ synthase, a microsomal glutathione-S-transferase, nucleophilic attack by glutathione at C$_6$ produces the sulphidopeptide LTC$_4$[54,55]. Sequential hydrolytic removal of glutamic acid and glycine by γ-glutamyl transpeptidase and dipeptidase results in the formation of LTC$_4$ metabolic products, LTD$_4$ and LTE$_4$, respectively which, together with LTC$_4$, comprise the so called SRS-A or sulphidopeptide leukotrienes.

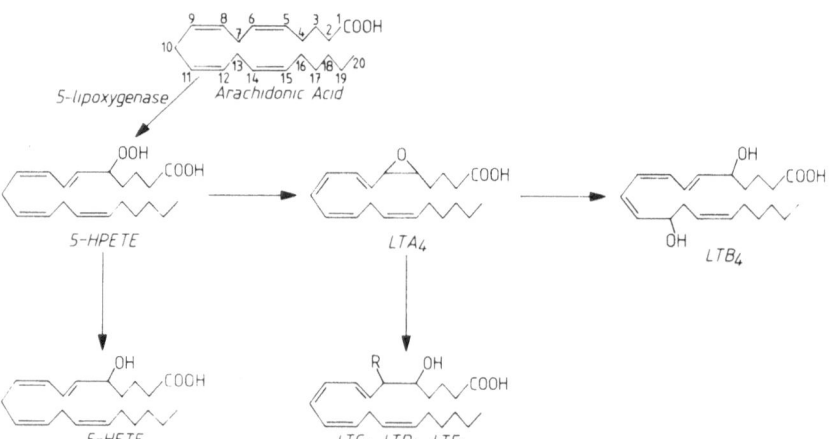

Figure 1.2 Generation of 5-HETE and leukotrienes from arachidonic acid. R = glutathione for LTC$_4$, cysteinylglycine for LTD$_4$ and cysteine for LTE$_4$

BIOLOGICAL EFFECTS OF EICOSANOIDS

Eicosanoids have a plethora of biological effects, influencing arterial and venous blood flow, capillary permeability, the tone of smooth muscle, cell chemotaxis/kinesis and the sensation of pain. Analysis of these effects is complex as eicosanoids may enhance or inhibit both each other's actions and the actions of other mediators released in inflammatory reactions.

In the lung, the cyclo-oxygenase products, PGG_2, PGH_2, $PGF_{2\alpha}$, PGD_2, TxA_2, the sulphidopeptide leukotrienes, LTC_4 and LTD_4, and lipoxin A are potent bronchoconstrictor agents. The most studied of these eicosanoids is $PGF_{2\alpha}$ which was originally reported to contract smooth muscle two decades ago[56,57]. When administered either intravenously or as an aerosol, $PGF_{2\alpha}$ causes an increase in airway resistance and a decrease in pulmonary compliance[58-61]. When administered to normal subjects by inhalation, $PGF_{2\alpha}$ causes an initial bronchoconstriction accompanied by irritation of the upper airways. With increasing concentrations, a recovery phase followed by a second dose-dependent bronchoconstriction ensues[62]. These two phases of bronchoconstriction have different mechanisms. The early phase, which is blocked by ipratropium bromide, is mediated by cholinergic reflexes, whilst the second, ipratropium bromide-resistant, phase is probably a direct action of $PGF_{2\alpha}$ on smooth muscle. Patients with asthma who show enhanced non-specific bronchial reactivity, are up to 1000 times more sensitive to the bronchoconstrictor effects of $PGF_{2\alpha}$ than normal subjects. This increase, which is greater than that occurring with histamine or methacholine, may be explained by the ability of $PGF_{2\alpha}$ to enhance lung responsiveness to other bronchoconstrictor agents[63,64].

The mast cell-generated prostaglandin, PGD_2, and its primary metabolite, $9\alpha,11\beta$-PGF, are 3.5 times more potent than $PGF_{2\alpha}$ and 30 times more potent than histamine in causing bronchoconstriction[65,66]. As 20–30 times more histamine than PGD_2 is released from lung mast cells on antigenic challenge[20], it would be expected that these mediators would contribute equally to the early asthmatic reaction. The prostaglandin endoperoxides, PGG_2 and PGH_2, are 5–10 times more potent than $PGF_{2\alpha}$ in causing smooth muscle contraction but their instability makes an evaluation of their biological role difficult. The availability of chemically synthesized endoperoxides will hopefully make this task easier. The association between the release of TxA_2 and bronchoconstriction in the guinea pig is well established[21]. However, its short half-life in aqueous solution, and the lack, until recently, of synthetic TxA_2 has prevented evaluation of exogenous TxA_2. Furthermore, the effects of TxA_2 in causing platelet aggregation are likely to preclude experiments with exogenous TxA_2 in man for ethical reasons.

In contrast to the bronchoconstrictor effects described above, some prostaglandins have bronchodilator effects, or act as functional antagonists of bronchoconstriction. PGE_2 has long been recognized as a bronchodilator both *in vitro*[57] and in man[67-69], although, in low concentrations, it may have some bronchoconstrictor action. Its effects on smooth muscle are mediated by its stimulation of receptors which activate adenylyl cyclase to elevate intracellular cyclic AMP[70]. The possible use of PGE_2 as a bronchodilator for asthma therapy is limited by its propensity to cause irritation of the upper respiratory tract causing coughing and transient bronchoconstriction[71], its diverse effects on other organs when absorbed systemically and its short biological half-life. PGI_2 is only a weak bronchodilator in the large diameter airways and its effects are only demonstrable in a small proportion of subjects who inhale it[72]. Interestingly, this prostaglandin, which also induces constriction of the small airways, appears to be functionally antagonistic in protecting the airways against the bronchoconstrictor effects of inhaled PGD_2.[73]

The original interest in the sulphidopeptide leukotrienes stemmed from their potent contractile effects on smooth muscle, particularly on the airways. Indeed, LTC_4 and LTD_4 are probably the most powerful bronchoconstrictors in man, being up to 100 times more potent than PGD_2 and 5000 times more potent than methacholine when inhaled by normal subjects. However, unlike histamine, methacholine, PGD_2 and $PGF_{2\alpha}$, where marked increases in sensitivity occur[74], the sensitivity to inhaled LTC_4 and LTD_4 is increased only marginally in asthma[75]. A further action of LTC_4 and LTD_4 which may be of relevance to asthma is their ability to increase bronchial mucus production[76].

The effect of eicosanoids on the microvasculature and their ability to cause the chemotactic accumulation of leukocytes are most easily demonstrated following their intradermal injection into the skin. In this situation, PGD_2 and $9\alpha,11\beta$-PGF_2 are weak vasodilators, but, unlike histamine, do not increase capillary permeability[77,78]. As such, they cause a flare reaction similar to that observed with histamine, albeit at concentrations some 50–100 times higher, but induce minimal wealing[77-79]. The ability of intradermal PGD_2 to cause a persistent erythema with neutrophil accumulation, but not cause a late reaction, as observed with antigen[77] indicates that this prostaglandin has either direct or indirect chemotactic activity but that it does not have the capacity to activate the influxed cells. Of the other prostanoids, PGE_2,[79,80] and PGI_2,[80] have both been reported to induce erythema on intradermal injection but their characteristics have been less well defined.

The lipoxygenase products also have potent effects on the microvasculature. LTC_4 and LTD_4, although causing vasoconstriction in the guinea pig[81], are vasodilatory in human skin and are equipotent with histamine in causing weal and flare reactions[82-84]. The ability to induce a marked weal also indicates that LTC_4 and LTD_4 increase capillary permeability allowing plasma exudation[81]. However, the sulphidopeptide leukotrienes are not chemotactic for leukocytes, as indicated by their failure to cause neutrophil or eosinophil accumulation locally after intradermal injection[77]. This is in contrast to LTB_4 whose actions in the skin appear to be entirely dependent upon leukocyte accumulation as a result of directed chemotaxis[77,82].

BIOLOGICAL SOURCES OF EICOSANOIDS

When considering the role of eicosanoids in inflammatory reactions, it is necessary to make three considerations. The first is the generation of eicosanoids from the cell which provides the initial trigger for the response, the effect of these mediators on the influx and activation of secondary inflammatory cells and their effects on the cells normally resident within the tissue. The second is the generation and effects of eicosanoids derived from the secondary inflammatory cells which include eosinophils, neutrophils, macrophages and platelets. The third is the stimulation of eicosanoid production by the cells normally resident within the tissue. Needless to say, the presence of disease means that the cells behaviour may be different from that predicted from a knowledge of their behaviour under normal conditions.

In vivo experiments or experiments using whole tissues, although giving a profile of eicosanoid production, do not throw light on the cellular source of the mediators. Knowledge of this is important to define the sequence of cell activation so that appropriate pharmacological intervention may be made. Likewise, histochemical studies, while giving an indication of the capacity of a cell to undertake lipid oxidation[85], do not define the products formed. Either cell culture or dispersion of tissues followed by purification of the individual cells liberated is necessary to localize eicosanoid production.

MAST CELLS

Cross-linkage of membrane bound IgE on the surface of the mast cell provides the initial trigger for the immediate hypersensitivity reaction. Mast cells obtained from the peritoneal cavity of the rat and those dispersed from human lung by proteolytic digestion and subsequently purified by countercurrent elutriation or density gradient centrifugation are the most extensively studied[80,87]. More recently, mast cells from human skin have been dispersed and purified[88]. With other tissues, studies have been performed on impure cell preparations containing less than 5% mast cells.

The most abundant cyclo-oxygenase product generated by mast cells is PGD_2. Indeed, the mast cell is the major source of this prostaglandin in allergic and inflammatory reactions. Maximal activation of human mast cells results in the generation of $50-100$ ng $PGD_2/10^6$ cells, $20-30$ times less than the amount of histamine released under the same conditions[20]. The major route for the primary metabolism of PGD_2 in man is its stereospecific 11-ketoreduction to $9\alpha,11\beta$-PGF_2[89,90]. This biologically active PGD_2 metabolite is then sequentially converted to the inactive compound, 13,14-dihydro-15-keto-$9\alpha,11\beta$-PGF_2 (see Chapter 5).

Antigen challenge of human lung fragments or dispersed but unpurified human lung cells leads to the generation of the sulphidopeptide leukotrienes, LTC_4, LTD_4 and LTE_4[91,92]. However, when purified lung mast cells are incubated with tritiated arachidonic acid, LTC_4 alone is released[93]. Similar results have been obtained using purified human skin mast cells (Robinson, Benyon and Church, unpublished observations). These observations imply that LTC_4 released by mast cells may be converted to LTD_4 by other cells within the lung[94]. However, the contribution of other cells to leukotriene production must not be ignored.

Mast cells isolated from BAL of man show quantitative differences in respect to eicosanoid generation. In comparison with mast cells dispersed

9

from human lung parenchyma, BAL cells release more PGD_2 (100–200 ng/10^6 mast cells) upon immunological activation[95], a finding supported by the 180-fold increase in PGD_2 in BAL fluid from asthmatic subjects after allergen challenge[96]. This finding suggests a heterogeneity of human mast cells with respect to eicosanoid generation. However, the similarity of eicosanoid production by lung- and skin-derived mast cells would argue against this. An alternative suggestion may be that the juxtaposition of BAL mast cells to antigen and irritant substances has resulted in them being in a constant state of activation.

The ability of mast cells to generate LTB_4 and the mono- and di-HETEs is less clear. 5-HETE and 12-HETE have been detected following calcium ionophore activation of rat serosal mast cells[97], mouse bone marrow-derived mast cells[98] and cultured murine MC9 mast cells[99]. Similarly, challenge of human lung mast cells yields small quantities[93] of 5-HETE and LTB_4. However, our recent experiments with human purified skin mast cells suggest that LTC_4 is the only mast cell-derived lipoxygenase product[24].

LEUKOCYTES

The next facet of the scenario to consider is the generation of eicosanoids from secondary inflammatory cells, including basophils, eosinophils, neutrophils, macrophages and monocytes, which accumulate at the site of an inflammatory reaction in response to the action of a variety of chemotactic factors, some of which may also cause their activation. Such factors include eosinophil chemotactic factors[100,101], neutrophil chemotactic factors[102], PAF-acether[103], PGD_2[77], histamine[104] and inflammatory factor of anaphylaxis[105]. An oligopeptide prostaglandin-generating factor of anaphylaxis (PGF-A) which has been described to be released from mast cells, induces the release of the prostanoids, $PGF_{2\alpha}$, PGE_2 and TxA_2 from guinea-pig and human lung tissue, and the lipoxygenase products, 5-HETE, 15-HETE and LTB_4 from human lung tissue[106–108]. This spectrum of lipoxygenase products has been associated with increased mucus secretion in human lung[108].

It is now becoming clear that leukocytes may be activated directly by antigen in a manner analogous to that of mast cells. The presence of high-affinity IgE-Fc receptors on basophils is well established. More recently, an IgE-Fc receptor with a lower affinity for IgE[109] has been demonstrated on a wide variety of leukocytes, including eosinophils[110], monocytes[111], macrophages[112] and lymphocytes[113,114]. Platelets also possess similar low-affinity IgE-Fc receptors[109]. It is tempting to speculate that the late reaction following antigen challenge results from the secondary activation by antigen of leukocytes accumulating in the tissues following their chemotactic attraction.

The leukocyte family have the capacity to generate a wide spectrum of eicosanoids, both prostanoids and lipoxygenase products, which may make significant contributions to both early- and late-onset allergic and inflammatory reactions.

Furthermore, it is now evident that the spectrum of eicosanoids produced by a cell may depend both qualitatively and quantitatively on the agent with which it is stimulated. In this short review, I have concentrated on which eicosanoids a cell type has the enzymatic capabilities of synthesizing rather than enter the wide and complex debate of differential cell stimulation.

Of the prostaglandins, PGE_2 is generated in large quantities by macrophages, monocytes, lymphocytes, neutrophils and eosinophils[115,116]. $PGF_{2\alpha}$ does not appear to be generated in significant quantities by any of the leukocyte family, including the basophil[117,118]. Although TxA_2 was originally recognized to be produced by the blood platelet[119], it is now clear that the macrophage may also generate large quantities of this eicosanoid[120]. Macrophages may also generate significant quantities of PGI_2[120].

Leukocytes may also generate substantial quantities of lipoxygenase products. The major product generated by neutrophils is LTB_4[121]. However, these cells also have the capacity to metabolize LTB_4, 20-hydroxy- and 20-carboxy-LTB_4 which have little biological activity[121]. These cells also generate LTC_4 in quantities amounting to about 10% of LTB_4[121]. Additional products, identified following stimulation of neutrophils, include 15-HPETE and 15-HETE, indicating the presence of a 15-lipoxygenase enzyme whose activity can be unmasked by cell damage[122]. Although they also have high 15-lipoxygenase activity, as demonstrated by their production of 15-HETE[126], the major eicosanoid product derived from eosinophils stimulated with calcium ionophore IgG or opsonized zymosan is LTC_4[123-126]. Eosinophils have also been recently recognized as synthesizing lipoxins on incubation with calcium ionophore. Monocytes also have both activities, stimulation with calcium ionophore producing LTB_4 as the major product with smaller amounts of 5- and 15-lipoxygenase, LTC_4 and 15-HETE[125-127]. The macrophage, in contrast, does not appear to have 15-lipoxygenase activity and produces mainly LTB_4 and 5-HETE[130-133]. Lipoxins derive from human leukocytes, but, although the eosinophil has been implicated, definitive evidence as to the source has yet to be published[49].

The third aspect of the scenario is the production of eicosanoids by the cells normally present in the target tissue in response to the inflammation. These responses, which are specific to particular tissues, are discussed in detail in the following chapters.

INHIBITION OF EICOSANOID SYNTHESIS OR ACTIONS AS A THERAPY FOR INFLAMMATORY DISORDERS

It is clear that eicosanoids have the capacity to make a significant contribution to the pathogenesis and symptoms of disease with an inflammatory basis. Our experiences with cyclo-oxygenase inhibitors have shown them to have a place in the management of inflammatory disorders of the joints but to be of little therapeutic benefit in asthma or skin diseases. During recent years, many effective inhibitors of lipoxygenase enzymes and antagonists of lipoxygenase products at their effector sites have been synthesized. Also, many claims of potential benefit to man have been made from results using isolated tissues and experimental animals. However, the only true test of a potential drug is in a clinical trial of its effectiveness in the disease state which it is intended to treat. Furthermore, it must also show demonstrable advantages over drugs currently in use to treat the disease.

Before reviewing our clinical knowledge of eicosanoid inhibition in disease, I would like to address briefly the problem of how to interpret a negative result. There are three main reasons why a potential drug may fail. First is that the mediator towards which the inhibitor or antagonist has been developed does not play a role in the clinical disease. Second, if it is involved, then its role is not large enough for significant benefit to accrue from its inhibition. Third, potency of the drug or the dose used may not be high enough to cause the desired inhibition of synthesis or receptor antagonism. This last point may be examined with antagonists by use of standard agonists. It is of particular relevance to synthesis inhibitors because there are, at present, no truly satisfactory methods for assaying sulphidopeptide leukotriene generation *in vivo* in man and, therefore, no way of telling why the drug did not work.

In mild seasonal asthma, particularly associated with rhinitis, bronchoconstriction is initiated by the release, from activated mast cells, of smooth muscle spasmogens, including histamine, prostaglandins and leukotrienes. Although antagonists of all these substances may have a partial protective role in the relief of symptoms, it is clear that a drug which would prevent mast cell mediator release or a functional antagonist of smooth muscle contraction would be more effective. The mast cell stabilizing drug, sodium cromoglycate[134], or β-adrenoceptor stimulants, which are both mast cell stabilizers and bronchodilators[134], are very effective drugs in immediate bronchoconstriction following exposure to allergen. The failure of piriprost to inhibit allergen- or exercise-induced asthma[135] and the weak efficacy of FPL-55712 and FPL-59257 in comparison with sodium cromoglycate in a variety of bronchial provocation experiments[136] suggests that lipoxygenase inhibitors and antagonists will have little place in the treatment of acute bronchoconstriction in asthma.

Of more relevance to chronic asthma is the ability of a drug to prevent late reactions and the onset of bronchial hyper-reactivity. Drugs available at present for the treatment of these phases of asthma include sodium cromoglycate, nedocromil sodium, methylxanthines and corticosteroids. Experiments in a sheep model of asthma have suggested that leukotrienes are of crucial importance in the development of late reactions; antigen-induced reactions being mimicked by inhalation of LTD_4[137]. In this model, corticosteroids, which would decrease arachidonic acid availability thereby decreasing leukotriene production[6] and the leukotriene antagonist, LY-171883, are both effective inhibitors of the late response. However, in man, inhalation of LTD_4, whilst causing an immediate bronchoconstriction, does not induce late reactions[138]. Also, piriprost does not block the onset of late reactions following allergen provocation[135]. In mild chronic asthma, however, the selective LTC_4/LTD_4 antagonist, LY-171883, caused a significant improvement in FEV_1 and a concomitant reduction in bronchodilator usage in a 6 week trial. Thus, lipoxygenase products may have a role in chronic asthma. However, the degree of benefit that would accrue from the use of effective lipoxygenase inhibitors or leukotriene antagonists in asthma has yet to be determined.

12

Although urticarial lesions in the skin may be treated with considerable success by histamine H_1-antagonists and corticosteroids, eczematous and psoriatic lesions are notoriously difficult to control with drugs. Psoriasis, in particular, is associated with increased levels of arachidonic acid together with its cyclo-oxygenase and lipoxygenase products[139,140]. As such, this condition may be amenable to treatment with drugs which reduce or antagonize these lipid mediators. In psoriasis, topical corticosteroids lower the amounts of free arachidonic acid, LTB_4 and 12-HETE but not PGE_2; anthralin (1,8,9-trihydroxyanthracine), a weak 5-lipoxygenase inhibitor but a potent 12-lipoxygenase inhibitor, lowers free arachidonic acid levels but not those of its metabolites; whereas etretinate, an aromatic retinoid, reduces levels of arachidonic acid and 12-HETE but not LTB_4 or PGE_2. All these changes are associated with a clinical improvement of psoriasis[141]. It will be interesting to see the effects of newer more potent lipoxygenase inhibitors in this condition for only then can it be decided which mediators are the cause of and which arise from the effect of the disease.

Unlike asthma or skin diseases, non-steroidal anti-inflammatory drugs, presumably acting as cyclo-oxygenase inhibitors, have a place in the treatment of rheumatic diseases. They provide relief from pain and swelling but do not control the progression of joint damage. Only the use of potent lipoxygenase inhibitors will illustrate the role of lipoxygenase products of arachidonic acid in this aspect of joint disease. As discussed by Henderson in Chapter 7, an interaction between the monokine, interleukin 1, and PGE_2 is considered to be of more importance in rheumatoid arthritis.

We are now entering a most fascinating stage of research with eicosanoids. The availability of inhibitors and antagonists of lipoxygenase and its products will give us the opportunity to put to the test the hypothesis that lipoxygenase products are of pivotal importance in inflammatory diseases. I await the results with interest although I am pessimistic about the usefulness of such drugs in the treatment of inflammatory diseases of the lung, skin and joints.

REFERENCES

1. Hutson, P.A., Church, M.K., Clay, T.P., Miller, P. and Holgate, S.T. (1987). Early and late phase bronchoconstriction following allergen challenge of non-anaesthetized guinea pigs: I. The association of disordered airway physiology to leucocyte infiltration. *Am. Rev. Respir. Dis.* (In press)
2. Dvorak, A.M., Dvorak, H.F., Peters, S.P., Schulman, E.S., MacGlashan, D.W., Pyne, K., Harvey, V.S., Galli, S.J. and Lichtenstein, L.M. (1983). Lipid bodies: cytoplasmic organelles important to arachidonate metabolism in macrophages and basophils. *J. Immunol.*, **131**, 2965–2976
3. Blackwell, G.J., Flower, R.J., Nijkamp, F.P. and Vane, J.R. (1978). Phospholipase A_2 activity of guinea-pig isolated perfused lungs: stimulation and inhibition by anti-inflammatory steroids. *Br. J. Pharmacol.*, **62**, 79–89
4. Blackwell, G.J., Carnuccio, R., Di Rosa, M., Flower, R.J., Parente, L. and Persico, P. (1980). Macrocortin: a polypeptide causing the antiphospholipase effect of glucocorticoids. *Nature (London)*, **287**, 147–149
5. Hirata, F. (1983). Lipomodulin: a possible mediator of the actions of glucocorticoids. *Adv. Prostagl. Thrombox. Leuk. Res.*, **11**, 73–78

6. Flower, R.J. (1985). The lipocortins and their role in controlling defense reactions. *Adv. Prostagl. Thrombox. Leuk. Res.*, **15**, 201–203
7. Kennerly, D.A., Sullivan, T.J. and Parker, C.W. (1979). Activation of phospholipid metabolism during mediator release from stimulated rat mast cells. *J. Immunol.*, **122**, 152–159
8. Ishizaka, T. and White, J.R. (1986). Triggering mechanisms of mast cells and basophils. In Reed, C.E. (ed.) *Proceedings of the XII International Congress of Allergy and Clinical Immunology. J. Allergy Clin. Immunol.*, pp.9–63. (St. Louis: CV Mosby)
9. Berridge, M.J. (1984). Inositol triphosphate and diacylglycerol as second messengers. *Biochem. J.*, **220**, 345–360
10. Hamberg, M. and Samuelsson, B. (1973). Detection and isolation of an endoperoxide intermediate of prostaglandin biosynthesis. *Proc. Natl. Acad. Sci. USA*, **70**, 899–903
11. Hamberg, M. and Samuelsson, B. (1974). Prostaglandin endoperoxides. VII. Novel transformations of arachidonic acid in guinea-pig lung. *Biochem. Biophys. Res. Commun.*, **61**, 942–949
12. Sun, F.F., Chapman, J.P. and McGuire, J.C. (1977). Metabolism of prostaglandin endoperoxide in animal tissues. *Prostaglandins*, **14**, 1055–1074
13. Hamberg, M., Svensson, J. and Samuelsson, B. (1975). Novel transformations of prostaglandin endoperoxides: formation of thromboxanes. In Samuelsson, B. and Paoletti, R. (eds.) *Advances in Prostaglandin and Thromboxane Research*, **1**, 19–27. (New York: Raven Press)
14. Piper, P.J. and Vane, J.R. (1969). Release of additional factors in anaphylaxis and its antagonism by anti-inflammatory drugs. *Nature (London)*, **223**, 29–35
15. Piper, P.J. and Walker, J.L. (1973). The release of spasmogenic substances from human chopped lung tissue and its inhibition. *Br. J. Pharmacol.*, **47**, 291–304
16. Mathé, A.A., Yen, S.S., Sohn, R. and Hedqvist, P. (1977). Release of prostaglandins and histamine from sensitized and anaphylactic guinea-pig lungs – changes in cyclic AMP levels. *Biochem. Pharmacol.*, **26**, 181–188
17. Gryglewski, R.J., Korbut, R., Ocetkiewicz, A., Splawinski, J., Wojtaszek, B. and Swies, J. (1978). Lungs as a generator of prostacyclin – hypothesis on physiological significance. *Naunyn-Schmeideberg's Arch. Pharmacol.*, **304**, 45–50
18. Schulman, E.S., Newball, H.H., Demers, L.M., Fitzpatrick, F.A. and Adkinson, N.F. (1981). Anaphylactic release of thromboxane A2, prostaglandin D2 and prostacyclin from human lung parenchyma. *Am. Rev. Respir. Dis.*, **124**, 402–406
19. Lewis, R.A., Holgate, S.T., Roberts, L.J., Oates, J.A. and Austen, K.F. (1981). Preferential generation of prostaglandin D2 by rat and human mast cells. In Austen, K.F., Becker, E.L. and Simon, A.L. (eds.) *Biochemistry of Acute Allergic Reactions*, pp. 239–254. (New York: Alan R. Liss)
20. Holgate, S.T., Burns, G.B., Robinson, C. and Church, M.K. (1984). Anaphylactic and calcium dependent generation of prostaglandin D2 (PGD2), thromboxane B2 and other cyclooxygenase products of arachidonic acid by dispersed human lung cells and relationship to histamine release. *J. Immunol.*, **133**, 2138–2144
21. Boot, J.R., Cockerill, A.F., Dawson, W., Mallen, D.N.B. and Osborne, D.J. (1978). Modification of prostaglandin and thromboxane release by immunological sensitization and successive immunological challenges by guinea-pig lung. *Int. Arch. Allergy Appl. Immunol.*, **57**, 159–164
22. Black, A.K., Fincham, N., Greaves, M.W. and Hensby, C.N. (1981). Changes in levels of arachidonic acid and prostaglandins D2, E2, F2 and 6-oxo-PGF1z in human skin within 48 hours following ultraviolet B radiation. *Br. J. Dermatol.*, **105**, 353–354
23. Oikarinen, A., Viinikka, L., Rytsala, H., Kiistla, U.and Ylikorkala, O. (1981). Prostacyclin, thromboxane and prostaglandin F2z in suction blister fluid of human skin: effectof systemic aspirin and glucocorticoid treatment. *Life Sci.*, **29**, 391–396
24. Benyon, R.C., Robinson, C., Holgate, S.T. and Church, M.K. (1987). Prostaglandin D2 release from human skin mast cells in response to ionophore A23187. *Br. J. Pharmacol.*, **92**, 635–638
25. Dawson, W., Boot, J.R., Cockerill, A.F., Mallen, D.N.B. and Osborne, D.J. (1976). Release of novel prostaglandins and thromboxanes after immunological challenge of guinea-pig lung. *Nature (London)*, **262**, 699–702

26. Al-Ubaidi, F. and Bakhle, Y.S. (1980). Differences in biological activation of arachidonic acid in perfused lungs from guinea-pig, rat and man. *Eur. J. Pharmacol.*, **62**, 89–96

27. Piper, P.J. and Samhoun, M.N. (1981). The mechanism of action of leukotrienes C_4 and D_4 in guinea-pig isolated perfused lung and parenchymal strips of guinea-pig, rabbit and rat. *Prostaglandins*, **21**, 793–803

28. Powell, W.S. and Solomon, S. (1978). Biosynthesis of prostaglandins and thromboxane B_2 by fetal lung homogenates. *Prostaglandins*, **15**, 351–364

29. Olley, P.M., Coceani, F., Rowe, R.D. and Swyver, P.R. (1980). Clinical use of prostaglandin synthetase inhibitors in cardiac problems of the newborn. In Samuelsson, B., Ramwell, P.W. and Paoletti, R. (eds.) *Advances in Prostaglandin and Thromboxane Research*, **7**, 913–916. (New York: Raven Press)

30. Bakhle, Y.S. and Zakrzewski, J.T. (1980). The influence of the oestrus cycle on the metabolism of exogenous arachidonate in rat isolated lung [Abstract]. *Br. J. Pharmacol.*, **70**, 83P–84P

31. Maggi, F.M., Tyrrell, N., Maddox, Y., Watkins, W., Remey, E.R. and Ramwell, P.W. (1980). Prostaglandin synthetase activity in vascular tissue of male and female rats. *Prostaglandins*, **19**, 985–993

32. Berti, F., Folco, G.C., Nicosai, S., Omini, C. and Pasargiklian, R. (1979). The role of histamine H1 and H2 receptors in the generation of thromboxane A_2 in perfused guinea-pig lungs. *Br. J. Pharmacol.*, **65**, 629–633

33. Platshon, L.F. and Kaliner, M. (1978). The effects of the immunological release of histamine upon human lung cyclic nucleotide levels and prostaglandin generation. *J. Clin. Invest.*, **62**, 1113–1121

34. Hardy, C.C., Holgate, S.T. and Robinson, C. (1986). Evidence against the formation of 13,14-dihydro-15-keto-prostaglandin F_2, following inhalation of prostaglandin D_2 in man. *Br. J. Pharmacol.*, **87**, 563–568

35. Kellaway, C.H. and Trethewie, E.R. (1940). The liberation of slow-reacting smooth muscle stimulating substances in anaphylaxis. *Q. J. Exp. Physiol.*, **30**, 121–145

36. Brocklehurst, W.E. (1981). Steps in the dark – an outline history of the study of SRS-A. In Piper, P.J. (ed.) *SRS-A and Leukotrienes*, pp.7–11. (Chichester: Wiley)

37. Editorial. (1955). Anti-histamines and asthma (annotation). *Lancet*, **2**, 1182

38. Murphy, R.C., Hammarström, S. and Samuelsson, B. (1979). Leukotriene C: a slow reacting substance from murine mastocytoma cells. *Proc. Natl. Acad. Sci. USA*, **76**, 4275–4279

39. Orange, R.P., Murphy, R.C., Karnovsky, M.L. and Austen, K.F. (1973). The physical characteristics and purification of slow reacting substance of anaphylaxis. *J. Immunol.*, **110**, 760–770

40. Jakschik, B.A., Falkenheim, S. and Parker, C.W. (1974). Precursor role of arachidonic acid in release of slow reacting substance from rat basophilic leukaemia cells. *Proc. Natl. Acad. Sci. USA*, **74**, 4577–4581

41. Borgeat, P. and Samuelsson, B. (1979). Transformation of arachidonic acid by rabbit polymorphonuclear leucocytes. Formation of a novel dihydroxyeicosatetraenoic acid. *J. Biol. Chem.*, **254**, 2643–2646

42. Samuelsson, B., Borgeat, P., Hammarström, S. and Murphy, R.C. (1979). Introduction of a nomenclature: leukotrienes. *Prostaglandins*, **17**, 785–787

43. Hammarström, S., Murphy, R.C., Samuelsson, B., Clark, D.A., Mioskowski, C. and Corey, E.J. (1979). Structure of leukotriene C_4. Identification of the amino acid part. *Biochem. Biophys. Res. Commun.*, **91**, 1266–1272

44. Morris, H.R., Taylor, G.W., Piper, P.J. and Tippins, J.R. (1980). The structure elucidation of slow-reacting substance of anaphylaxis, SRS-A from guinea pig lung. *Nature (London)*, **285**, 104–106

45. Orning, L., Hammarström, S. and Samuelsson, B. (1980). Leukotriene D: A slow reacting substance from rat basophilic leukemia cells. *Proc. Natl. Acad. Sci. USA*, **77**, 2014–2017

46. Drazen, J.M., Lewis, R.A., Austen, K., Toda, M., Brion, F., Marfat, A. and Corey, E.J. (1981). Contractile activities of structural analogs of leukotrienes C and D: Necessity for a hydrophobic region. *Proc. Natl. Acad. Sci. USA*, **78**, 3195–3198

47. Lewis, R.A., Drazen, J.M., Austen, K.F., Clark, D.A. and Corey, E.J. (1980). Identification of the C(6)-S-conjugate of leukotriene A with cysteine as a naturally occurring slow

reacting substance of anaphylaxis (SRS-A). Importance of the 11-cis-geometry for biological activity. Biochem. Biophys. Res. Commun., 96, 271–277

48. Hammarström, S. (1983). Leukotrienes. Annu. Rev. Biochem., 52, 355–377
49. Serhan, C.N., Hamberg, M. and Samuelsson, B. (1984). Trihydroxytetraenes: a novel series of compounds formed from arachidonic acid in human leukocytes. Biochem. Biophys. Res. Commun., 118, 943–949
50. Fitzsimmons, B.J., Adams, J., Leblanc, Y., Girard, Y., Evans, J.F. and Rokach, J. (1986). The lipoxins: synthesis and identification of the natural products. In Piper, P.J. (ed.) The Leukotrienes: Their Biological Significance, pp. 41–57. (New York: Raven Press)
51. Adams, J., Fitzsimmons, B.J., Girard, Y., Leblanc, Y., Evans, J.F. and Rokach, J. (1985). Enantiospecific and sterospecific synthesis of lipoxin A. Stereochemical assignment of the natural lipoxin A and its possible biosynthesis. J. Am. Chem. Soc., 107, 464–469
52. Shimizu, T., Izumi, T., Seyama, Y., Tadkoro, K., Rådmark, O. and Samuelsson, B. (1986). Characterization of leukotriene A_4 synthase from murine mast cells: evidence for its identity to arachidonate 5-lipoxygenase. Proc. Natl. Acad. Sci. USA, 83, 4175–4179
53. Ueda, N., Kaneko, S., Yoshimoto, T. and Yamamoto, S. (1986). Purification of arachidonate 5-lipoxygenase from porcine leukocytes and its reactivity with hydroperoxy acids. J. Biol. Chem., 261, 7982–7988
54. Bach, M.K. and Brashler, J.R. (1985). A comparison of the leukotriene synthesizing ability of subfractions of rat liver glutathione-S-transferases. Prostagl. Leuk. Med., 17, 125–136
55. Bach, M.K., Brashler, J.R., Peck, R.E. and Morton, D.R. (1984). Leukotriene C synthetase, a special glutathione S-transferase: properties of the enzyme and inhibitor studies with special reference to the mode of action of U-60,257, a selective inhibitor of leukotriene synthesis. J. Allergy Clin. Immunol., 74, 353–357
56. Horton, E.W. and Main, I.H.M. (1965). A comparison of the actions of prostaglandins F_2 and E_1 on smooth muscle. Br. J. Pharmacol., 24, 470–476
57. Sweatman, W.J.F. and Collier, H.O.J. (1968). Effects of prostaglandins on human bronchial muscle. Nature (London), 217, 69–76
58. Smith, A.P. and Cuthbert, M.F. (1972). The antagonistic action of prostaglandin F_2 and E_2 aerosols on bronchial muscle tone in man. Br. Med. J., 2, 212–214
59. Drazen, J.M. and Austen, K.F. (1974). Effects of intravenous administration of slow reacting substance of anaphylaxis, histamine, bradykinin and prostaglandin F_{2}, on pulmonary mechanism in the guinea-pig. J. Clin. Invest., 53, 1679–1685
60. Wasserman, M.A. (1976). Bronchopulmonary responses to prostaglandin F_{2}, histamine and acetylcholine in the dog. Eur. J. Pharmacol., 32, 146–155
61. Newball, H.H., Keiser, H.R. and Lenfant, C. (1980). Prostaglandin F_2 functions as a local hormone on human airways. Respir. Physiol., 41, 183–197
62. Lewis, R.A., Hardy, C. and Tattersfield, A.E. (1982). Low and high dose response to prostaglandin F_{2z} in normal subjects. Clin. Sci., 63, 7P
63. Kitamura, S., Ishiharu, Y., Yotsumoto, H., Sasaki, K. and Kudoh, S. (1978). Effect of prostaglandin F_{2z} on the contractile responses of guinea-pig tracheal tissues induced by various bronchoconstrictors. Jpn. J. Thorac. Dis., 16, 315–319
64. Walters, E.H., Parrish, R.W., Bevan, C. and Smith, A.P. (1981). Induction of bronchial hypersensitivity: evidence for a role of prostaglandins. Thorax, 36, 571–574
65. Hardy, C.C., Robinson, C., Tattersfield, A.E. and Holgate, S.T. (1984). The bronchoconstrictor effect of inhaled prostaglandin D_2 in normal and asthmatic men. N. Engl. J. Med., 311, 209–213
66. Beasley, C.R.W., Robinson, C., Featherstone, R.L., Varley, J.G., Hardy, C.C., Church, M.K. and Holgate, S.T. (1987). $9\alpha,11\beta$-Prostaglandin F_2, a novel metabolite of prostaglandin D_2, is a potent contractile agonist of human and guinea pig airways. J. Clin. Invest. 79, 978–983
67. Cuthbert, M.F. (1969). Effect on airways resistance of prostaglandin E_1 given by aerosol to healthy and asthmatic subjects. Br. Med. J., 4, 723–727
68. Cuthbert, M.F. (1971). Bronchodilator activity of aerosols of prostaglandin E_1 and E_2 in asthmatic subjects. Proc. R. Soc. Med., 64, 15–18
69. Smith, A.P., Cuthbert, M.F. and Dunlop, L.S. (1975). Effects of inhaled prostaglandins E_1, E_2 and F_{2z} on the airway resistance of normal and asthmatic man. Clin. Sci. Mol. Med., 48, 421–430

16

70. Weinryb, I., Michel, I.M. and Hess, S.M. (1973). Adenylate cyclase from ginea-pig lungs: further characterization and inhibitory effects of substrate analogs and cyclic nucleotides. *Arch. Biochem. Biophys.*, **154**, 240–249

71. Seth, R.V., Clarke, V.S., Lewis, R.A. and Tattersfield, A.E. (1981). Effect of propranolol on the airway response to prostaglandin E_2 in normal man. *Br. J. Clin. Pharmacol.*, **12**, 731–735

72. Hardy, C.C., Robinson, C., Lewis, R.A., Tattersfield, A.E. and Holgate, S.T. (1985). The airway and cardiovascular responses to inhaled prostaglandin I_2 in normal and asthmatic man. *Am. Rev. Respir. Dis.*, **131**, 18–21

73. Hardy, C.C., Robinson, C., Bradding, P. and Holgate, S.T. (1984). Prostacyclin: a functional antagonist of prostaglandin D_2-induced bronchoconstriction [Abstract]. *Thorax*, **39**, 696

74. Mathé, A.A., Hedqvist, P., Strandberg, K. and Leslie, C.A. (1977). Aspects of prostaglandin function in the lung. *N. Engl. J. Med.*, **296**, 850–855

75. Adelroth, E., Morris, M.M., Hargreave, F.E. and O'Byrne, P.M. (1984). Airway responsiveness to leukotrienes C_4 and D_4 and to methacholine in patients with asthma and normal controls. *N. Engl. J. Med.*, **315**, 480–484

76. Marom, Z., Shelhamer, J.H., Bach, M.K., Morton, D.R. and Kaliner, M. (1982). Slow reacting substances, leukotrienes C_4 and D_4, increase the release of mucus from human airways in vitro. *Am. Rev. Respir. Dis.*, **126**, 449–451

77. Soter, N.A., Lewis, R.A., Corey, E.J. and Austen, K.F. (1983). Local effects of synthetic leukotrienes (LTC_4, LTD_4, LTE_4 and LTB_4) in human skin. *J. Invest. Dermatol.*, **80**, 115–119

78. Beasley, R., Hovell, C., Mani, R., Robinson, C. and Holgate, S.T. (1987). The comparative vascular effects of histamine, prostaglandin (PG) D_2, its metabolite $9\alpha,11\beta$-PGF_2 and $PGF_{2\alpha}$ in human skin. Manuscript submitted

79. Flower, R.J., Harvey, E.A. and Kingston, W.P. (1976). Inflammatory effects of prostaglandin D_2 in rat and human skin. *Br. J. Pharmacol.*, **56**, 229–233

80. Williams, T.J. (1979). Prostaglandin E_2, prostaglandin I_2 and the vascular changes in inflammation. *Br. J. Pharmacol.*, **65**, 517–524

81. Peck, M.J., Piper, P.J. and Williams, T.J. (1981). The effect of leukotrienes C_4 and D_4 on the microvasculature of guinea-pig skin. *Prostaglandins*, **21**, 315–321

82. Camp, R.D.R., Coutts, A.A., Greaves, M.W., Kay, A.B. and Walport, M.J. (1983). Responses of human skin to intradermal injection of leukotrienes C_4, D_4 and B_4. *Br. J. Pharmacol.*, **80**, 497–502

83. Bisgaard, H., Lerche, A. and Kristensen, J.K. (1985). Leukotriene- and histamine-induced vascular permeability and interstitial transport in the skin. *J. Invest. Dermatol.*, **84**, 427–429

84. Bisgaard, H. (1987). Vascular effects of leukotriene D_4 in human skin. *J. Invest. Dermatol.*, **88**, 109–114

85. Ryan, J.W. and Ryan, U.S. (1977). Pulmonary endothelial cells. *Fed. Proc.*, **36**, 2683–2691

86. Church, M.K., Pao, G.J-K. and Holgate, S.T. (1982). Characterization of histamine secretion from dispersed human lung mast cells: effects of anti-IgE calcium ionophore A23187, compound 48/80 and basic polypeptides. *J. Immunol.*, **129**, 2116–2121

87. Schleimer, R.P., MacGlashan, D.W., Peters, S.P., Pinckard, R.N., Adkinson, N.F. and Lichtenstein, L.M. (1986). Characterization of inflammatory mediator release from purified human lung mast cells. *Am. Rev. Respir. Dis.*, **133**, 614–617

88. Benyon, R.C., Lowman, M.A. and Church, M.K. (1987). Human skin mast cells: their dispersion, purification and secretory characterization. *J. Immunol.*, **138**, 861–867

89. Liston, T.E. and Roberts, L.J. (1985). Metabolic fate of radiolabelled prostaglandin D_2 in a normal human male volunteer. *J. Biol. Chem.*, **260**, 13172–13180

90. Liston, T.E. and Roberts, L.J. (1985). Transformation of prostaglandin D_2 to $9\alpha,11\beta$-(15S)-trihydroxy-prosta-(5Z,13E)-dien-1-oic acid ($9\alpha,11\beta$-prostaglandin F_2): a unique biologically active prostaglandin produced enzymatically in vivo in humans. *Proc. Natl. Acad. Sci. USA*, **82**, 6030–6034

91. Harvey, J., Holgate, S.T., Peters, B.J., Robinson, C. and Walker, J.R. (1985). Oxidative transformations of arachidonic acid in human dispersed lung cells: disparity between utilization of endogenous and exogenous substrate. *Br. J. Pharmacol.*, **86**, 417–426

92. Lewis, R.A., Austen, K.F., Drazen, J.M., Clark, D.A. and Corey, E.J. (1980). Slow reacting substance of anaphylaxis: identification of leukotrienes C-1 and D from human and rat sources. *Proc. Natl. Acad. Sci. USA*, **77**, 3710–3714

93. Peters, S.P., MacGlashan, D.W., Schulman, E.S., Schleimer, R.P., Hayes, E.C., Rokach, J., Adkinson, N.F. and Lichtenstein, L.M. (1984). Arachidonic acid metabolism in purified human lung mast cells. *J. Immunol.*, **132**, 1972–1979

94. Sirois, P., Brousseau, Y., Chagnon, M., Gentile, J., Gladu, M., Salari, H. and Borgeat, P. (1985). Metabolism of leukotrienes by adult and fetal human lungs. *Exp. Lung Res.*, **9**, 17–30

95. Flint, K.C., Hudspith, B.N., Leung, K.B.P., Pearce, F.L., Seiger, K., Hammond, M.D.H., Brostoff, J. and Johnson, N.McI. (1985). IgE-dependent release of leukotriene C_4 and prostaglandin D_2 from human bronchoalveolar cells [Abstract]. *Thorax*, **40**, 716

96. Murray, J.J., Tonel, A.B., Brash, A.R., Roberts, L.J., Gosset, P., Workman, R., Capron, A. and Oates, J.A. (1986). Release of prostaglandin D_2 into human airways during acute antigen challenge. *N. Engl. J. Med.*, **315**, 800–804

97. Roberts, L.J., Lewis, R.A., Oates, J.A. and Austen, K.F. (1979). Prostaglandin, thromboxane and 12-hydroxy-5,8,10,14-eicosatetraenoic acid production by ionophore-stimulated rat serosal mast cells. *Biochim. Biophys. Acta*, **575**, 185–192

98. Wei, Y., Heghinian, K., Bell, R.L. and Jakschik, B.A. (1986). Contribution of macrophages to immediate hypersensitivity reaction. *J. Immunol.*, **137**, 1993–2000

99. Musch, M. W., Bryant, R.W., Coscolluella, C., Myers, R.F. and Siegel, M.I. (1985). Ionophore-stimulated lipoxygenase activity and histamine release in a clone murine mast cell, MC-9. *Prostaglandins*, **29**, 405–430

100. Kay, A.B., Stechschulte, D.J. and Austen, K.F. (1971). An eosinophil leukocyte chemotactic factor of anaphylaxis. *J. Exp. Med.*, **133**, 602–619

101. Goetzl, E.J. and Austen, K.F. (1980). Natural eosinophilotactic peptides: evidence of heterogeneity and studies of structure and function. In Mahmoud, A.A.F. and Austen, K.F. (eds.) *The Eosinophil in Health and Disease*, pp. 149–165. (New York: Grune and Stratton)

102. Kay, A.B. and Lee, T.H. (1982). Neutrophil chemotactic factor of anaphylaxis. *J. Allergy Clin. Immunol.*, **70**, 317–320

103. Wardlaw, A.J. and Kay, A.B. (1986). PAF-acether is a potent chemotactic factor for human eosinophils [Abstract]. *J. Allergy Clin. Immunol.*, **77** (Suppl), 236

104. Turnbull, L.W. and Kay, A.B. (1976). Eosinophils and mediators of anaphylaxis. Histamine and imidazole acetic acid as chemotactic agents for human eosinophil leukocytes. *Immunology*, **31**, 797–802

105. Oertel, H.L. and Kaliner, M. (1981). The biologic activity of mast cell granules. III. Purification of inflammatory factors of anaphylaxis (IF-A) responsible for causing late-phase reactions. *J. Immunol.*, **127**, 1398–1402

106. Steel, L.K. and Kaliner, M.A. (1981). Prostaglandin generating factor of anaphylaxis. Identification and isolation. *J. Biol. Chem.*, **256**, 12692–12698

107. Steel, L.K., Bach, D. and Kaliner, M.A. (1982). Prostaglandin-generating factor of anaphylaxis. II. Characterization of activity. *J. Immunol.*, **129**, 1233–1238

108. Marom, Z., Shelhamer, J.H., Steel, L., Goetzl, E.J. and Kaliner, M. (1984). Prostaglandin generating factor of anaphylaxis induces mucus glycoprotein release and the formation of lipoxygenase products of arachidonate from human airways. *Prostaglandins*, **28**, 79–91

109. Capron, A., Dessaint, J.P., Capron, M., Joseph, M., Ameisen, J.C. and Tonnel, A.B. (1986). From parasites to allergy: the second receptor for IgE (FcE R2). *Immunol. Today*, **7**, 15–18

110. Capron, M., Capron, A., Dessaint, J.P., Torpier, G., Gunnar, S., Johansson, O. and Prin, A. (1981). Fc receptors for IgE on human and rat eosinophils. *J. Immunol.*, **126**, 2087–2092

111. Melewicz, F.M. and Spiegelberg, H.L. (1980). Fc receptors for IgE on a subpopulation of human peripheral blood monocytes. *J. Immunol.*, **125**, 1026–1031

112. Dessaint, J.P., Torpier, G., Capron, M., Bazin, H. and Capron, A. (1979). Cytophilic binding of IgE to the macrophage. I. Binding characteristics of IgE on the surface of macrophages in the rat. *Cell. Immunol.*, **46**, 12–23

113. Gonzalez Molina, A. and Spiegelberg, H.L. (1977). A sub-population of normal peripheral B lymphocytes that bind IgE. *J. Clin. Invest.,* **59**, 616–624

114. Yodoi, J. and Ishizaka, K. (1979). Lymphocytes bearing Fc receptors for IgE. 1. Presence of human and rat T-lymphocytes with Fc receptors. *J. Immunol.,* **122**, 2577–2583

115. Parker, C.W. (1986). Leukotrienes and prostaglandins in the immune system. In Zor, U., Naor, Z. and Koehn, F. (eds.) *Advances in Prostaglandin. Thromboxane and Leukotriene Research,* **16**, 113–134. (New York: Raven Press)

116. Hubscher, T. (1975). Role of the eosinophil in allergic reactions. II. Release of prostaglandins from human eosinophil leukocytes. *J. Immunol.,* **114**, 1389–1393

117. Adkinson, N.F., Barron, T., Powell, S. and Cohen, S. (1977). Prostaglandin production by human peripheral blood cells in vitro. *J. Lab. Clin. Med.,* **90**, 1043–1053

118. Tolone, G., Bonasera, L., Brai, M. and Tolone, C. (1977). Prostaglandin production by human polymorphonuclear leukocytes during phagocytosis in vitro. *Experientia,* **33**, 961–962

119. Hamberg, M., Svensson, J. and Samuelsson, B. (1975). Thromboxanes: a new group of biologically active compounds derived from prostaglandin endoperoxides. *Proc. Natl. Acad. Sci. USA,* **72**, 2994–2998

120. Foegh, M., Maddox, Y.T., Winchester, J., Rakowski, T., Schreiner, G. and Ramwell, P.W. (1983). Prostacyclin and thromboxane release from human peritoneal macrophages. In Samuelsson, B., Ramwell, P.W. and Paoletti, R. (eds.) *Advances in Prostaglandin, Thromboxane and Leukotriene Research,* **12**, 45–49. (New York: Raven Press)

121. Braquet, M., Garay, R., Ducousso, R., Borgeat, P., De Feudis, F.V. and Braquet, P. (1984). Transmembrane potassium movements and arachidonic acid cascade. I. A study in A23187-stimulated human leukocytes. In Braquet, P. *et al.* (eds.) *Prostaglandins and Membrane Ion Transport.* (New York: Raven Press)

122. Fruteau de Laclos, B., Braquet, P. and Borgeat, P. (1984). Characteristics of leukotriene (LT) and hydroxyeicosatetraenoic acid (HETE) synthesis in human leukocytes in vitro: effect of arachidonic acid concentration. *Prostgl. Leuk. Med.,* **13**, 47–52

123. Weller, P.F., Lee, C.W., Foster, D.W., Corey, E.J., Austen, K.F. and Lewis, R.A. (1983). Generation and metabolism of 5-lipoxygenase pathway leukotrienes by human eosinophils: predominant production of leukotriene C$_4$. *Proc. Natl. Acad. Sci. USA,* **80**, 7626–7630

124. Shaw, R.J., Walsh, G.M., Cromwell, O., Moqbel, R., Spry, C.J.F. and Kay, A.B. (1985). Activated human eosinophils generate SRS-A leukotrienes following IgG-dependent stimulation. *Nature (London).* **316**, 150–152

125. Borgeat, P., Rabinovitch, H., Fruteau de Laclos, B., Picard, S., Braquet, P., Herbert, J. and Laviolette, M. (1984). Eosinophil-rich human polymorphonuclear leukocyte preparations characteristically release leukotriene C$_4$ on ionophore A23187 challenge. *J. Allergy Clin. Immunol.,* **74**, 310–315

126. Henderson, W.R., Harley, J.B. and Fauci, A.S. (1984). Arachidonic acid metabolism in normal and hypereosinophilic syndrome eosinophils: generation of leukotrienes B$_4$, C$_4$ and D$_4$ and 15-lipoxygenase products. *Immunology,* **51**, 679–686

127. Goldyne, M.E., Burrish, G.F., Poubelle, P. and Borgeat, P. (1984). Arachidonic acid metabolism among human mononuclear leukocytes: lipoxygenase-related pathways. *J. Biol. Chem.,* **259**, 8815–8819

128. Pawlowski, N.A., Kaplan, G., Hamill, A.L., Cohn, Z.A. and Scott, W.A. (1983). Arachidonic acid metabolism by human monocytes: studies with platelet depleted cultures. *J. Exp. Med.,* **158**, 393–412

129. Poubelle, P., Beaulieu, A.D. and Borgeat, P. (1985). Leukotriene synthesis by synovial fluid and blood polymorphonuclear leukocytes (PMNL) and monocyte-macrophages of rheumatoid arthritis (RA). *Adv. Inflamm. Res.,* **10**, 156–159

130. Fels, A.O., Pawlowski, N.A., Cramer, E.B., King, T.K.C., Cohn, Z.A. and Scott, W.A. (1982). Human alveolar macrophages produce LTB$_4$. *Proc. Natl. Acad. Sci. USA,* **79**, 7866–7870

131. MacDermot, J., Kelsey, C.R., Waddell, K.A., Richmond, R., Knight, R.K., Cole, P.J., Dollery, C.T., Landon, D.N. and Blair, I.A. (1984). Synthesis of leukotriene B$_4$ and prostanoids by human alveolar macrophages analysed by gas chromatography/mass spectrometry. *Prostaglandins.* **27**, 163–179

19

132. Martin, T.R., Altman, L.T., Albert, R.C. and Henderson, W.R. (1984). Leukotriene B₄ production by the human alveolar macrophage: a potential mechanism for amplifying inflammation in the lung. *Am. Rev. Respir. Dis.*, **129**, 106–111

133. Braquet, P., Borgeat, P., Etienne, A. and Braquet, M. (1985). Stimulus–secretion coupling and leukotriene formation in the triggering of immediately hypersensitivity reactions. *Ann. Inst. Past. Immunol.*, **136D**, 186–203

134. Howarth, P.H., Durham, S.R., Lee, T.H., Kay, A.B., Church, M.K. and Holgate, S.T. (1985). Influence of albuterol, cromolyn sodium and ipratropium bromide on the airway and circulating mediator responses to antigen bronchial provocation in asthma. *Am. Rev. Respir. Dis.*, **132**, 986–992

135. Mann, J.S., Robinson, C., Sheridan, A.Q., Clement, P., Bach, M.K. and Holgate, S.T. (1986). Effect of piriprost (U-60,257) a novel leukotriene inhibitor on allergen and exercise induced bronchoconstriction in asthma. *Thorax*, **41**, 746–752

136. Holroyd, M.C. cited in Massicot, J.G., Soberman, R.J., Ackerman, N.R., Heavey, D., Roberts, L.J. and Austen, K.F. (1987). Workshop: Potential therapeutic uses of inhibitors of leukotriene generation and function. *Prostaglandins*, **32**, 480–494

137. Abraham, W.M. (1987). The importance of lipoxygenase products of arachidonic acid in allergen-induced late responses. *Am. Rev. Respir. Dis.*, **135**, S49–53

138. Higgins, D.A. and O'Byrne, P.M. (1987). Inhaled leukotriene D₄ does not cause a late asthmatic response in atopic subjects [Abstract]. *J. Allergy Clin. Immunol.*, **79**, 141

139. Hammarström, S., Hamberg, M., Samuelsson, B., Duell, E.A., Stawski, M. and Vorhees, J.J. (1975). Increased concentrations of nonesterified arachidonic acid, 12L-hydroxyeicosatetraenoic acid, prostaglandin E₂, and prostaglandin F₂ₓ in the epidermis of psoriasis. *Proc. Natl. Acad. Sci. USA*, **72**, 5130–5134

140. Brain, S.D., Camp, R.D.R., Kobza Black, A., Dowd, P.M., Greaves, M.W., Ford-Hutchinson, A.W. and Charleson, S. (1985). Leukotrienes C₄ and D₄ in psoriatic skin lesions. *Prostaglandins*, **26**, 611–619

141. Barr, R.M. cited in Massicot, J.G., Soberman, R.J., Ackerman, N.R., Heavey, D., Roberts, L.J. and Austen, K.F. (1987). Workshop: Potential therapeutic uses of inhibitors of leukotriene generation and function. *Prostaglandins*, **32**, 480–494

20

2
Contribution of Eicosanoids to the Immediate and Late Inflammatory Responses

O. CROMWELL

INTRODUCTION

Early- and late-phase reactions (EPR, LPR) occur in the skin, nasal passages and lungs of subjects with specific immunoglobulin E (IgE) antibody to the reaction-provoking antigen. Late phase reactions are, however, restricted to a subset of individuals. It is the study of this group in particular that has attracted most attention in recent years since the realization that the features of the late response more closely resemble those of allergic diseases than do those of early reactions. In the case of asthma, in particular, the LPR, unlike the EPR, is only partially reversed by sympathomimetic drugs and is completely blocked by corticosteroids, observations akin to those seen in the day-to-day course of the disease[1]. Warner et al.[2] showed that immunotherapy with *Dermatophagoides pteronyssinus* in a group of asthmatic children had no effect on the early asthmatic reaction (EAR), but the late asthmatic reaction (LAR) was inhibited in approximately 50% of the children. These patients also showed the greatest improvement in symptoms. Difficulties in obtaining human tissue and the ethical problems associated with conducting experiments in man have forced researchers to turn to animal models in order to gain insight into the mechanisms of the responses (see Chapter 9). Whilst much valuable information has been, and continues to be, obtained from animal models of the EPR and LPR, great care must always be taken in interpreting the relevance of the findings to man. There are many instances which highlight this problem. For example, leukotriene B_4 (LTB_4) is a potent chemotactic agent for human neutrophils[3] which suggests that it might be an important factor in the recruitment of inflammatory cells into the extravascular tissues. However, in the case of rat neutrophils, this leukotriene has little or no chemotactic activity[4]. The sulphidopeptide leukotrienes are contractile agonists

21

of human airway smooth muscle with a potency up to 1000 times greater than that of histamine[5], yet they are far less potent on the airway tissue of several animal species[6].

In recent years, significant progress in the development of techniques for cell isolation, purification and culture have enhanced our understanding of the contributions of various human cell types to hypersensitivity and inflammatory reactions. Furthermore, refinements in methods for measurement of several of the putative mediators of these processes, together with the development of safe procedures for *in vivo* skin, nasal and lung provocation testing[7], have facilitated progress towards an understanding of the mechanisms of EPR and LPR in man.

Variations of Koch's original postulates can be applied usefully in the evaluation of the contribution of different mediators to EPR and LPR. Firstly, the mediator must reproduce some of the pathophysiological features of the reactions when administered to man. Secondly, the mediator should be identified in body fluids in temporal association with one or both of the reactions, and either the tissues or any inflammatory cells that may infiltrate should be recognized as having the capacity to produce that mediator. Thirdly, the actions of the putative mediators should be diminished by specific antagonists[8]. These basic postulates will be applied when considering the possible roles of specific eicosanoids in EPR and LPR.

CLINICAL AND HISTOLOGICAL SEQUELAE OF EPR AND LPR

The administration of antigen intradermally, intrabronchially or intranasally induces physiological reactions in atopic individuals, that is those with antigen-specific IgE antibodies. The EPR will normally occur within minutes of provocation, peaking between 5 and 20 min, and resolves within 60 min. This reaction may then be followed by an LPR which peaks between 6 and 9 h and resolves within 24 h, although in some individuals resolution may take considerably longer.

Skin

In man, the early cutaneous response to antigen challenge is characterized by a weal and flare reaction. A central pale swelling, attributable to increased vascular permeability and tissue oedema, is surrounded by a region of erythema due to vasodilatation and increased blood flow. In rodents, the reaction is restricted to induration at and around the injection site. Cutaneous LPRs begin to develop clinically 1–2 h after the EPR and manifest themselves in humans by erythema, a burning sensation, tenderness, induration and pruritis. The reactions are IgE-dependent, but are independent of immune complex formation and complement activation. Early studies in patients sensitive to *Aspergillus* led to the hypothesis that late reactions were attributable to a Type III response[9] (Arthus type immune complex reaction) involving deposition of IgG and the complement component, C3, in the skin[10]. Later studies found no evidence of IgG, IgA, IgM or complement deposition following antigen challenge[11,12], and indeed it has been shown recently that immunotherapy with ragweed extract suppresses late-phase skin reactions, the degree of suppression correlating with the level of IgG antibody[13]. Solley *et al.*[12] established the importance of IgE in the cutaneous EPR and LPR when they showed that transfer of these reactions by atopic sera was blocked either by heating the serum or by removing IgE with specific immunoadsorbents. Histologically, the late reaction is characterized by infiltration of neutrophils, eosinophils and, later, mononuclear cells, whilst mast cell numbers apparently decrease, presumably because the cells degranulate and can no longer interact with metachromatic stains[14].

Lung

There are close parallels between the events in the skin and those in the lung, and indeed skin reactivity to allergen challenge is usually a reliable indicator of airway sensitivity and EAR. However, cutaneous LPRs are not a good indicator of LAR[15]. Inhalation of specific antigen by atopic individuals may activate mast cells via an IgE-dependent mechanism resulting in mediator release, whilst a non-specific stimulus, such as exercise, may precipitate a similar reaction. The EAR is rapid in onset and characterized by an increase in airway resistance. The transient nature of the reaction suggests that bronchospasm due to smooth muscle contraction is the major contributory factor rather than inflammatory events. The increase in airway resistance is paralleled by increases in plasma histamine and high molecular weight chemotactic activity (HMW–NCA)[16]. Histamine is probably responsible for a large proportion of the EAR, either through direct action on smooth muscle or via vagal reflexes, since astemizole, a selective H_1-antagonist, attenuates the reaction[17]. The initial release of mast cell-associated mediators is followed by recruitment of inflammatory cells. Neutrophils and monocytes which are activated in terms of increased expression of IgG (Fc) and complement (C3b) receptors appear in the circulation in increasing numbers up to 60 min[18]. The activation of these membrane receptors and the bronchospasmic response are both blocked by prior administration of sodium cromoglycate (SCG).

In patients with severe asthma, a strong provoking stimulus may result in the development of LARs which are generally more severe and more protracted than EARs, being slow to evolve and resolve. The small peripheral airways are more susceptible to local inflammatory reactions, particularly vasodilatation, increased vascular permeability and tissue oedema. The subacute or chronic phase of the asthmatic response, which may persist after the LPR, probably involves mucus hypersecretion and gross infiltration of inflammatory cells[19]. This is suggested by the autopsy findings after asthma death which reveal a large number of eosinophils and mononuclear cells, principally lymphocytes, in the airways and in the surrounding tissue[20]. There is extensive epithelial shedding and thickening of the basement membrane, the latter consistent with rapid turnover of the epithelial layer. The airways are often totally occluded with mucus containing substantial cell debris, and this mucus plugging results in air trapping in the parenchyma and hyperinflation of the lung. The involvement of peripheral small airways in the late phase of the asthmatic response is supported by the results of gas density/flow rate studies during the course of the response to antigen provocation. In patients breathing a mixture of helium and oxygen, a decrease in the density dependence of gas flow during the LAR pointed to the involvement of small airways[21] where both bronchoconstriction and local inflammation may contribute to the obstruction.

Animal models have made important contributions towards an understanding of the pathogenesis of the pulmonary response. Whether or not the LAR is similar to the cutaneous reaction, regarding involvement of IgE as opposed to IgG and histological changes, has been tested with a model of asthma in rabbits immunized with *Alternaria tenius*[22,23]. Animals with IgE antibody alone developed both early and late reactions. The reactivity could be transferred by intravenous injection of serum, and there was no evidence of complement or immune-complex deposition. Antigen challenge elicited vasodilatation and inflammatory cell infiltration during the EAR, whilst oedema and inflammatory cell infiltration were associated with the LAR. Neutrophils predominated at 6 h, but these were outnumbered by mononuclear cells as the reaction began to subside.

Direct evidence of inflammatory cell involvement in the LAR in man has only been obtained very recently by performing bronchoalveolar lavage (BAL) during the course of the reaction. Influx of neutrophils[24–26], eosinophils[24,25,27] and lymphocytes[25] has been observed together with an apparent decrease in the number of mast cells[25] and degranulation of eosinophils[27,28]. An increase in the number of peripheral blood eosinophils has been observed 24 h after antigen challenge in those patients experiencing an LAR, but not in those with an isolated EAR[29]. There was a reverse correlation between baseline eosinophil counts and airway hyperreactivity expressed in terms of methacholine PC_{20}, and a similar correlation in the case of the change in the eosinophil count at 24 h. This prompted the suggestion that there may be a direct association between eosinophils and bronchial hyperreactivity in subjects who develop late reactions.

The concept of hyperreactivity is an important one in determining the pattern of early and late asthmatic reactions (Figure 2.1). Hyperreactivity is associated with LAR but not isolated EAR, and is inhibited by prior administration of SCG or corticosteroids[30]. β-Adrenoceptor agonists, such as salbutamol, inhibit the EAR but not the LAR or the increase in bronchial hyperreactivity, suggesting that the mast cell, which is stabilized by β-agonists[31], is not as important to the LAR as the EAR. Airway hyperreactivity has been shown to have developed within 3 h of bronchial provocation, that is after the EAR but before the LAR, suggesting that the latter may be a consequence of a hyperreactive state[32].

The ability of exercise and other non-specific stimuli to precipitate EAR and LAR is dependent upon a hyperreactive state. The mechanisms by which these non-specific stimuli are effective are unclear, but temporal associations between rises in plasma histamine and serum HMW–NCA and exercise-induced early and late reactions suggest that the mast cell may be implicated[19].

24

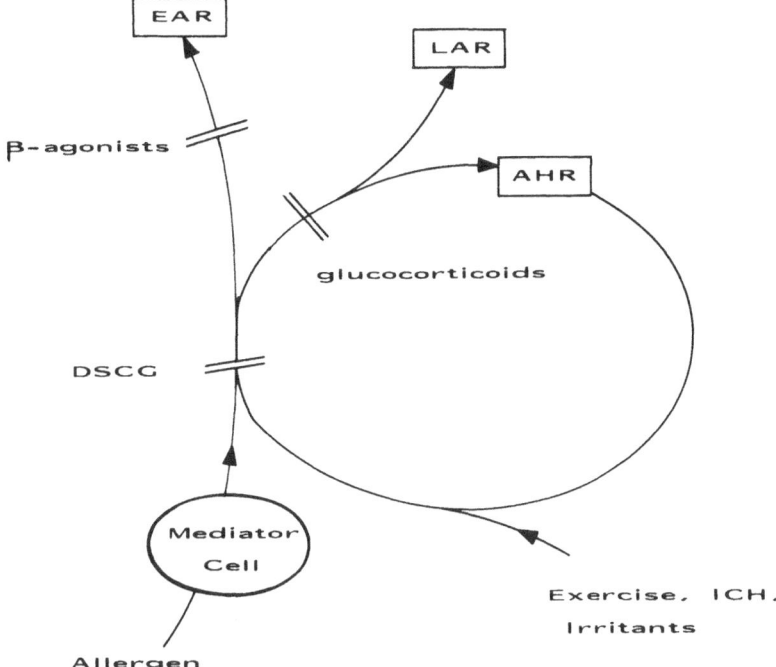

Figure 2.1 The interrelationship between the early asthmatic response (EAR), the late asthmatic response (LAR) and airway hyperreactivity (AHR)

Nose

The nose and paranasal sinuses serve to humidify, warm and filter inspired air which is en route to the lungs. Rhinitis is particularly prevalent, affecting as much as 15% of the general population, yet study of the mechanisms of nasal disease has attracted little attention until recent years. Even then, much of that interest has stemmed from the fact that the nasal mucosa has several features in common with the lung mucosa and is therefore likely to provide information to improve the understanding of pulmonary events.

Allergic rhinitis, of either the perennial or seasonal type, is triggered by inhalation of allergen. This reacts with specific IgE antibody bound to mediator secreting cells, particularly mast cells and basophils, and this, in turn, elicits the generation of various vasoactive, chemotactic and enzymatic mediators. The principal features of allergic rhinitis are sneezing, itching, congestion due to vasodilation, enhanced vascular permeability and oedema, cell infiltration, and increased nasal secretion (rhinorrhoea)[33]. The nasal mucosa is characteristically pale, blue, oedematous and covered with thin clear secretions. Nasal symptoms are often accompanied by production of tears, conjunctivitis and a sensation of an itchy palate. As in the asthmatic response, the clinical, pathological and pharmacological features of the disease can be divided into three principal phases, namely a rapid early reaction, a late sustained phase and a subacute/chronic inflammatory phase. The early reaction is particularly associated with sneezing, rhinorrhoea, and the sudden paroxysm (fit of disease) experienced during the pollen season by hay fever sufferers. The response is largely blocked by prior administration of SCG or histamine H_1-antagonists, and, as with EAR, corticosteroids are not effective inhibitors of the early reaction in the nose[34]. The LPR is associated with nasal blockage due to mucosal oedema, and mucus hypersecretion. There is a dramatic infiltration of both neutrophils and particularly eosinophils. These cells, together with mononuclear cells, feature in the chronic phase of the disease, which is also characterized by partial or total nasal obstruction and a mucopurulent discharge.

THE CONTRIBUTIONS OF EICOSANOIDS TO THE PATHOGENESIS OF EPR AND LPR

In recent years it has become increasingly apparent that the pathogenesis of diseases of the skin and upper and lower airways in which inflammation is a significant factor may involve the direct actions of many mediators and other agents, and also interrelationships between mediators. The concept of diseases such as asthma and rhinitis being attributable to a single mediator, or indeed the mediators from one cell type, is no longer tenable.

In the skin, nose and lungs, both EPRs and LPRs involve the same basic inflammatory processes. The contribution of eicosanoids to these responses is far from understood. There is strong indirect evidence for their involvement from the well-documented comprehensive range of pharmacological actions. Furthermore, the relative potentials of those cells involved in inflammatory events to generate specific eicosanoids is increasingly well appreciated. Animal models of these diseases have delineated specific roles for various eicosanoids which are integral to the mechanisms leading to the overall responses. However, these findings do not necessarily apply to man where direct evidence for the involvement of specific eicosanoids is only now beginning to emerge, particularly from studies in the skin and nose.

The demonstration of pharmacologically active levels of mediators in association with EPRs and LPRs is difficult for many reasons. The quantities in which they are produced are likely to reflect their potency in particular systems, and, as these are high in many human tissues, the *in vivo* concentrations will be low, particularly outside the immediate environment of the inflammatory focus. Furthermore, out of necessity, the body is able to metabolize rapidly the biologically potent mediators to relatively inactive metabolites. These problems are particularly apparent with the lung where sampling from the immediate environment of the asthmatic reaction is virtually impossible.

The recent availability of several 5-lipoxygenase inhibitors and leukotriene antagonists should facilitate the acquisition of a better understanding of events, particularly as these drugs become available for clinical studies.

26

Skin

The initial erythema apparent after antigen provocation in the skin of sensitive individuals is attributable to vasodilatation, increased blood flow and the recruitment of new vessels. The wealing reaction, which usually accompanies the erythema, reflects local tissue oedema which is a consequence of increased vascular permeability and the extravasation of plasma proteins. The increased vascular permeability also facilitates the efflux of inflammatory cells from the blood vessels into the surrounding tissues in response to chemotactic and chemokinetic stimuli. Several studies have suggested that PGD_2, PGE_2 and PGI_2, together with various products of the lipoxygenase pathway, may play a role as mediators of vascular events and inflammatory cell infiltration in the skin[35,36].

Prostaglandin E_2 and PGI_2 produce a prolonged erythema when injected intradermally[37], and LTC_4 and LTD_4 cause a dose-related erythema and weal formation in man[38]. Direct measurement of blood flow using a laser–Doppler technique showed that both LTC_4 and LTD_4 increased flow at a point 5 mm from the injection site[39]. The presence of a weal precluded measurements being made closer to the injection site. The erythema induced by intracutaneous injections[40] of 1 nmol of LTC_4, D_4 or E_4 persisted for up to 6 h, whereas weals resolved within 2 h. The effects of PGD_2 were shorter-lived[40,41], and LTB_4 produced only a transient weal and flare followed by induration with infiltration of neutrophils after 3–4h. Similar induration and perivascular neutrophil infiltrates were observed[38] after intradermal injections of LTB_4. The combination of LTB_4 and PGD_2 amplified induration with an increase in neutrophil infiltration[40].

Vasodilator mediators, including PGE_2 and PGI_2, which themselves have no direct vasopermeability effects, can promote vascular leakage through their effect in increasing postcapillary hydrostatic pressure[36]. Evidence from studies with LTD_4 on the hamster cheek pouch showed that the leakage was at the level of the postcapillary venules[42]. In this same model, LTC_4 and LTD_4 were shown to induce a transient constriction of arterioles. Leukotriene B_4 promotes white cell adhesion to endothelial surfaces and extravasation *in vivo*[43-45], and neutrophil chemotaxis *in vitro*[3,46].

Increased vascular permeability may be the result of one of three mechanisms. Firstly, direct action of an agonist via its specific receptors. The action of histamine is likely to be through specific receptors which are localized predominantly in the postcapillary venules[36], and sulphidopeptide leukotrienes may also act via specific receptors. Secondly, induction of leakage may result from the action of a secondary mediator. For example, it has been suggested that C3a and C5a stimulate mast cells to secrete histamine[47]; PGI_2 production by endothelial cells[48] is promoted by LTD_4 and LTE_4; and PAF-acether promotes leukotriene production in isolated rat lung[49] (see below). The third alternative involves neutrophils as intermediaries[50]. Under normal conditions, a pool of leukocytes is associated with the endothelial surface; the cells are propelled along the surface and constitute a marginating pool which is in dynamic equilibrium with the circulating cells. Chemotactic factors released as a consequence of an inflammatory trigger influence this marginating pool and promote adhesion of the cells to the endothelium. Co-operation between these adhering cells and the endothelium promotes an increase in vascular permeability and inflammatory cell exudation into the extra-vascular tissue. Chemotactic factors which may promote this series of events include LTB_4 (neutrophils and, to a lesser extent, eosinophils[51]) and PAF-acether (eosinophils[52]).

The principal primary mediator-producing cell in the skin is likely to be the mast cell which is activated via an IgE antibody specific reaction. Secondary sources may indicate the keratinocyte, which is a cell of monocyte/macrophage lineage in the epidermis, vascular endothelial cells and leukocytes in the inflammatory cell infiltrate. Mast cells are a potential source of a number of 'newly-generated' mediators, including LTC_4, 5-HETE, PGD_2 and possibly LTB_4, derived from the arachidonic acid pool incorporated in membrane phospholipids, as well as preformed granule-associated mediators, including histamine. The action of these mediators on secondary mediator cells may, in addition, promote generation of other eicosanoids; for example human keratinocytes have the capacity[53] to produce LTB_4, whilst endothelial cells from various species may produce PGI_2 (human)[54], TxA_2 (TxB_2) (bovine)[55], PGE_2 and $PGF_{2\alpha}$ (human)[56], LTB_4 and LTE_4 (porcine)[57].

Direct evidence of eicosanoid production in association with cutaneous EPR and LPR following antigen challenge in man has been obtained from skin window[58] and skin blister studies[59 61] whilst measurements in plasma from the venous drainage of challenge sites have been conducted in studies of physical urticarias[62]. Talbot and co-workers[58] used skin chambers located over denuded skin to compare the effects of ragweed and grass pollen epicutaneous challenge with buffer controls in a group of atopic individuals. The histamine concentration following antigen challenge peaked during the first hour at a level significantly greater than control, and then progressively declined. The generation of LTC_4 followed a different time-course. Samples collected hourly following antigen challenge showed elevated levels of LTC_4 at all time points compared with the parallel buffer controls. Maximal levels occurred between 2 and 4 hours after challenge and LTC_4 concentrations correlated with antigen dose. There were no significant changes in LTB_4 levels throughout the time-course of the investigation. As the flare associated with the development of a weal induced by intracutaneous injection of LTC_4 persists[40] for up to 6 h, it is perhaps unfortunate that this study was not extended beyond that time point. Nonetheless, the findings support the view that LTC_4 may be important in the pathogenesis of allergic skin reactions. Measurements of sulphidopeptide leukotrienes and LTB_4 in skin blister fluid following Prausnitz-Küstner reactions in peanut-sensitive subjects were made 30 min after challenge by ingestion of peanuts[59]. There was a significant increase in the concentration of LTC_4 immunoreactive material, and LTB_4 concentrations increased in 9 out of the 12 subjects tested. It was concluded that LTC_4 was contributing to the allergic cutaneous reaction, but it was felt unlikely that LTB_4 was involved in the response, presumably because the increases in concentrations were small and only observed in some patients. Although both these studies failed to identify LTB_4 in association with either the EPR or the LPR, it is premature to dismiss LTB_4 as a mediator of the reactions before making a full appraisal of the assay technology, particularly with regard to its recovery from the samples, and giving full consideration to the metabolic fate of the mediator *in vivo*. There is evidence that PGD_2 is produced, together with histamine, by patients with cold urticaria, a significant rise in the concentration of this eicosanoid being detected 12 min after challenge[62].

The likely sorces of LTC_4 are the resident mast cells and eosinophils which begin to accumulate from 2 h onwards. PGD_2 may also be produced by the mast cells. Monocytes and basophils do not begin to accumulate in the cellular infiltrate until later and therefore are unlikely to contribute to these LTC_4 concentrations.

The demonstration of increased concentrations of a mediator in association with a response does not answer the question of whether that mediator is a cause or a consequence of the response. This point arises from a study conducted by Dorsch and Ring[60], in which skin blister fluid recovered at progressive time intervals from the sites of dual cutaneous reactions was injected into separate sites on the donor and thereby elicited LPR. Fluid collected at 30 min, in association with an EPR, induced an LPR at a separate site, whereas fluid collected at 180 or 300 min had a lesser effect. The possible involvement of residual antigen was discounted. These observations suggest that the mediators formed during the early response are necessary for the full expression of an LPR. In a subsequent study, this same group identified peak concentrations of histamine during the EPR (30 min) and raised concentrations of TxB_2 in association with the LPR (6 h)[63]. The full significance of such observations will only become clear when data for other potential mediators are available together with data from studies involving specific antagonists and/or inhibitors of mediator synthesis. Studies with specific histamine H_1 and H_2 antagonists revealed that the EPR was significantly inhibited by an H_1, but not an H_2 antagonist. Neither antagonist alone had an effect on the LPR, but in combination they obliterated the LPR in most subjects. Histamine alone does not produce a late response, and therefore the data suggest either involvement of mast cell mediators other than histamine or mediators such as arachidonic acid metabolites generated secondary to mast cell activation[64]. Acetylsalicylic acid was without effect, thus raising doubts as to a role for prostaglandins. The efficacy of a locally administered β_2-adrenoceptor agoniser, terbutaline, in blocking allergic cutaneous reactions testifies to the importance of the mast cell[65].

Lung

The oxidative metabolism of arachidonic acid by human pulmonary tissue generates a spectrum of pharmacological mediators including, via the cyclo-oxygenase pathway, PGD_2, PGE_2, $PGF_{2\alpha}$, PGI_2 and TxA_2, and, via lipoxygenase pathways, LTC_4, LTD_4, LTE_4, LTB_4 and various mono-HETEs[66-68]. Inflammatory cells that infiltrate into the extravascular tissues in association with the LAR are an additional potential source of some of these mediators.

Bronchoconstrictor activity is associated with PGD_2, $PGF_{2\alpha}$, TxA_2, LTC_4, LTD_4, LTE_4 and LTB_4. Prostaglandin D_2 may exert some of its effect through one of its immediate metabolites[69], $9\alpha,11\beta$-PGF_2, and any action on the part of LTB_4 would be through its ability to cause TxA_2 release from lung parenchyma[70].

Inhalation of aerosolized LTC_4 and LTD_4 by normal human volunteers revealed that they had approximately 4000 and 6000 times the potency of histamine respectively when measuring $\dot{V}_{30}$ (flow at 30% of vital capacity)[71,72]. The measurement of $\dot{V}_{30}$ is thought to reflect changes in calibre of small airways. The maximal effects produced by optimal concentrations of LTC_4 and LTD_4 were comparable, but the time course of their effects differed. The response time to LTC_4 was slower than to LTD_4, a maximal effect[71,72] being seen between 12 and 17 min as opposed to 2 and 7 min. The effect produced by LTC_4 was slower to resolve than that due to LTD_4. Later studies which compared measurements of $\dot{V}_{30}$ and specific airway conductance, which is thought to reflect effects on large airways, failed to distinguish a preferential effect on small peripheral airways, but did confirm the potency and time-course of action of these leukotrienes. The time-course is consistent with changes in lung function associated with the EAR. The EAR is thought to reflect bronchospastic changes in larger, more central airways, whilst the LAR involves the more peripheral, small airways[19]. Measurement of $\dot{V}_{30}$ in asthmatics[73] did not reveal hypersensitivity to LTC_4 and LTD_4, but measurement of airway resistance, which is dependent on central airway function, did reveal hyper-reactivity[74,75] in proportion to histamine reactivity.

Leukotriene E_4 has been shown to induce bronchoconstriction in normal subjects, and, whilst its activity is less than that of LTC_4 or LTD_4, it is still 100 times more active than histamine[76].

Inhalation of an aerosolized solution of synthetic LTD_4 by sheep with a documented history of LAR to *Ascaris suum* produced both early and late reactions as measured by changes in specific airway resistance[77]. The leukotriene antagonist FPL 55712 reversed both LTD_4-induced responses when given as a 1% w/v aerosolized solution. It blocked only the LAR induced by antigen provocation whereas SCG was effective against both EAR and LAR[78]. Indomethacin had no effect on either reaction[79]. These data suggested a prominent role for sulphidopeptide leukotrienes in the LAR in sheep.

Mast cells are undoubtedly the principal potential source of LTC_4 in EAR. Allergen challenge of bronchial strips from asthmatic subjects sensitive to birch pollen triggered smooth muscle contraction which was related to LTC_4 production[80]. In a separate study using human bronchial smooth muscle spirals, an IgE-mediated contraction was not blocked by any one of diphenhydramine, indomethacin or the 5-lipoxygenase inhibitor U-60257 (piriprost), or combinations of any two drugs, although all three together caused significant inhibition of contraction[81]. Dazoxiben, a thromboxane-synthesis inhibitor, had no effect on contraction when tested alone. In combination with diphenhydramine and U-60257, it inhibited contraction by more than 60%, suggesting that at least part of the contractile response is due to TxA_2.

Macrophages and eosinophils, which also have IgE (Fc) receptors, albeit of lower affinity than those on mast cells, could also contribute following IgE-dependent activation[82,83]. The large numbers of eosinophils migrating into the extravascular pulmonary tissue and the airways during the course of the LAR and in chronic asthma are a potential source of LTC_4. Various studies[84-86] have shown that these cells can produce LTC_4 in pharmacologically active amounts following stimulation with the calcium ionophore, A23187, but, more importantly, following reaction of IgG with membrane-associated Fc receptors[87].

Prostaglandin D_2 is the principal cyclo-oxygenase product of human lung parenchymal mast cells[68,88], and $PGF_{2\alpha}$ is produced in lesser amounts. Measurement of specific airway conductance showed that PGD_2 had broncho-constrictor properties in both normal and asthmatic subjects, but $PGF_{2\alpha}$ was active only in the asthmatic group at the concentrations used. Both prostaglandins produced maximal effects within 3 min, PGD_2 being 3.5 times more active[89] than $PGF_{2\alpha}$. The time-course of release of PGD_2 from purified human lung mast cells in vitro[68] is faster than that of LTC_4 and achieves 50% within 5 min. PAF-acether, on the other hand, is synthesized rapidly and levels are maximal at 2 min. However, there is little solid evidence that PAF-acether is released extracellularly in significant quantities. The kinetics of generation of all three mediators are compatible with their playing a role in EAR. Mast cell-associated chemotactic factors, such as LTB_4 and HMW-NCA, can enhance the numeric expression of membrane receptors for IgG (Fc) and complement (C3b) on neutrophils, eosinophils and monocytes[19,90], as judged by using a rosette technique. This may have biological significance as time-dependent increases in the percentages of neutrophil and monocyte rosettes have been observed in vivo in association with both exercise- and specific allergen-induced asthma[18,91]. The increase in complement receptors was seen to continue through into the LPR following antigen provocation[92]. Leukotriene B_4 will enhance the cytotoxic capacity of neutrophils, and to a lesser extent eosinophils, towards opsonized helminthic larvae in vitro (schistosomula of Schistosomula mansoni)[93]. This increased cytotoxic capacity has been shown to be manifested by neutrophils following exercise-induced asthma[94] and is thought to reflect an increased functional expression of receptors. Inflammatory cells, activated according to these criteria, may be recruited to the lung and participate in LPR.

One manifestation in the LAR is bronchoconstriction, and the capacities of various eicosanoids to induce this have been discussed earlier. Various mediators could theoretically contribute to the inflammatory components of the LAR, and are probably similar to those which promote haemodynamic changes, increases in vascular permeability and inflammatory cell exudation in the skin. An important consideration is that many of these mediators may be derived from the infiltrating leukocytes and these could serve to perpetuate the response. Neutrophils, for example, may be recruited into the extravascular pulmonary tissue by chemotactic agents such as LTB_4, 5-HETE and PGD_2, generated in association with EAR. These cells may then generate LTB_4 to continue the recruitment. Leukotriene B_4 is also chemotactic for eosinophils, but its activity is overshadowed by that of PAF-acether[95]. Indirect evidence to support a role for neutrophils in LAR comes from a rabbit model of an allergen-induced LPR, in which chemical depletion of neutrophils abrogated the response[96]. The reaction was restored after reconstitution of the neutrophils[97].

Bronchorrhoea or excess bronchial secretion is associated with various pulmonary diseases, including asthma[98], and is a feature of LAR, but more particularly, chronic asthma. The main component of the secretions is produced by the serous and mucous cells in the submucosal glands and by goblet cells. The submucosal glands are under parasympathetic nerve control, unlike goblet cells, which may respond independently to non-specific irritants, such as sulphur dioxide and smoke, or to specific inflammatory mediators. Using cultured human respiratory mucosa and the ability of this tissue to incorporate radio-isotopically labelled sugars and amino acids into newly-synthesized mucous glycoproteins, several mucus secretagogues have been identified. These include arachidonic acid and several of its cyclo-oxygenase and lipoxygenase metabolites, notably PGE_1, $PGF_{2\alpha}$, PGD_2, PGI_2, LTC_4, LTD_4 and the 5-, 8-, 9-, 11-, 12- and 15-monoHETEs[98]. Conversely, PGE_2 inhibits mucus secretion as do eicosatetraenoic acid (ETYA), U-60,257 and other lipoxygenase inhibitors, and corticosteroids. Mucus hypersecretion and mucus plugging, which are features of chronic and severe asthma, may be due in part to one or more of these mediators. The eosinophil, which features prominently in the vasculature, extravascular tissue and airways may contribute to events by generating LTC_4 and 15-HETE. The latter is also produced by pulmonary epithelial cells[99]. The effectiveness of lipoxygenase inhibitors in reducing secretion lends further support to the suggestion that these mediators may be important *in vivo*.

Whilst, on the one hand, several eicosanoids may influence mucus production, on the other they may play a significant role in the control of mucociliary clearance. In patients with allergic bronchial asthma, involuntary clearance is impaired and a further decrease in tracheal mucus transport is seen in association with EAR[100]. *In vitro* studies with sheep tracheal epithelial cells showed that LTC_4, PGE_1, and PGE_2 within the range $10^{-8}-10^{-6}$ mol L^{-1}, all increased ciliary beat frequency. In these experiments, $PGF_{2\alpha}$ had no effect[101].

Direct evidence to implicate specific mediators with EAR and LPR is difficult to obtain. Concentrations of the mast cell-associated mediators histamine and high molecular weight neutrophil chemotactic activity (HMW–NCA) have been shown to be raised during both EAR and LAR following antigen challenge[102], but, for many reasons, it has proved difficult to demonstrate parallel increased concentrations of eicosanoids in association with these responses, always supposing they do occur. Sampling from the peripheral venous circulation remote from the site of mediator production is far from ideal because of dilution throughout the body and rapid metabolism. Furthermore, the assay of lipid mediators from plasma requires a preliminary extraction which invariably results in some loss. Radioimmunoassay supported by high performance liquid chromatography (HPLC) verification is satisfactory for determination of leukotriene concentrations[103] and some cyclo-oxygenase metabolites, but gas chromatography–mass spectrometry (GC–MS) is the method of choice for many of the eicosanoids.

Challenge of asthmatic lung tissue with specific antigen clearly demonstrated its capacity to generate sulphidopeptide leukotrienes[80]. The measurement of LTC_4 immunoreactivity in the blood of asthmatic children suggested that

32

there was an association between eicosanoid concentration and severity of the asthma[104]. There was, however, considerable overlap between the asymptomatic, slight to moderate, and severe asthma groups. Also, the control group of five healthy adult males was inappropriate. A similar investigation in our laboratory has failed to distinguish between these groups of patients in terms of 'resting' plasma LTC_4 concentrations (unpublished data). An investigation of three asthmatics who developed both EAR and LAR revealed no significant changes in HMW–NCA, LTB_4 or LTC_4 immunoreactivity over a 12 h period following methacholine bronchial provocation. After antigen challenge, increases in LTB_4 and HMW–NCA corresponded with early and late reactions. Concentrations of LTB_4 ($ng\,ml^{-1}$) were 1.2, 0.5 and 1.1 during the early response and 1.0, 0.8 and 1.8 during the late reaction. Changes in LTC_4 concentrations were small and inconsistent[105]. However, subsequent studies in our laboratory using improved extraction techniques together with HPLC and radioimmunoassay, suggest that LTC_4 is released in significant amounts in association with EAR (unpublished data). Data obtained in another laboratory[106] comparing normal volunteers and asthmatics during a severe attack, showed increased levels of venous plasma LTB_4, 4.1 ± 0.7 vs $8.4 \pm 1.8\,pmol\,ml^{-1}$.

Plasma levels of TxB_2, which reflect TxA_2 production, have been shown to rise in association with the EAR following antigen challenge in subjects with single EAR or dual reactions[107]: indomethacin pretreatment suppressed the LAR. Increases in TxB_2 were blocked by the indomethacin but at the same time PGI_2 levels were increased. Shepard et al. suggested that this indomethacin-dependent production of PGI_2, which has smooth muscle relaxing properties[107], and inhibition of TxB_2, contributed to the suppression of the LAR. This supports the view of Schellenberg et al.[81] that TxA_2 may contribute to the contractile response in lung.

It is to be hoped that BAL performed in asthmatics in association with EAR and LAR will prove to be rewarding but it remains to be seen whether the mediator concentrations reflect the product of lumenal cells alone or a contribution from pulmonary tissue as well.

Nose

The nose is arguably the most appropriate organ for the study of EPR and LPR as the nasal passages are easily accessible for studying cytological changes and the release of inflammatory mediators during the course of the response to antigen challenge. The nasal secretions can be harvested rapidly, so minimizing the chances for their metabolism, and the nature of the secretions is such that the recovery of lipid mediators is far less problematical than is the case with plasma.

One of the first reported studies that attempted to identify the mediators involved in the pathogenesis of allergic rhinitis was that of Dolovich et al.[108] who identified kinin-like activity in the nasal secretions of atopic subjects following specific antigen challenge. The first evidence of eicosanoid generation came from a study of the nasal secretions of symptomatic hay fever subjects. Prostaglandin E was found in the secretions obtained from six of the twelve patients studied[109]. The first study to demonstrate a clear association between mediator release and the physiological changes of allergic rhinitis, produced following insufflation of allergen into the nose, identified histamine, TAME-esterase and PGD_2 in nasal lavage[110]. Nasal airway resistance was assessed by anterior rhinomanometry but did not accurately reflect the nasal response. Repeated washing with warm saline was found to be necessary in order to reduce the background levels of mediators so that subsequent allergen-associated concentration changes could be fully appreciated. Allergen-induced responses frequently led to mucosal oedema and reduced nasal capacity which hampered recovery of nasal lavage fluid. Nevertheless increases in histamine, TAME-esterase and PGD_2 were shown to accompany the allergen-induced physiological changes in the nose as reflected by the number of sneezes. All three mediators were considered to be mast cell associated, and released or generated through the involvement of IgE-mediated mechanisms[111].

Subsequent studies identified a significant correlation between the clinical response to ragweed antigen and the production of sulphidopeptide leukotrienes[112,113]. There was a dose-dependent relationship between the quantity of antigen insufflated into the nose and the amount of immunoreactive LTC_4 produced. Reversed-phase HPLC revealed a mixture of LTC_4, D_4 and E_4, indicating enzymatic degradation of LTC_4. The maximum concentration of LTC_4 was recovered in the 7.5 min nasal lavage. Control nasal challenges were performed with methacholine[113], which acts directly on glandular cholinoceptors to promote nasal secretion[114]. There were no significant amounts of sulphidopeptide leukotrienes either before or after methacholine challenge, indicating that it was not the production of nasal secretions *per se* that stimulated mediator generation. LTB_4 was also produced following antigen challenge but it was found in smaller quantities than LTC_4 (4.3 pmol (range 2.7–6.4) LTB_4 against 21.0 pmol (9.6–27.9) LTC_4).

The nasal LPR manifests itself by a recurrence of symptoms 3 to 11 h after challenge. Whereas EPR was associated[115] with increases in the concentrations of histamine, TAME-esterases, kinins and PGD_2, PGD_2 was not produced during the LPR. In man, PGD_2 is a mast cell product and its absence from nasal secretions prompted the suggestion that basophils in the late phase cellular infiltrate were partly responsible for the LPR. Evidence for basophil infiltration in association with LPRs in man is weak but an analogy can be made with the late phase of cutaneous basophil hypersensitivity in animal models[116].

The nasal LPR is characterized by a massive infiltration of neutrophils and eosinophils, and LTB_4 could be one chemotactic agent that promotes this. However, oral administration of the corticosteroid prenisolone did not block LTB_4 production following antigen nasal challenge[117] despite the fact that the corticosteroid abrogated the LPR, the inflammatory cell infiltrate[118] and the release of histamine, TAME-esterase and kinins[119].

The study of mucus secretion by cultured nasal turbinate tissue suggests that the number of agents able to promote secretion is relatively restricted compared with that for lung mucosa[95]. Neither arachidonic acid nor any of its cyclo-oxygenase and lipoxygenase metabolites were effective, in contrast to findings with lung mucosa.

Leukotriene D_4 applied topically to nasal mucosa produced a dose-dependent increase in blood flow over the range 0.063–4.0 nmol as assessed by laser-Doppler measurement[120]. This observation is supported by similar findings in human skin[39].

In vitro studies to assess the likely potential of nasal tissue for generating mediators of inflammation can be performed most conveniently using nasal polyp tissue, which contains essentially the same cellular constituents as the nasal mucosa. Specific allergen challenge of chopped nasal polyp tissue, passively sensitized with serum from an allergen-sensitive subject, resulted[121] in histamine release, maximal at approximately 5 min, and generation of sulphidopeptide leukotrienes and LTB_4 which were detected after 30 min.

Eye

Tears from subjects with grass pollen rhinoconjunctivitis, obtained after specific allergen challenge, have been shown to contain LTC_4 immunoreactivity[122]. The EPR, characterized by intense redness, swelling and itching of the conjunctivi, occurred after 5–10 min. Formal identification of the leukotrienes by reversed-phase HPLC was not possible for individual samples, but pooled material was found[59] to contain LTC_4, LTD_4 and LTE_4. There was no indication of a rise in LTB_4 levels following antigen challenge[59].

CONCLUSIONS

The investigation of EPRs, and particularly LPRs, has revealed the importance of inflammation in the pathogenesis of these diseases with an allergic background. The success of glucocorticosteroids in inhibiting the LPR, but not the EPR, is reflected in their ability to block the inflammatory cell infiltrate and the release of mediators. The side-effects produced by the use of glucocorticosteroids on a continuing day-to-day basis for the control of those diseases associated with LPRs merits the investigation of alternative anti-inflammatory therapy.

The control of eicosanoid production through the inhibition of phospholipase activity may be a significant factor in the modulation of inflammatory reactions by glucocorticosteroids, which may act via the endogenous phospholipase inhibitor, lipocortin. Non-steroidal anti-inflammatory drugs can block the cyclo-oxygenase activity, the first step in the generation of the prostaglandins. A number of drugs showing specificity for the 5-lipoxygenase pathway are now becoming available for evaluation. One study has called into doubt a possible role for leukotrienes in the pathogenesis of exercise- and allergen-induced asthma[123]. Piriprost U-60,257, a 5-lipoxygenase inhibitor with some leukotriene antagonist properties[124], had no protective effect against changes in FEV_1 following either exercise- or antigen-induced EAR or antigen-induced LPR[123]. The inhibition of one pathway, either lipoxygenase or cyclo-oxygenase, may cause an imbalance between pro- and anti-inflammatory properties of various eicosanoids. This is particularly so in the case of cyclo-oxygenase inhibition in some asthmatic subjects in whom a worsening of symptoms occurs. This could be explained in terms of reduced levels of the bronchodilator prostaglandins, PGE_2 and PGI_2, which may be essential to counter the bronchoconstrictor properties of other prostaglandins, leukotrienes and non-lipid mediators, so maintaining 'airway tone' - the *status quo*. The leukotriene pathway has greater potential for control because it involves a number of enzyme-specific steps at which drugs would intervene. Furthermore, specific receptors for sulphidopeptide leukotrienes on both vascular and non-vascular smooth muscle, and for LTB_4 on neutrophils, offer potential scope for specific receptor antagonists.

The evidence for the pro-inflammatory activities of eicosanoids is substantial and there is a considerable amount of data suggesting that various of these mediators are involved with EPR, LPR and hyperreactivity, and in turn with associated disease. There is therefore good cause for developing the means of controlling the biosynthesis and functional activity of these mediators.

REFERENCES

1. Durham, S.R., Carroll, M., Lee, T.H., Cromwell, O., Graneek, B., Newman-Taylor, A.J. and Kay, A.B. (1986). Mechanisms of early and late asthmatic reactions. In Reed, E. (ed.) *Proceedings of the XII International Congress of Allergy and Clinical Immunology*, pp. 229–236. (St. Louis, Missouri: C.V. Mosby)
2. Warner, J.O., Price, J.F., Soothill, J.F. and Hey, E.N. (1978). Controlled trial of hypersensitization to *Dermatophagoides pteronyssinus* in children with asthma. *Lancet*, **2**, 912–915
3. Goetzl, E.J. and Pickett, W.C. (1980). The human PMN leucocyte chemotactic activity of complex hydroxyeicosatetraenoic acids (HETEs). *J. Immunol.*, **125**, 1789–91
4. Kopp, D.E., Esser, B., Tashoff, T., Goldman, D.W., Goetzl, E.J. and Lemanske, R.F. (1986). In vivo and in vitro assessment of the role of leukotriene B_4 as a mediator of rat cutaneous late-phase reactions. *J. Allergy Clin. Immunol.*, **77**, 302–8
5. Dahlén, S.E., Hedqvist, P., Hammarström, S. and Samuelsson, B. (1980). Leukotrienes are potent constrictors of human bronchi. *Nature*, **288**, 484–86
6. Krell, R.D., Osborn, R., Vickery, L., Falcone, K., O'Donnell, M., Gleason, J., Kinzig, C. and Bryan, D. (1981). Contraction of isolated airway smooth muscle by synthetic leukotrienes C_4 and D_4. *Prostaglandins*, **22**, 387–409
7. Cromwell, O., Durham, S.R., Shaw, R.J., Mackay, J.A. and Kay, A.B. (1986). Provocation tests and measurements of mediators from mast cells and basophils in asthma and allergic rhinitis. In Weir, D.M., Blackwell, C.C. and Herzenberg, L.A. (eds.) *Handbook of Experimental Immunology*, 4th Edn. Vol. 4, pp. 127–127.51. (Edinburgh: Blackwell Scientific Publications)
8. Editorial (1983). Inflammatory mediators of asthma. *Lancet*, **2**, 829–831
9. Coombs, R.R.A. and Gell, P.G.H. (1968). Classification of allergic reactions responsible for clinical hypersensitivity and disease. In Gell, P.G.H. and Coombs, R.R.A. (eds.) *Clinical Aspects of Immunology*, 2nd Edn. pp. 575–596. (Oxford: Blackwell Scientific Publications)
10. Pepys, J., Turner-Warwick, M., Dawson, P.L. and Hinson, K.F.W. (1986). Arthus (type III) skin test reactions in man. Clinical and immunopathological features. In Rose, B., Richter, M., Sehon, A. and Frankland, A.W. (eds.) *Allergology*. Proceedings of the Sixth Congress of the International Association of Allergology, pp. 221–235. (Amsterdam: Excerpta Medica Foundation)
11. Dolovich, J., Hargreave, F.E., Chalmers, R., Shier, K.J., Gauldie, J. and Bienenstock, J. (1973). Late cutaneous allergic responses in IgE-dependent reactions. *J. Allergy Clin. Immunol.*, **52** 38–46

12. Solley, G.O., Gleich, G.J., Jordan, R.E. and Schroeter, A.L. (1976). The late phase of the immediate wheal and flare skin reaction: its dependence upon IgE antibodies. *J. Clin. Invest.*, **58**, 408–20
13. Pienkowski, M.M., Norman, P.S. and Lichtenstein, L.M. (1985). Suppression of late-phase skin reactions by immunotherapy with ragweed extract. *J. Allergy Clin. Immunol.*, **76**, 729–34
14. Atkins, P.C., Green, G. and Zweiman, B. (1973). Histologic studies on human skin test responses to ragweed, compound 48/80, and histamine. *J. Allergy Clin. Immunol.*, **51**, 263–73
15. Price, J.F., Hey, E.N. and Soothill, J.F. (1982). Antigen provocation to the skin, nose and lung in children with asthma: immediate and dual hypersensitivity reactions. *Clin. Exp. Immunol.*, **47**, 587–94
16. Kay, A.B. and Lee, T. (1982). Neutrophil chemotactic factor of anaphylaxis. *J. Allergy Clin. Immunol.*, **70**, 317–20
17. Holgate, S.T., Emanuel, M.B. and Howarth, P.H. (1985). Astemizole and other H_1 antihistaminic drug treatment of asthma. *J. Allergy Clin. Immunol.*, **76** (Suppl.), 375–80
18. Carroll, M., Durham, S.R., Walsh, G.M. and Kay, A.B. (1985). Activation of neutrophils and monocytes after allergen- and histamine-induced bronchoconstriction. *J. Allergy Clin. Immunol.*, **75**, 290–296
19. Kay, A.B. (1986). Mediators and inflammatory cells in asthma. In Kay, A.B. (ed.) *Asthma: Clinical Pharmacology and Therapeutic Progress*, pp. 1–10. (Oxford: Blackwell Scientific Publications)
20. Hogg, J.C. (1985). The pathology of asthma. *Clin. Chest Med.*, **5**, 567–71
21. Metzger, W.J., Nugent, K. and Richerson, H.B. (1985). Site of airflow obstruction during early and late phase asthmatic responses to allergen bronchoprovocation. *Chest*, **88**, 369–75
22. Behrens, B.L., Clark, R.A.F., Feldsein, D.C., Presley, D.M., Glezen, L.S., Groves, J.P. and Larsen, G.L. (1985). Comparison of the histopathology of the immediate and late asthmatic and cutaneous responses in a rabbit model. *Chest*, **87**, 153S
23. Larsen, G.L., Shampain, M.P., Marsh, W.R. and Behrens, B.L. (1984). An animal model of the late asthmatic response to antigen challenge. In Kay, A.B., Austen, K.F. and Lichtenstein, L.M. (eds.) *Asthma: Physiology, Pharmacology and Treatment*, pp. 245–262. (London: Academic Press)
24. Metzger, W.J., Nugent, K., Richerson, H.B., Moseley, P., Larkin, R., Zavala, D. and Hunninghake, G.W. (1985). Methods of bronchoalveolar lavage in asthmatic patients following bronchoprovocation and local antigen challenge. *Chest*, **87**, 16S–19S
25. Diaz, P., Gonzalez, C., Galleguillos, F., Ancic, P. and Kay, A.B. (1986). Eosinophils and macrophages in bronchial mucus and bronchoalveolar lavage during allergen induced late-phase asthmatic reactions. *J. Allergy Clin. Immunol.*, **77**, 244 (Abst.)
26. Boschetto, P., Zocca, E., Milani, G.F., Licata, B., Pivirotto, F., Mapp, C.E. and Fabbri, L.M. (1986). Bronchoalveolar neutrophilia during late, but not early, asthmatic reactions induced by toluene diisocyanate (TDI). *J. Allergy Clin. Immunol.*, **77**, 244 (Abst.)
27. de Monchy, J.G.R., Kauffman, H.F., Venge, P., Koeter, G.H., Jansen, H.M., Sluiter, H.J. and de Vries, K. (1985). Bronchoalveolar eosinophilia during allergen-induced late asthmatic reactions. *Am. Rev. Respir. Dis.*, **131**, 373–6
28. Worden, K., Metzger, W.J., Kopp, W., Richerson, H.B. and Hunninghake, G.W. (1983). Dissolution of eosinophil granules in bronchial lavage obtained from allergic asthmatics during bronchoprovocation and seasonal exposure. *Proc. Ann. EMSA*, **41**, 798
29. Durham, S.R. and Kay, A.B. (1985). Eosinophils, bronchial hyperreactivity and late-phase asthmatic reactions. *Clin. Allergy*, **15**, 411–18
30. Cockroft, D.W. and Murdock, K.Y. (1986). Protective effect of inhaled Albuterol, Cromolyn, Beclamethasone and placebo on allergen-induced early asthmatic response (EAR), late asthmatic response (LAR), and allergen induced increase in bronchial responsiveness to inhaled histamine. *J. Allergy Clin. Immunol.*, **77**, 122 (Abst.)
31. Holgate, S.T., Benyon, R.C., Howarth, P.H., Agius, R., Hardy, C., Robinson, C., Durham, S.R., Kay, A.B. and Church, M.K. (1985). Relationship between mediator release from human lung mast cells in vitro and in vivo. *Int. Arch. Allergy Appl. Immunol.*, **77**, 47–48
32. Durham, S.R., Graneek, B., Hawkins, R. and Newman-Taylor, A. (1986). Increases in non-specific bronchial responsiveness precede the late asthmatic reaction induced by occupational agents. *J. Allergy Clin. Immunol.*, **77**, 173 (Abst.)

33. Wasserman, S.I. (1982). Immunology and pathophysiology of allergic rhinitis. In Goetzl, E.J. and Kay, A.B. (eds.) *Current Perspectives in Allergy*, pp. 40–51. (Edinburgh: Churchill Livingstone)

34. Mygind, N. (1979). *Nasal Allergy*, 2nd Edn. (Oxford: Blackwell Scientific Publications)

35. Camp, R.D.R. (1982). Prostaglandins, hydroxy fatty acids, leukotrienes and inflammation of the skin. *Clin. Exp. Dermatol.*, **7**, 435–44

36. Smedegard, G. and Björk, J. (1985). Inflammation and the microvascular endothelium. In Venge, P. and Lindbaum, A. (eds.) *Inflammation*, pp. 25–46. (Stockholm: Almqvist and Wiksell International)

37. Solomon, L.M., Juhlin, L. and Kirschenbaum, M.B. (1968). Prostaglandins on cutaneous vasculature. *J. Invest. Dermatol.*, **51**, 280–282

38. Camp, R.D.R., Coutts, A.A., Greaves, M.W., Kay, A.B. and Walport, M.J. (1983). Responses of human skin to intradermal injection of leukotrienes C_4, D_4 and B_4. *Br. J. Pharmacol.*, **80**, 497–502

39. Bisgaard, H., Kristensen, J. and Sondergaard, J. (1982). The effect of leukotriene C_4 and D_4 on cutaneous blood flow in humans. *Prostaglandins*, **23**, 797–801

40. Soter, N.A., Lewis, R.A., Corey, E.J. and Austen, K.F. (1983). Local effects of synthetic leukotrienes (LTC_4, LTD_4 and LTB_4) in human skin. *J. Invest. Dermatol.*, **80**, 115–119

41. Flower, R.J., Harvey, E.A. and Kington, W.P. (1976). Inflammatory effects of prostaglandin D_2 in rat and human skin. *Br. J. Pharmacol.*, **56**, 229–33

42. Dahlén, S-E., Björk, J., Hedqvist, P., Arfors, K.-E., Hammarström, S., Lindgren, J-A. and Samuelsson, B. (1981). Leukotrienes promote plasma leakage and leukocyte adhesion in postcapillary venules: *in vivo* effects with relevance to the acute inflammatory response. *Proc. Natl. Acad. Sci. USA*, **78**, 3887–91

43. Lindbom, L., Hedqvist, P., Dahlén, S.-E., Lindgren, J.-A. and Arfors, K.-E. (1982). Leukotriene B_4 induces extravasation and migration of polymorphonuclear leukocytes *in vivo. Acta Physiol. Scand.*, **116**, 105–108

44. Bray, M.A., Ford-Hutchinson, A.W. and Smith, M.J.H. (1981). Leukotriene B_4: an inflammatory mediator *in vivo. Prostaglandins*, **22**, 213–222

45. Lewis, R.A., Goetzl, E.J., Drazen, J.M., Soter, N.A., Austen, K.F. and Corey, E.J. (1981). Functional characterization of synthetic leukotriene B and its stereochemical isomers. *J. Exp. Med.*, **154**, 1243–48

46. Ford-Hutchinson, A.W., Bray, M.A., Doig, M.V., Shipley, M.E. and Smith M.J.H. (1980). Leukotriene B: A potent chemokinetic and aggregating substance released from polymorphonuclear leukocytes. *Nature*, **286**, 264–65

47. Holgate, S.T., Hardy, C.C., Robinson, C., Agius, R.M. and Howarth, P.H. (1986). The mast cell as a primary effector cell in the pathogenesis of asthma. *J. Allergy Clin. Immunol.*, **77**, 274–82

48. Pologe, L.G., Cramer, E.B., Pawlowski, N.A., Abraham, E., Cohn, Z.A. and Scott, W.A. (1984). Stimulation of human endothelial cell prostacyclin synthesis by select leukotrienes. *J. Exp. Med.*, **160**, 1043–53

49. Voelkel, N.F., Worthen, S., Reeves, J.T., Henson, P.M. and Murphy, R.C. (1982). Non-immunological production of leukotrienes induced by platelet activating factor. *Science*, **218**, 286–88

50. Wedmore, C.V. and Williams, T.J. (1981). Control of vascular permeability by polymorphonuclear leucocytes in inflammation. *Nature*, **289**, 646–650

51. Björk, J., Dahlén, S.E., Hedqvist, P. and Afors, K.-E. (1983). Leukotrienes B_4 and C_4 have distinct microcirculatory action *in vivo*. In Samuelsson, B., Ramwell, P.W. and Paoletti, R. (eds.) *Advances in Prostaglandin, Thromboxane and Leukotriene Research*, **12**, 1–6. (New York: Raven Press)

52. Björk, J. and Smedegard, G. (1983). Acute microvascular effects of PAF-acether, as studied by intravital microscopy. *Eur. J. Pharmacol.*, **96**, 87–94

53. Grabbe, J., Rosenbach, T. and Czornetzki, B.M. (1985). Production of LTB_4-like chemotactic arachidonate metabolites from human keratinocytes. *J. Invest. Dermatol.*, **85**, 527–30

54. Weksler, B.B., Marcus, A.J. and Jaffe, E.A. (1977). Synthesis of prostaglandin I_2 (prostacyclin) by cultured human and bovine endothelial cells. *Proc. Natl. Acad. Sci. USA*, **74**, 3922–6

55. Ingerman-Wojenski, C., Silver, M.J., Smith, J.B. and Macarak, E. (1981). Bovine endothelial cells in culture produce thromboxane as well as prostacyclin. *J. Clin. Invest.*, **67**, 1292–96

56. Alhenc-Gelas, F., Tsai, S.J., Callahan, K.S., Campbell, W.B. and Johnson, A.R. (1982). Stimulation of prostaglandin formation by vasoactive mediators in cultured human endothelial cells. *Prostaglandins*, **24**, 723–4

57. Piper, P.J. and Galton, S.A. (1984). Generation of leukotriene B_4 and leukotriene E_4 from porcine pulmonary artery. *Prostaglandins*, **28**, 905–14

58. Talbot, S.F., Atkins, P.C., Goetzl, E.J. and Zweiman, B. (1985). Accumulation of leukotriene C_4 and histamine in human allergic skin reactions. *J. Clin. Invest.*, **76**, 650–56

59. Bisgaard, H., Ford-Hutchinson, A.W., Charleson, S. and Taudorf, E. (1985). Production of leukotrienes in human skin and conjunctival mucosa after specific allergen challenge. *Allergy*, **40**, 417–23

60. Dorsch, W. and Ring, J. (1981). Induction of late cutaneous reactions by skin blister fluid from allergen-tested and normal skin. *J. Allergy Clin. Immunol.*, **67**, 117–23

61. Dorsch, W., Ring, J., Weber, P.C. and Strasser, T. (1985). Detection of immunoreactive leukotrienes LTC_4/D_4 in skin-blister fluid after allergen testing in patients with late cutaneous reactions (LCR). *Arch. Dermatol. Res.*, **277**, 400–401

62. Heavey, D., Kobza-Black, A., Barrow, S.E., Chappell, C.G., Greaves, M.W. and Dollery, C.T. (1985). Prostaglandin D_2 and histamine release in cold urticaria. *Br. J. Clin. Pharmacol.*, **20**, 270P

63. Dorsch, W., Ring, J., Reimann, H.J. and Geiger, R. (1982). Mediator studies in skin blister fluid from patients with dual skin reactions after intradermal antigen challenge. *J. Allergy Clin. Immunol.*, **70**, 236–42

64. Smith, J.A., Mansfield, L.E., de Shazo, R.D. and Nelson, H.S. (1980). An evaluation of the pharmacologic inhibition of the immediate and late cutaneous reaction to allergen. *J. Allergy Clin. Immunol.*, **65**, 118–21

65. Ting, S., Zweiman, B. and Lavker, R. (1983). Terbutaline modulation of human allergic skin reactions. *J. Allergy Clin. Immunol.*, **71**, 437–41

66. Adkinson, N.F. Jr., Schulman, E.S. and Newball, H.H. (1983). Anaphylactic release of arachidonic acid metabolites from the lung. In Newball, H.H. (ed.) *Immunopharmacology of the Lung*, pp. 55–72. (New York: Marcel Dekker, Inc.)

67. Lewis, R.A., Austen, K.F., Drazen, J.M., Clark, D.A., Marfat, A. and Corey, E.J. (1980). Slow reacting substance of anaphylaxis: Identification of leukotrienes C-1 and D from human and rat sources. *Proc. Natl. Acad. Sci. USA*, **77**, 3710–14

68. Schleimer, R.P., MacGlashan, D.W., Peters, S.P., Pinckard, R.N., Adkinson, N.F. and Lichtenstein, L.M. (1986). Characterisation of inflammatory mediator release from purified human lung mast cells. *Am. Rev. Respir. Dis.*, **133**, 614–617

69. Beasley, C.R.W., Featherstone, R.L., Church, M.K. and Holgate, S.T. (1986). 11-Epi-prostaglandin F_{2alpha} is a potent contractile agonist of human airways. *J. Allergy Clin. Immunol.*, **77**, 155 (Abst.)

70. Piper, P.J. and Samhoun, M.N. (1982). Stimulation of arachidonic acid metabolism and generation of thromboxane A_2 by leukotriene B_4, C_4 and D_4 in guinea pig lung *in vitro*. *Br. J. Pharmacol.*, **77**, 267–275

71. Weiss, J.W., Drazen, J.M., Coles, N., McFadden, E.R., Weller, P., Corey, E.J., Lewis, R.A. and Austen, K.F. (1982). Bronchoconstrictor effects of leukotriene C in humans. *Science*, **216**, 196–198

72. Weiss, J.W., Drazen, J.M., McFadden, E.R., Weller, P., Corey, E.J., Lewis, R.A. and Austen, K.F. (1983). Airway constriction in normal humans produced by inhalation of leukotriene D. Potency, time course, and effect of aspirin therapy. *J. Am. Med. Assoc.*, **249**, 2814–2817

73. Griffin, M., Weiss, J.W., Leitch, A.G., McFadden, E.R., Corey, E.J., Austen, K.F. and Drazen, J.M. (1983). *N. Engl. J. Med.*, **308**, 436–439

74. Smith, L.J., Greenberger, P.A., Patterson, R., Krell, R.D. and Bernstein, P.R. (1985). The effect of inhaled leukotriene D_4 in humans. *Am. Rev. Respir. Dis.*, **131**, 368–372

75. Bisgaard, H., Groth, S., Taudorf, E. and Madsen, F. (1984). Hyperreactive airway response to LTD_4 in exogenous asthmatics compared to non-atopics. *Prostaglandins*, **28**, 635

76. Barnes, N.C. and Costello, J.F. (1986). Leukotrienes and Asthma. In Kay, A.B. (ed.) *Asthma: Clinical Pharmacology and Therapeutic Progress*, pp. 194–204. (Oxford: Blackwell Scientific Publications)

77. Abraham, W.M., Delehunt, J.C., Russi, E., Wanner, A., Yerger, L. and Chapman, G.A. (1983). Inhalation of leukotriene D₄ produces both early and late bronchoconstriction in allergic sheep. *Am. Rev. Respir. Dis.*, **127**, 65 (Abst.)

78. Russi, E.W., Perruchoud, A.P., Yerger, L.D., Stevenson, J.S., Tabak, J., Marchette, B. and Abraham, W.M. (1984). Late phase bronchial obstruction following non-immunologic mast cell degranulation. *J. Appl. Physiol.*, **57**, 1182–1188

79. Abraham, W.M. and Perruchoud, A.P. (1986). Allergen induced late bronchial responses: Physiologic and pharmacologic studies in allergic sheep. In Kay, A.B. (ed.) *Asthma: Clinical Pharmacology and Therapeutic Progress*, pp. 11–22. (Oxford: Blackwell Scientific Publications)

80. Dahlén, S.E., Hansson, G., Hedqvist, P., Björck T., Granström, E. and Dahlén, B. (1983). Allergen challenge of lung tissues from asthmatics elicits bronchial contraction that correlates with the release of leukotrienes C₄, D₄ and E₄. *Proc. Natl. Acad. Sci. USA*, **80**, 1712–1716

81. Schellenberg, R.R. (1986). Role of Thromboxane A₂ in anti-IgE challenged human bronchus. *J. Allergy Clin. Immunol.*, **77**, 123 (Abst.)

82. Melewicz, F.M., Kline, L.E., Cohen, A.B. and Spiegelberg, H.L. (1982). Characterization of Fc receptors for IgE on human alveolar macrophages. *Clin. Exp. Immunol.*, **49**, 364–370

83. Capron, M., Kusnierz, J.-P., Prin, L., Spiegelberg, H.L. Ovlaque, G., Gosset, P., Tonnel, A.-B. and Capron, A. (1985). Cytophilic IgE on human blood and tissue eosinophils: Detection by flow microfluorometry. *J. Immunol.*, **134**, 3013–18

84. Shaw, R.J., Cromwell, O. and Kay, A.B. (1984). Preferential generation of leukotriene C₄ by human eosinophils. *Clin. Exp. Immunol.*, **56**, 716–722

85. Weller, P.F., Lee, C.W., Foster, D.W., Corey, E.J., Austen, K.F. and Lewis, R.A. (1983). Generation and metabolism of 5-lipoxygenase pathway leukotrienes by human eosinophils: Predominant production of leukotriene C₄. *Proc. Natl. Acad. Sci. USA*, **80**, 7626–7630

86. Henderson, W.R., Harley, J.B. and Fauci, A.S. (1984). Arachidonic acid metabolism in normal and hypereosinophilic syndrome human eosinophils: generation of leukotrienes B₄, C₄, D₄ and 15-lipoxygenase products. *Immunology*, **51**, 679–686

87. Shaw, R.J., Walsh, G.M., Cromwell, O., Moqbel, R., Spry, C.J.F. and Kay, A.B. (1985). Activated human eosinophils generate SRS-A leukotrienes following IgG-dependent stimulation. *Nature*, **316**, 150–52

88. Holgate, S.T., Burns, G.B., Robinson, C. and Church, M.K. (1984). Anaphylactic- and calcium-dependent generation of prostaglandin D₂ (PGD₂), thromboxane B₂ and other cyclooxygenase products of arachidonic acid by dispersed human lung cells and relationship to histamine release. *J. Immunol.*, **133**, 2138–44

89. Hardy, C.C., Robinson, C., Tattersfield, A.E. and Holgate, S.T. (1984). The bronchoconstrictor effect of inhaled prostaglandin D₂ in normal and asthmatic men. *N. Engl. J. Med.*, **311**, 209–13

90. Kay, A.B. and Walsh G.M. (1984). Chemotactic factor-induced enhancement of the binding of human immunoglobulin classes and subclasses to neutrophils and eosinophils. *Clin. Exp. Immunol.*, **57**, 729–734

91. Papageorgiou, N., Carroll, M., Durham, S.R., Lee, T.H., Walsh, G.M. and Kay, A.B. (1983). Complement receptor enhancement as evidence of neutrophil activation after exercise-induced asthma. *Lancet*, **2**, 1220–1223

92. Durham, S.R., Carroll, M., Walsh, G.M. and Kay, A.B. (1984). Leucocyte activation in allergen-induced late-phase asthmatic reactions. *N. Engl. J. Med.*, **311**, 1398–1402

93. Moqbel, R., Sass-Kuhn, S.P., Goetzl, E.J. and Kay, A.B. (1983). Enhancement of neutrophil- and eosinophil-mediated complement-dependent killing of schistosomula of *Schistosoma mansoni in vitro* by leukotriene B₄. *Clin. Exp. Immunol.*, **52**, 519–527

94. Moqbel, R., Durham, S.R., Shaw, R.J., Walsh, G.M., MacDonald, A.J., Mackay, J., Carroll, M.P. and Kay, A.B. (1986). Enhancement of leucocyte cytotoxicity after exercise-induced asthma. *Am. Rev. Respir. Dis.*, **133**, 609–613

95. Wardlaw, A.J. and Kay, A.B. (1986). PAF-acether is a potent chemotactic factor for human eosinophils. *J. Allergy Clin. Immunol.*, **77**, 236 (Abst.)

96. Murphy, K.R., Wilson, M.C., Irvin, C.G., Glezen, L.S., Marsh, W.R., Haslett, C., Henson, P.M. and Larsen, G.L. (1986). The requirement for polymorphonuclear leukocytes in the

late asthmatic response and heightened airways reactivity in an animal model. *Am. Rev. Respir. Dis.*, **134**, 62–68

97. Larsen, G.L., Wilson, M.C., Marsh, W.R., Haslett, C. and Murphy, K.E. Neutrophils and late-phase reactions. In Kay, A.B. (ed.) *Allergy and Inflammation*, pp. 225–244. (London: Academic Press)

98. Kaliner, M., Marom, Z., Patow, C. and Shelhamer, J. (1984). Human respiratory mucus. *J. Allergy Clin. Immunol.*, **73**, 318–23

99. Hunter, J.A., Finkbeiner, W.E., Nadel, J.A., Goetzl, E.J. and Holtzman, M.J. (1985). Predominant generation of 15-lipoxygenase metabolites of arachidonic acid by epithelial cells from human trachea. *Proc. Natl. Acad. Sci. USA*, **82**, 4633–37

100. Mezey, R.J., Cohn, M.A., Fernandez, R.J., Januszkiewicz, A.J. and Wanner, A. (1978). Mucociliary transport in allergic patients with antigen-induced bronchospasm. *Am. Rev. Respir. Dis.*, **118**, 677 (Abst.)

101. Wanner, A., Mauren, D., Abraham, W.M., Szepfalusi, Z. and Sielczak, M. (1983). Effects of chemical mediators of anaphylaxis on ciliary function. *J. Allergy Clin. Immunol.*, **72**, 663–67

102. Durham, S.R., Lee, T.H., Cromwell, O., Shaw, R.J., Merrett, T.G., Merrett, J., Cooper, P. and Kay, A.B. (1984). Immunological studies in allergen-induced late-phase asthmatic reactions. *J. Allergy Clin. Immunol.*, **74**, 49–60

103. Heavey, D.J., Richmond, R., Turner, N., Kobza-Black, A., Taylor, G.W., Chappell, C.G., Barrow, S.E. and Dollery, C.T. (1986). Measurement of leukotrienes C_4 and D_4 in inflammatory fluids. In Piper, P.J. (ed.) *Leukotrienes – Their Biological Significance*, pp. 185–198 (New York: Raven Press)

104. Isono, T., Koshihawa, Y., Murota, S., Fukuda, Y. and Furukawa, S. (1985). Measurement of immunoreactive LTC_4 in blood of asthmatic children. *Biochem. Biophys. Res. Commun.*, **130**, 486–92

105. Cromwell, O., Shaw, R.J., Durham, S.R. and Kay, A.B. (1984). Plasma LTB_4 concentrations during early and late phase antigen-induced asthmatic reactions. *J. Allergy Clin. Immunol.*, **73**, 147 (Abst.)

106. Zakrzewski, J.T., Barnes, N.C., Piper, P.J. and Costello, J.F. (1985). Measurement of leukotrienes in arterial and venous blood from normal and asthmatic subjects by radioimmunoassay. *Br. J. Clin. Pharmacol.*, **19**, 574P

107. Shepard, E., Malan, L., MacFarlane, C.M., Morton, W. and Joubert, J.R. (1985). Lung function and plasma levels of thromboxane B_2, 6-ketoprostaglandin F_{1alpha} and beta-thromboglobulin in antigen induced asthma before and after indomethacin pretreatment. *Br. J. Clin. Pharmacol.*, **19**, 459–70

108. Dolovich, J., Bach, N. and Arbesman, C. (1970). Kinin-like activity in nasal secretions of allergic patients. *Int. Arch. Allergy Appl. Immunol.*, **38**, 337–44

109. Okazaki, T., Reisman, R. and Arbesman, C. (1977). Prostaglandin E in the secretions of allergic rhinitis. *Prostaglandins*, **13**, 681–90

110. Naclerio, R.M., Meier, H.L., Kagey-Sobotka, A., Adkinson, N.F., Meyers, D.A., Norman, P.S. and Lichtenstein, L.M. (1983). Mediator release after nasal airway challenge with antigen. *Am. Rev. Respir. Dis.*, **128**, 597–602

111. Norman, P.S., Naclerio, R.M., Creticos, P.S., Togias, A. and Lichtenstein, L.M. (1985). Mediator release after physical and nasal challenges. *Int. Arch. Allergy Appl. Immunol.*, **77**, 57–63

112. Creticos, P.S., Peters, S.P., Adkinson, N.F., Naclerio, R.M., Hayes, E.C., Norman, P.S. and Lichtenstein, L.M. (1984). Peptide leukotriene release after antigen challenge in patients sensitive to ragweed. *N. Engl. J. Med.*, **310**, 1620–30

113. Shaw, R.J., Fitzharris, P., Cromwell, O., Wardlaw, A.J. and Kay, A.B. (1985). Allergen-induced release of sulphidopeptide leukotrienes (SRS-A) and LTB_4 in allergic rhinitis. *Allergy*, **40**, 1–6

114. Borum, P. (1979). Nasal methacholine challenge. A test for the measurement of nasal activity. *J. Allergy Clin. Immunol.*, **63**, 253–57

115. Meyers, D.A., Kagey-Sobotka, A., Plaut, M., Norman, P.S. and Lichtenstein, L.M. (1985). Inflammatory mediators in late antigen-induced rhinitis. *N. Engl. J. Med.*, **313**, 65–70

116. Askenase, P.W. (1973). Cutaneous basophil hypersensitivity in contact sensitized guinea pigs. I. Transfer with immune sera. *J. Exp. Med.*, **138**, 1144

117. Freeland, H.S., Pipkorn, U., Naclerio, R.M., Adkinson, N.F. and Lichtenstein, L.M. (1986). The role of leukotriene B_4 (LTB_4) in human allergic late phase reactions: lack of LTB_4 inhibition by systemic glucocorticoids. *J. Allergy Clin. Immunol.*, **77**, 244 (Abst.)
118. Bascom, R., Pipkorn, U., Gleich, G., Lichtenstein, L.M. and Naclerio, R.M. (1986). Effect of systemic steroids on eosinophils (EOS) and major basic protein (MBP) during nasal antigen challenge. *J. Allergy Clin. Immunol.*, **77**, 246 (Abst.)
119. Pipkorn, U., Proud, D., Schleimer, R.P., Peters, S.P., Adkinson, N.F. Jr., Kagey-Sobotka, A., Norman, P.S., Lichtenstein, L.M. and Naclerio, R.M. (1986). Effect of systemic glucocorticoid treatment on human nasal mediator release after antigen challenge. *J. Allergy Clin. Immunol.*, **77**, 180 (Abst.)
120. Bisgaard, H., Olsson, P. and Bende, M. (1984). Leukotriene D_4 increases nasal blood flow in humans. *Prostaglandins*, **27**, 599–604
121. Salari, H., Borgeat, P., Steffenrud, S., Richard, J., Bédard, P.M., Hébert, J. and Pelletier, G. (1986). Immunological and non-immunological release of leukotrienes and histamine from human nasal polyps. *Clin. Exp. Immunol.*, **63**, 711–717
122. Bisgaard, H., Ford-Hutchinson, A.W., Charleson, S. and Taudorf, E. (1984). Detection of leukotriene C_4-like immunoreactivity in tear fluid from subjects challenged with specific allergen. *Prostaglandins*, **27**, 369–74
123. Mann, J.S., Robinson, C., Sheridan, A.Q., Clement, P., Bach, M.K. and Holgate, S.T. (1986). Effect of inhaled Piriprost (U-60, 257) a novel leukotriene inhibitor, on allergen and exercise induced bronchoconstriction in asthma. *Thorax*, **41**, 746–752
124. Bach, M.K., Brashler, J.R., Smith, H.W., Fitzpatrick, F.A. and McGuire, J.C. (1982). 6,9-Deepoxy-6,9-(phenylimino)-$\Delta^{6,8}$-prostaglandin I_1, (U60,257) a new inhibitor of leukotriene C and D synthesis: in vitro studies. *Prostaglandins*, **23**, 759–77

3
Interactions Between Eicosanoids and Other Mediators of Inflammation

P. G. HELLEWELL and T. J. WILLIAMS

INTRODUCTION

The characteristic features of an acute inflammatory response are local vasodilatation, increased microvascular permeability, accumulation of leuko- cytes and pain. These phenomena occur as a result of the local generation of mediators in response to a stimulus. However, as will become clear in this chapter, the action of a given mediator alone is often insufficient to induce an overt inflammatory response and is dependent on an interaction, or synergism, with another mediator to produce the features described above.

Historically, the first example of synergism between eicosanoids and other mediators was the observation of Goldblatt[1] that the adrenaline-induced contractions of guinea-pig seminal vesicles *in vitro* were markedly enhanced in the presence of seminal fluid, a rich source of prostaglandins (PGs). Later studies showed that purified PGE_1 and PGE_2 were capable of sensitizing guinea- pig uterus to the contractile actions of spasmogens, such as vasopressin[2]. Similar observations demonstrating the sensitizing properties of PGs to the effects of other mediators were made on other smooth muscle preparations, such as the rat stomach[3] and the rabbit aorta[4]. The importance of these interactions with respect to smooth muscle function *in vivo* is unclear; however, with respect to inflammatory reactions, the results of *in vivo* experiments suggest that these interactions play a fundamental role.

After the first demonstration of E-type prostaglandins in inflammatory exudates[5], it was not long before PGs, particularly PGE_1, were reported to induce most of the features of an inflammatory response, vasodilatation, increased vascular permeability and leukocyte accumulation[6-8]. With evidence that the anti-inflammatory activity of aspirin and indomethacin was due to inhibition of PG synthesis[9-11], PGs were regarded as the all-important inflammatory mediators. In retrospect, early observations on the effects of

PGs on vascular permeability and leukocyte accumulation were probably of limited importance for several reasons: when injected intradermally in rats, large doses ($>0.1\ \mu g$) of PGE_1 and PGE_2 were required to induce changes in vascular permeability and these effects were apparently mediated through release of histamine and 5-hydroxytryptamine from skin mast cells[8]. More recent work in guinea-pig and rabbit skin has shown that PGs (unlike histamine and bradykinin) are poor inducers of plasma exudation when injected[12,13]. When compared with, for example, activated serum as a chemotactic stimulus *in vitro* and *in vivo*, PGE_1, at concentrations too high to be of biological significance, is extremely weak[7,14]. Thus, it is generally accepted that PGs have little direct effect on vascular permeability and leukocyte accumulation, although, in human studies, some individuals do respond to intradermal injections of E-type prostaglandins with a weal and flare reaction, perhaps because of histamine release.

It is with another feature of inflammation, pain, that the first clear-cut role for PGs in inflammation became apparent. Intradermal administration of PGs into human skin was shown to induce hyperalgesia[15,16], but the importance of this observation was not realized until after the discovery of inhibition of cyclo-oxygenase by non-steroid anti-inflammatory drugs (NSAIDs) when Ferreira[17] made an important observation that prostaglandins could act synergistically with other mediators to cause pain. Prevention of the development of hyperalgesia by blockade of prostaglandin synthesis was suggested to be the mechanism of the analgesic action of NSAIDs[17].

Since this observation, it has become clear that mediator synergism is an important component of inflammation, not only in terms of pain but also in the induction of oedema and leukocyte accumulation.

INTERACTIONS OF PROSTAGLANDINS WITH KININS AND AMINES

In 1972, Ferreira showed that PGs, particularly PGE_1 and PGE_2, produced hyperalgesia in man[17]. Subdermal infusion of histamine, bradykinin or PGs did not produce pain; however, addition of PG to the bradykinin or histamine infusion induced an extremely painful response, while infusion of bradykinin plus histamine did not produce pain. The potentiation of histamine-induced itch by PGs has also been demonstrated[18]. Various studies have extended these findings[19], including the observation that PGI_2 can also synergize with other mediators to produce pain[19,20]. The mechanism of prostaglandin-induced hyperalgesia is not clear but probably involves a lowering of the threshold of sensory pain fibres[19].

The ability of NSAIDs to inhibit vasodilatation in certain types of inflammation can be explained by the many observations showing that certain PGs (PGE_2 and PGI_2) have powerful vasodilator effects on the microvasculature[21-24]. However, PGs are weak at inducing oedema formation when injected into the skin of rabbits and guinea-pigs[12,13,25], yet, in the same animals, administration of a NSAID can effectively suppress the oedema induced by intradermal injection of micro-organisms[25]. It was then realized

44

that, as with pain responses, PGs have a modulatory role in oedema formation. In guinea-pig[12], rabbit[25] and rat[26], PGs produced a marked potentiation of the oedema responses induced by agents such as histamine and bradykinin and the potentiating ability of PGs was directly proportional to their ability to induce vasodilatation as measured using a [133]Xenon clearance technique[13,25,27]. The most potent vasodilators (PGE$_1$, PGE$_2$ and PGI$_2$) exhibited the most marked synergism[27], although other PGs (D$_2$, F$_{2\alpha}$, G$_2$) and arachidonic acid all possessed oedema-potentiating activities[13,25,27]. From these observations, a two mediator hypothesis of inflammation was proposed[28]. This states that the magnitude of oedema in an inflammatory reaction is dependent both on the permeability of the venules and the tone of the arterioles, and that these events can be induced by two different mediators. Thus, histamine increases venular permeability[29], causing plasma protein leakage and this is markedly enhanced by certain PGs, probably as a consequence of increased hydrostatic pressure within the venule lumen. The original observation in guinea-pig by Williams and Morley[12] showing synergism between bradykinin or histamine and PGs has been made in several species, including man[30–33]. Additionally, synergism between 5-hydroxytryptamine (5-HT) and PGE$_2$ has been observed but only in the rat[34]. In species other than rodents, 5-HT is inactive at increasing microvascular permeability.

Vasodilator substances, other than PGs, can also potentiate oedema; agents such as adenosine[25], vasoactive intestinal peptide (VIP)[35], calcitonin gene-related peptide (CGRP)[36] and isoprenaline[13] can synergize with bradykinin and histamine, and other mediators of increased vascular permeability, leading to oedema formation. An example of synergism between bradykinin and several vasodilators leading to oedema formation in rabbit skin is shown in Figure 3.1. In support of the modulatory role of blood flow in oedema formation are the observations in rabbit skin that vasoconstrictors, such as noradrenaline and angiotensin II, reduce exudation and blood flow in parallel[13,37].

Synergism appears to be important in a low perfusion tissue such as rabbit skin. In a tissue with a higher basal blood flow, such as the rabbit peritoneum, inhibition of prostaglandin synthesis by indomethacin makes relatively little difference to plasma protein leakage which occurs following intraperitoneal injection of zymosan[38]. This may be relevant to situations in which indomethacin and other NSAIDs are weak at suppressing oedema clinically.

The proposed mechanism underlying the synergistic action of PGs in inflammation, i.e. through vasodilatation, has been challenged recently on the basis of experiments performed with PGE$_1$ in the dog forelimb[39,40]. To eliminate the vasodilator action of PGE$_1$, the tissue was perfused at a constant flow rate. Infusion of PGE$_1$ or bradykinin alone induced only a little oedema formation (assessed by limb weight) while a combined infusion produced marked oedema. The mechanism proposed for this synergism was one of receptor sensitization[40], analogous to the pain-enhancing properties of certain PGs[17]. However, the effect of a combined infusion, but not of PGE$_1$ or bradykinin alone, was abolished in the presence of diphenydramine, a histamine H$_1$-antagonist[40]. Thus, as seen in early experiments in the rat[8], PGE$_1$ at the high doses used (4 μg min^{-1} infused intra-arterially) may well have been acting

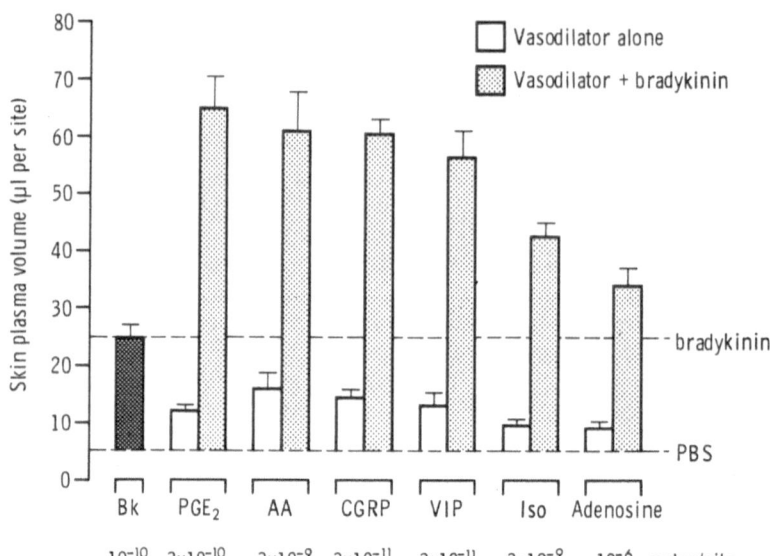

Figure 3.1 Oedema formation in rabbit skin induced by a synergism between bradykinin and a range of vasodilators. Oedema was assessed as the local accumulation of intravenously injected ^{125}I-albumin in response to intradermal injection of bradykinin (Bk) alone, vasodilators alone or combinations of bradykinin + vasodilators. Agents were injected (0.1 ml volumes) at the doses shown and after 30 min the animal was killed, injection sites were punched out and counted in an automatic gamma-counter together with plasma samples. Oedema is expressed in terms of an equivalent plasma volume for each skin site. Results are expressed as the mean ± SEM of 6 replicate injections per treatment. (Iso = isoprenaline)

to induce mast cell degranulation and the observed enhancing action of PGE$_1$ was due to endogenous histamine release. Other vasodilator PGs, PGE$_2$ or PGI$_2$, were not tested in these experiments so it is unclear as to whether or not the phenomenon was unique to PGE$_1$.

In addition to increasing microvascular permeability, bradykinin and histamine possess some intrinsic vasodilator activity which is detectable using ^{133}Xenon clearance[25]. When compared with PGE$_2$, however, they are far less potent at increasing blood flow. Nevertheless, injection of either bradykinin or histamine alone leads to significant oedema formation in guinea-pigs and rabbits[12,14], but these responses are markedly enhanced by addition of vasodilator PGs. Using bradykinin as a vasodilator in rabbit skin, Higgs and colleagues demonstrated synergism with LTB$_4$ leading to oedema formation[14,41]. When compared with PGs, e.g. PGE$_2$ and PGI$_2$, and peptides, e.g. VIP and CGRP, the role of bradykinin and histamine as vasodilators in inflammation may be of limited importance.

The overt pro-inflammatory properties of PGs are complicated by observations that PGE$_1$ and PGE$_2$ at high doses can reduce inflammation, such as in adjuvant arthritis and carageenan oedema, in the rat[42-44]. These observations have been extended primarily by Fantone and colleagues[45], who have

46

demonstrated that in the rat the oedema responses induced by intradermal injection of histamine, bradykinin and 5-HT are suppressed by systemic treatment of the animals with high doses of PGE_1 or a stable derivative, 15-methyl-PGE_1. The mechanism of this inhibition was attributed to inhibition of endothelial cell functions by PGs. However, recent observations in the rabbit have demonstrated that the degree of suppression of oedema formation induced by intradermal injection of bradykinin using systemic treatment with PGs was related to the extent of PG-induced vasodepression[46]. Interestingly, when a subvasodepressor dose of 15-methyl-PGE_1 or PGI_2 was administered systemically, such that oedema responses to intradermal bradykinin and histamine were unaffected, oedema responses to intradermal injection of polymorphonuclear (PMN) leukocyte chemoattractants were selectively suppressed[46]. This is discussed further in the section on interactions of prostaglandins with complement and bacterial-derived peptides.

INTERACTIONS OF PROSTAGLANDINS WITH PLATELET ACTIVATING FACTOR

Inflammatory changes in the cutaneous microvasculature

Platelet activating factor (PAF-acether) was originally described as a substance that was released from sensitized rabbit basophils upon exposure to antigen, and which activated rabbit platelets[47]. It is now clear that this compound has many powerful actions besides platelet activation in a variety of species, including man[48,49].

The ability of PAF-acether to increase microvascular permeability was first shown by Vargaftig and Ferreira in the rat paw[50]. PAF-acether was also shown to induce hyperalgesia in this species. Intradermal injection of PAF-acether induces an increase in microvascular permeability in the rabbit, and synergism with PGE_2 leading to oedema formation has been demonstrated[51]. Similar observations with PAF-acether and vasodilator PGs have been made in guinea-pig[52,53], rat[53] and man[49,54]. Intradermal injection of PAF-acether alone can induce a small but significant increase in vascular permeability in rabbit skin[51,55,56] although this response is small when compared with the response obtained in the presence of a vasodilator PG, such as PGE_2. An example is shown in Figure 3.2 which also illustrates the dose-dependence of the response.

Intradermal injection of PAF-acether in rabbits also induces the local accumulation of polymorphonuclear (PMN) leukocytes as assessed histologically[57]. Similar experiments have been carried out in our laboratory demonstrating the accumulation of intravenously injected [111]Indium-labelled PMNs at sites of PAF-acether injection (Rampart and Williams, unpublished observations). Interestingly, synergism with PGE_2 leading to further PMN accumulation was also observed, suggesting that both oedema formation and PMN leukocyte accumulation are dependent on local blood flow, which not only increases hydrostatic pressure in the venule, but also increases the supply of cells to the venule. Despite observations that intradermal injection of PAF-acether can induce PMN leukocyte accumulation, cutaneous oedema responses

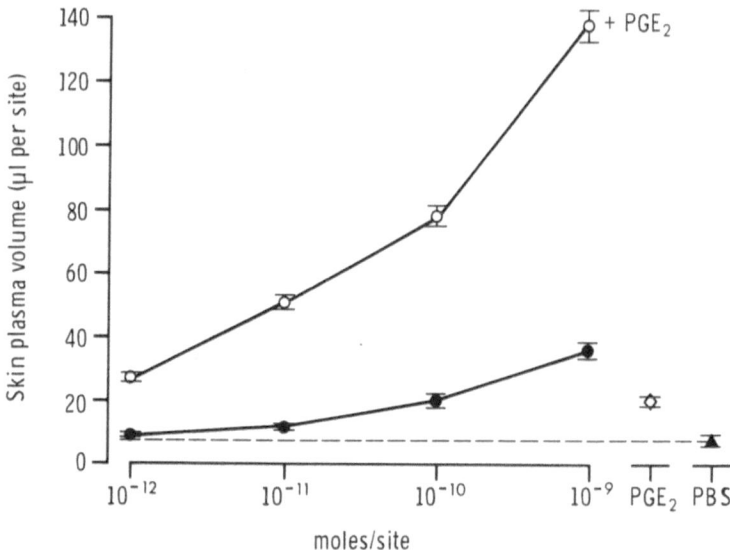

Figure 3.2 Dose-dependent oedema formation induced by a synergism between PAF and PGE$_2$ in rabbit skin. The experimental procedure was the same as that described in Figure 3.1. Responses to PAF alone (●), PAF + PGE$_2$ (○), and PGE$_2$ alone (◇) are shown. A fixed dose of PGE$_2$ (3 x 10^{-10} mol/site) was used throughout. Results are expressed as mean ± SEM of 6 replicate injections

are not suppressed in rabbits depleted of their circulating PMN leukocytes[51], unlike responses to other leukocyte chemoattractants such as C5a des Arg (see later). Oedema responses to PAF-acether also seem to be independent of circulating platelets[58].

In the hamster cheek pouch microcirculation, there is evidence that some of the permeability-increasing action of PAF-acether is PMN leukocyte dependent. By monitoring the leakage of intravenously injected fluorescein-labelled dextran, Björk and colleagues showed that the response to topically applied PAF-acether (20 nmol L^{-1}) was reduced in magnitude and duration in hamsters depleted of their circulating PMN leukocytes[59]. We have performed similar experiments in rabbit skin, measuring the duration of the permeability response to intradermal injection of PAF-acether. However, using the doses of PAF-acether shown in Figure 3.2, we were unable to detect any difference between the responses to PAF-acether in normal and neutropaenic animals (Hellewell and Williams, unpublished observations).

Inflammatory changes in the pulmonary microcirculation

Synergism between PAF-acether and PGs has also been reported in pulmonary microcirculation. Worthen and colleagues injected PAF-acether intravenously into anaesthetized rabbits and after one hour measured the number of PMN leukocytes in lavage fluid and the proportion of intravenously injected

[^{125}I]albumin that had accumulated in the air spaces[60]. Injection of PAF-acether alone induced minimal neutrophil emigration and accumulation of [^{125}I]albumin measured one hour after challenge. However, a concomitant infusion of PGE_2 with PAF-acether resulted in marked neutrophil emigration, the increase being proportional to the rate of PGE_2 infusion. When given by itself, PGE_2 did not cause accumulation of neutrophils or [^{125}I]albumin. Interestingly, despite the enhancement of neutrophil emigration by PGE_2, the accumulation of [^{125}I]albumin in air spaces was not significantly different from controls[61]. Thus, in the lung, PGE_2 can synergize with PAF-acether leading to neutrophil emigration, yet, in contrast to the observations made in the cutaneous vasculature, this does not correlate with an increase in plasma protein leakage.

INTERACTIONS OF PROSTAGLANDINS WITH COMPLEMENT-DERIVED AND BACTERIAL-DERIVED PEPTIDES

Permeability changes in the cutaneous microvasculature

The two-mediator hypothesis of inflammation was proposed based on the results of experiments in rabbit skin with vasodilator PGs and the permeability-increasing substances, histamine and bradykinin[28]. Experiments involving the intradermal injection of certain bacteria or yeast cell walls (zymosan), in which oedema formation was suppressed by local injection of indomethacin[25,62], suggested synergism between locally-generated vasodilator PGs and a locally-generated permeability-increasing mediator. Since inhibitors of histamine or kinin formation did not suppress zymosan-induced oedema formation[62], experiments were carried out in order to identify the unknown permeability-increasing mediator. It was found that incubation of bacteria, zymosan or immune complexes with samples of plasma, serum or lymph resulted in the generation of such a mediator[62–64]. When these samples were injected alone into rabbit skin, little oedema formation was observed. However, mixing with PGE_2 prior to injection resulted in marked oedema responses. Histamine H_1-receptor antagonists were ineffective in suppressing these responses[62,64]. The permeability-increasing activity was subsequently attributed to the complement fragment, C5a, following purification of the activity from zymosan-activated rabbit plasma[62].

C5a has also been detected in peritoneal inflammatory exudate following intraperitoneal injection of zymosan in the rabbit, using a specific radioimmunoassay[65]. For many years, the mechanism of action of C5a in inflammation was considered to be through its histamine-releasing or 'anaphylatoxic' activity[66]. In biological fluids, C5a is rapidly converted[66] to the more physiologically stable form, C5a des Arg, by the action of plasma carboxypeptidase N. Since human C5a des Arg is devoid of histamine-releasing activity[66], the observation that human C5a and C5a des Arg are approximately equipotent in increasing vascular permeability in rabbit skin[67] is of some significance because it dissociates histamine release from C5a-induced permeability changes. Similar observations have been made in rabbit skin using rabbit C5a and C5a des Arg (Jose and Williams, unpublished).

The mechanism of action of C5a or C5a des Arg in increasing vascular permeability was discovered to be different from mediators such as bradykinin and histamine when it was observed that, following intradermal injection in rabbit skin, the response to C5a was slightly delayed when compared with these other mediators[68]. Because C5a and C5a des Arg are powerful PMN leukocyte chemoattractants, the ability of C5a to induce leakage of plasma proteins in rabbits depleted of their circulating PMN leukocytes was investigated. The result was striking in that responses to C5a were abolished, while responses to bradykinin or histamine were unaffected[68]. Thus, the mechanism of C5a-induced permeability changes appears to involve a rapid interaction (detectable within 6 min of intradermal injection) between circulating PMN leukocytes and venular endothelium, resulting in an increased permeability to plasma proteins. The exact nature of the interaction remains to be established. Release of PAF-acether from PMN leukocytes was suggested as a possible mechanism since in vitro experiments[69] have shown that PAF-acether is secreted by PMN leukocytes in response to C5a. However, this would not seem to be the case since a specific PAF antagonist, L-652,731, was found to be without effect[56,70,71] on oedema responses to intradermal injection of C5a + PGE$_2$. Neither does the potential release of LTB$_4$ from PMN leukocytes seem to be involved in the response to C5a as LTB$_4$ also requires the presence of circulating PMN leukocytes to increase vascular permeability[68]. Furthermore, intradermal injection of C5a and PGE$_2$ with BW755C, a dual cyclo-oxygenase and lipoxygenase inhibitor, did not reduce the subsequent oedema response while responses to C5a and AA were abolished[72]. Whatever the underlying mechanism of the PMN leukocyte endothelial cell interaction, it is clear that it results in an extremely protracted response to intradermal C5a ($t_{1/2} \simeq 100$ min)[62,68].

Similar findings have been made with the bacterial-derived peptides, of which N-formyl-methionyl-leucyl-phenylalanine (FMLP) is the most extensively studied. It was realized in 1975 that bacteria in culture secrete N-formylated peptides which are powerful chemoattractants for PMN leukocytes[73]. Various N-formylated peptides were synthesized and tested[74] for chemotactic potency and the most active was FMLP. Only in 1984, when enough material was obtained from Escherichia coli culture filtrates, did structural analysis demonstrate[75] that the major chemotactic peptide secreted by the bacteria was indeed FMLP. When injected intradermally in rabbit skin, FMLP is equivalent to C5a in increasing microvascular permeability, and synergism with PGE$_2$ leading to oedema formation is observed[68] (see Figure 3.3). Both chemoattractants are 100–1000 times more potent than histamine. Additionally, responses to FMLP are dependent on circulating PMN leukocytes, and the ability of various formyl peptides to increase permeability correlates with their activity as leukocyte chemoattractants[76] (and Hellewell, Yarwood and Williams, unpublished).

As discussed briefly in the section describing interactions with kinins and amines, there are situations in which systemic treatment of animals with PGs results in suppression of inflammation, rather than enhancement. Many of the earlier studies, however, can be explained by the very high doses of PGs that were required to observe suppression. These doses undoubtedly induced severe hypotension[42-44]. In rats, oedema responses[45] to the complement

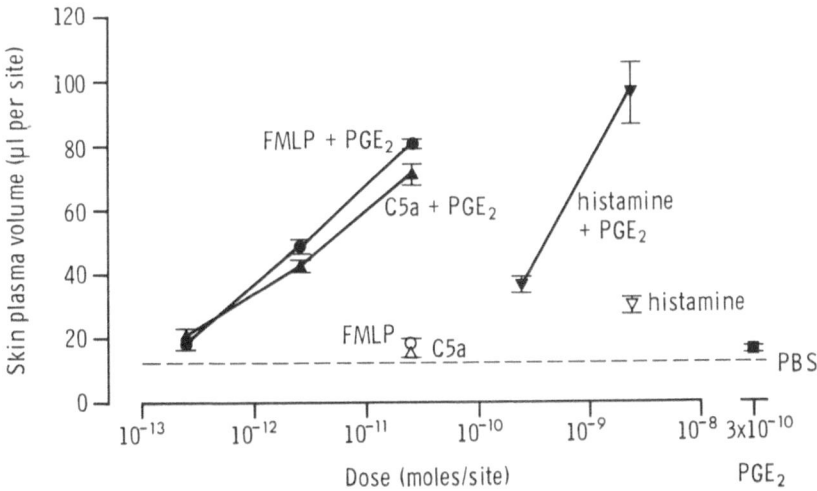

Figure 3.3 A comparison of the ability of C5a, FMLP and histamine to induce oedema formation in rabbit skin. Responses to agonists alone (open symbols) and in the presence of PGE_2 (closed symbols) are shown. PGE_2 was used at a dose of 3×10^{-10} mol/site throughout. When tested in the presence of PGE_2, FMLP and C5a were equipotent at increasing permeability, and were 100–1000 times more potent than histamine. Results are expressed as mean $\pm$ SEM of 6 replicate injections

fragment, C3a, and in a reversed passive Arthus reaction[77] (C5a dependent), have been reported to be suppressed by systemic treatment with up to 1 mg of PGE_1 injected subcutaneously. In the former publication the authors reported that there was no change in skin blood flow as inferred from skin temperature and suggested that the mechanism of action of systemic PGs was on the venular endothelium in the microvasculature. However, Rampart and Williams[46] have shown that systemic administration of 60 μg kg^{-1} of 15-methyl-PGE_1 to rabbits induced a significant fall in systemic blood pressure yet no change in skin temperature was detected using surface thermistors. Accompanying the blood pressure fall was a non-selective suppression of oedema formation, i.e. responses to C5a administered with PGE_2 and bradykinin administered with PGE_2 were suppressed. If a lower dose of PG was used, such that no change in systemic blood pressure was detected, then only responses to the combination of C5a and PGE_2 were suppressed. Similar findings were made using a systemic infusion of PGI_2. The attenuating effect was not restricted to C5a, responses to other PMN leukocyte chemoattractants, e.g. FMLP and LTB_4 also being suppressed while responses to histamine and PAF-acether were unaffected. The mechanism of the suppressant action of systemic PGs in unknown, but, since it can be demonstrated that only responses to leukocyte chemoattractants are affected, it probably involves an inhibitory effect on the PMN leukocyte. It is apparent that in the rabbit skin model, the effect of PGs can be pro- or anti-inflammatory depending on the route of administration. These observations may help to explain why, in situations such as experimentally-induced myocardial infarction, treatment with indomethacin can enhance the extent of tissue damage[78]. In this case, indomethacin may increase PMN leukocyte infiltration by preventing the negative feedback effect of PGI_2 secreted by endothelial cells into the lumen of coronary microvessels.

Cell accumulation in the cutaneous microvasculature

Intradermal injection of purified C5a into rabbit skin produces a dense infiltration of PMN leukocytes, as assessed histologically[62]. Similar observations have been made using ^{51}Cr-labelled leukocytes[79] and ^{111}In-labelled leukocytes (Rampart and Williams, unpublished). FMLP shows similar activity.

The concept that PGs may modulate chemotactic factor-induced migration of PMN leukocytes was suggested by Van Epps and colleagues[80]. They demonstrated that, in vitro, PGE_1, but not PGA_1 or $PGF_{1\alpha}$, at low concentrations (10^{-10}–10^{-7} mol L^{-1} enhanced leukocyte migration in responses to zymosan-activated serum and bacterial culture supernatants. Higher concentrations of PGE_1 decreased the chemotactic responses. As seen with intradermal injections of PAF-acether, PMN leukocyte accumulation in response to intradermal injection of C5a (and zymosan-activated plasma) and FMLP was markedly enhanced[81,82] by the simultaneous administration of a vasodilator PG, such as PGE_1, PGE_2 or PGI_2 (Rampart and Williams, unpublished). Injection of PG alone did not induce significant leukocyte accumulation and other dilators (e.g. VIP and CGRP) exerted similar actions (Rampart and Williams, unpublished) suggesting that the mechanism of action of the PG was not via a direct action on the leukocytes; rather, in a manner analogous to oedema responses, the effect of extravascular PG was on local blood flow, to increase the supply of leukocytes to the venules and therefore the number of cells that could emigrate in response to an extravascular chemotactic stimulus.

Inflammatory changes in the pulmonary microvasculature

Accumulation of PMN leukocytes in the air spaces of the lung appears to be common in many forms of lung injury[61]. Extravascular C5a has been strongly implicated in inducing pulmonary leukocyte emigration. Indeed, intratracheal administration of C5a and C5a des Arg in the rabbit causes PMN leukocytes to accumulate in the alveoli accompanied by histological evidence of oedema[83,84]. Analogous to the observations made in the cutaneous vasculature, intratracheal administration of C5a to rabbits depleted of their circulating PMN leukocytes does not lead to increases in vascular permeability[83]. Thus, a potential role for extravascular C5a in producing significant lung injury is apparent, although a possible modulatory action of extravascular PGs on plasma protein leakage and leukocyte emigration does not seem to have been investigated in this model.

Some recent observations have implicated intravascular C5a as an important component contributing to lung damage. Intravascular complement activation can occur during haemodialysis[85] and in patients at risk of developing adult respiratory distress syndrome (ARDS)[86]. The latter group of individuals are usually suffering from systemic disorders, such as sepsis, pancreatitis or burns[61]. Intravenous administration of the complement activator, cobra venom factor (CVF), to rats has been reported to induce lung injury[87]. In rabbits, however, intravenous infusion of C5a, zymosan-activated plasma or CVF was unable to induce changes in vascular permeability despite causing PMN leukocyte sequestration in pulmonary capillaries[88]. It was reported that a second insult to the lung, such as hypoxia, in combination with CVF was required to induce significant lung injury[89]. Rabbits receiving CVF alone or exposed to hypoxia for 12 min alone did not accumulate significant amounts of plasma [^{125}I]albumin or large numbers of PMN leukocytes in lavage fluid. Combining CVF and hypoxia had a synergistic effect such that the lavage:plasma [^{125}I]albumin ratio was markedly enhanced, as was the number of emigrating PMN leukocytes. The response to CVF and hypoxia was dependent on circulating leukocytes, since, in animals treated with nitrogen mustard, no significant accumulation of [^{125}I]albumin was observed. Lavage leukocytes and [^{125}I]albumin, but interestingly not interstitial [^{125}I]albumin, were suppressed by systemic treatment with a NSAID, meclofenamate. This, and the observation that hypoxia leads to PG generation[90], suggested that a cyclo-oxygenase product was involved in mediating the movement of albumin, and possibly neutrophils, across the alveolar epithelium[89]. In support of such a conclusion, a combined intravenous infusion of CVF with PGE$_2$ resulted in marked synergism leading to increases in lavage [^{125}I]albumin and PMN leukocytes[88]. This latter observation contrasts with the synergistic effect of PGE$_2$ with PAF-acether in the lung where only PMN leukocyte emigration, and not [^{125}I]albumin accumulation, was enhanced[60,61] (see earlier).

Synergism between chemotactic factors and agents other than PGs or hypoxia can also result in lung vascular injury. In the Schwartzman reaction in rabbits, intravenous administration of two doses of endotoxin 24 h apart results in symptoms of shock that can be fatal. Fehr and colleagues demonstrated that intravenous injection of FMLP into rabbits, followed 24 h later by injection of endotoxin or FMLP, did not result in death. In contrast, pretreatment with endotoxin, followed 24 h later by FMLP, was fatal[91]. In a similar manner, Worthen and colleagues showed that a low dose of LPS combined with N-formyl-norleucyl-leucyl-phenylalanine (FNLP) resulted in significant accumulation of [^{125}I]albumin in lavage fluid and retention of intravenously-injected [^{111}In] labelled PMN leukocytes in the pulmonary microcirculation[92]. Injection of saline, FNLP or LPS alone did not result in lung injury. The mechanism of this synergism remains unclear, but it may be important in the pathogenesis of ARDS where C5a, formyl peptides and endotoxins may be present in the circulation.

INTERACTIONS OF PROSTAGLANDINS WITH LEUKOTRIENES

Slow-reacting substance of anaphylaxis (SRS-A)[93], an activity generated during immediate type hypersensitivity reactions[94], is now known[95] to be composed of a mixture of leukotrienes, mainly LTC$_4$ and LTD$_4$ (see Chapter 1). SRS-A was first described because of its smooth muscle-contracting activity[93]. It was later found to increase vascular permeability when injected into guinea-pig skin; however, relatively high doses of SRS-A were required[96]. The latter observation can now be explained on the basis that SRS-A has two different activities when injected intradermally in the guinea-pig; it induces vasoconstriction and increases microvascular permeability[97,98]. When chemically-pure SRS-A, derived from antigen-challenged sensitized guinea-pig lungs, was tested in guinea-pig skin, it induced a small histamine-dependent increase in oedema formation as assessed using the local accumulation of intravenously injected [^{125}I]albumin. Addition of PGE$_1$ or PGE$_2$ greatly enhanced the responses to SRS-A, yet induced only a modest increase in plasma exudation due to injection of histamine[97]. When tested for its ability to influence local cutaneous blood flow using the ^{133}Xe clearance technique, SRS-A was found to be a powerful vasoconstrictor while histamine was a weak vasodilator[97]. Later experiments using chemically-synthesized LTC$_4$ and LTD$_4$ showed that both substances were vasoconstrictors in guinea-pig skin, LTC$_4$ being more potent and having a steeper dose-response curve[99]. When tested for their ability to induce plasma exudation, LTD$_4$ induced small oedema responses while responses to LTC$_4$ were undetectable. When mixed with PGE$_1$ or PGE$_2$ before injection, LTD$_4$ was more potent than LTC$_4$ in inducing oedema responses[99].

The vasoconstrictor action of LTC$_4$ is extremely powerful. Figure 3.4 shows the results of an experiment in the guinea-pig in which plasma exudation was

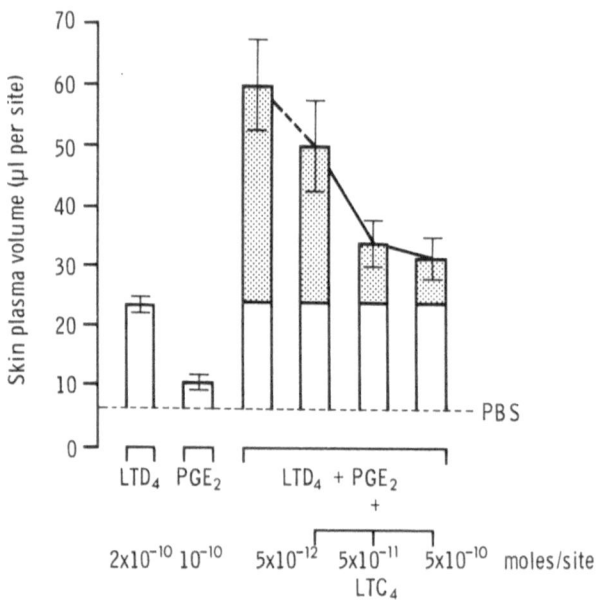

Figure 3.4 Oedema formation induced by a synergism between LTD$_4$ (2×10^{-10} mol/site) and PGE$_2$ (10^{-10} mol/site), and attenuation by LTC$_4$ (5×10^{-12}–5×10^{-10} mol/site), in guinea-pig skin. Results are expressed as means ± SEM of the mean of duplicate injections in 4 guinea-pigs

induced by intradermal injection of fixed doses of LTD_4 combined with PGE_2 in the presence of increasing doses of LTC_4. It is apparent that LTC_4 acting as a vasoconstrictor, is able to reduce blood flow and therefore oedema formation even in the presence of the vasodilator, PGE_2. LTC_4 and LTD_4 also induce vasoconstriction and plasma extravasation when applied topically to the microvasculature of the hamster cheek pouch[100]. In this preparation, LTC_4 was more effective at increasing vascular permeability, being approximately 5 times more potent than LTD_4, and about 5000 times more potent than histamine.

There appear to be marked species differences in the cutaneous responses to sulphidopeptide LTs. While LTC_4 and LTD_4 have powerful actions in guinea-pig and rat skin[99,101], in the rabbit, intradermal injection of LTs either alone or in combination with PGE_2, does not induce significant oedema formation[101] (Williams, unpublished). In humans, intradermally injected LTC_4 and LTD_4 caused dose-related erythema and wealing[102,103] although at the doses of LT used, no evidence of synergism with PGE_2 was detected[102].

In contrast, LTB_4 has properties quite different from LTC_4 and LTD_4. LTB_4 is highly chemotactic for PMN leukocytes in vitro[104]. It also causes extravasation of PMN leukocytes following injection into rabbit[41,105,106], monkey[107] and human skin[102,103] and following superfusion over the hamster cheek pouch[100,108] and rabbit skeletal muscle[109]. As found with the chemotactic agents, C5a and FMLP, LTB_4 induced an increased in vascular permeability in rabbit skin that was dependent on the presence of circulating PMN leukocytes[68]. A similar PMN-dependent mechanism of action of LTB_4 has also been observed in the hamster cheek pouch[108]. In guinea-pig skin, LTB_4 has relatively little activity[97,119]. Alone, LTB_4 does not influence cutaneous blood flow in the rabbit[110] but synergises with PGE_2 leading to oedema formation[68,105,110]. The LTB_4-induced accumulation of PMN leukocytes is also potentiated[105,106] by the injection of PGE_2 (Rampart and Williams, unpublished).

In human skin, injection of LTB_4 causes areas of induration accompanied by PMN leukocyte infiltration[102,103]. Furthermore, marked synergism with PGD_2, leading to a more intense leukocyte accumulation[103], and slight synergism with PGE_2, leading to enhancement of swelling, have been reported[102]. It was also noticed that LTB_4-induced lesions in human skin were tender[102,103]. Hyperalgesia induced by LTB_4 has been observed in rats[111]. The hyperalgesia was not affected by treatment of the rats with indomethacin but it was virtually abolished in animals depleted of their circulating PMN leukocytes. Hyperalgesia was not produced by LTD_4. This observation in rats has now been substantiated by experiments in humans[112] showing that injection of LTB_4 produces cutaneous hyperalgesia, the effect corresponding with the influx of PMN leukocytes. Thus, accumulation of PMN leukocytes in response to intradermal injection of LTB_4 leads, not only to increases in vascular permeability, but also to increases in sensitivity to pain.

INTERACTIONS OF EICOSANOIDS AND OTHER MEDIATORS IN ANIMAL MODELS OF ACUTE INFLAMMATION

Zymosan-induced oedema formation in rabbit skin can be effectively suppressed by indomethacin[25,62]. However, indomethacin has no effect on zymosan-induced oedema[25,62] when the cutaneous microvascular bed is maximally dilated using exogenous PGE_2. This has been taken as evidence of synergism between endogenous vasodilator PGs and a permeability-increasing agent, now known to be C5a. The analysis of the response to zymosan has allowed us to discover the mediators involved in a model of non-allergic inflammation. A similar approach has been taken to analyse the mediators responsible for inducing local oedema formation in two models of allergic inflammation, the passive cutaneous anaphylactic (PCA) reaction and the reversed passive Arthus (RPA) reaction. These are examples of type I and type III hypersensitivity reactions, respectively. The effects of local administration of indomethacin or PGE_2 on oedema formation in a PCA reaction and a RPA reaction in rabbit skin are shown in Figure 3.5. As with zymosan-induced oedema the response in the RPA reaction (Figure 3.5a) was effectively reduced by local indomethacin and this effect was reversed by local injection of PGE_2 (not shown here but see ref. 113). Also illustrated in Figure 3.5a, is the dramatic oedema-enhancing effect of PGE_2 when injected into RPA sites in the absence of indomethacin. These and other observations in the rabbit and other species[114-117] support the concept that, in the Arthus reaction, a vasodilator PG, such as PGE_2 or PGI_2, is acting synergistically with mediator(s) of increased microvascular permeability to induce oedema.

In contrast in the PCA reaction, oedema was not suppressed by local injection of indomethacin nor was oedema substantially enhanced by local

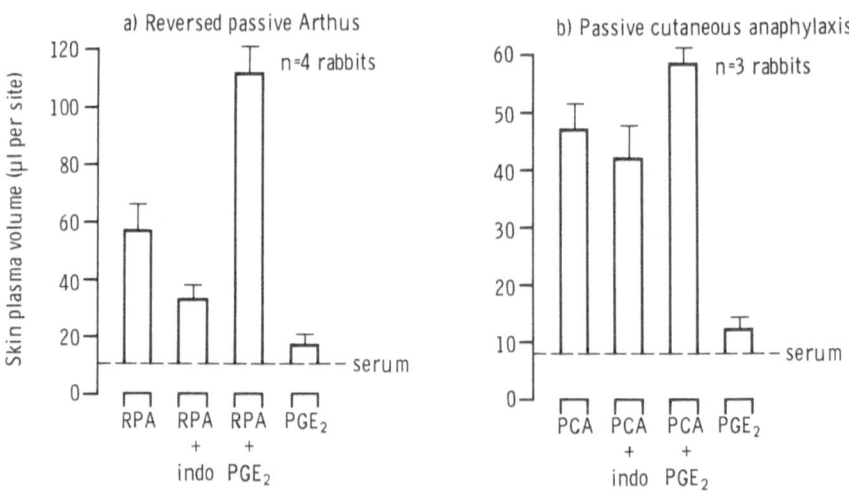

Figure 3.5 Effect of indomethacin and PGE_2 on oedema formation in a reversed passive Arthus reaction (RPA) and a passive cutaneous anaphylactic (PCA) reaction in rabbit skin. In the RPA reaction, indomethacin (10^{-8} mol/site) and PGE_2 (3×10^{-10} mol/site) were injected with antiserum (anti-bovine gamma globulin, anti-BGG) followed by an intravenous injection of antigen (BGG, 5 mg kg⁻¹). Oedema formation was measured over 2 h. In the PCA reaction, agents were injected locally with antigen (100 μg/site) into sites injected 48 h previously with antibody (IgE, 1/10 dilution). Oedema formation was measured over 30 min. Results show the mean ± SEM of the means of 6 replicate injections in n rabbits

PGE$_2$ (Figure 3.5b). These observations suggest that in the PCA reaction, endogenous PGs are not responsible for inducing the vasodilatation which is important for plasma extravasation to occur in rabbit skin. The fact that oedema could not be further enhanced by exogenous PGE$_2$ suggests that either the microcirculation was maximally dilated or that the tissue was rendered insensitive to vasodilator PGs. A similar lack of oedema-potentiating activity of PGs in this type of allergic inflammation has been observed in a PCA reaction in the rat paw[118].

The mediators of increased vascular permeability, with which endogenous PGs synergize, in the RPA reaction have been the subject of a recent investigation[113]. The Arthus reaction is characterized by immune complex formation and deposition in the walls of microvessels. This leads to activation of the complement system in tissue fluid via the classical pathway and the generation of the leukocyte chemoattractant, C5a. Since depletion of circulating complement and circulating PMN leukocytes is known to suppress oedema formation in Arthus reactions in a number of species[119], a central role for C5a in mediating oedema formation has been proposed[113]. This hypothesis is further supported by two observations. Firstly, incubation of immune complexes in plasma or serum leads to C5a generation which induces oedema formation when mixed with PGE$_2$ and injected intradermally in the rabbit[113]. Secondly, in an Arthus-type reaction in the peritoneal cavity of the rabbit, direct evidence of C5a generation has been obtained using a specific radioimmunoassay[65,113,120]. In this model, protein leakage is closely associated with C5a generation[113,120]. Evidence for a role of PAF-acether in synergizing with vasodilator PGs and thereby contributing to oedema formation in the RPA reaction has also been obtained[56,70,71]. This observation has recently been confirmed in the rabbit[121] and in the guinea-pig[122]. The work is based on the use of specific antagonists of PAF-acether that have recently become available[123,124]. The underlying mechanism is suggested to be that the PMN leukocytes, which have emigrated in response to extravascular C5a, secrete PAF-acether during phagocytosis of the immune complexes deposited in the microvessel wall[56,113].

MODULATION OF ACUTE INFLAMMATORY RESPONSES

The effects of inhibition of eicosanoid synthesis on inflammation are dealt with in detail in other chapters. In this section, we have included some illustrations of modulation of inflammatory responses by drugs acting on the responses of venular endothelial cells and PMN leukocytes to a given inflammatory mediator.

There is evidence that some drugs inhibit mediator-induced increases in microvascular permeability by a direct effect on the venular endothelial cells[125]. This is a mechanism that is distinct from a constrictor effect on arteriolar smooth muscle which would reduce inflammation by decreasing microvascular blood flow. The most commonly studied drugs in this respect are the β-adrenoceptor agonists such as isoprenaline, terbutaline and salbutamol[125]. Obviously, there are species and vascular-site differences in the effects of the agonists on permeability responses. For example, in rabbit skin, isoprenaline is a vasodilator and can therefore synergize with other mediators leading to oedema formation (see Figure 3.1). However, in other vascular beds, β-receptor agonists appear to inhibit venular permeability. The majority of observations have been made in the hamster cheek pouch[126], although it has also been shown in the canine perfused forelimb that an infusion of isoprenaline or terbutaline can inhibit bradykinin-induced oedema formation, despite inducing an increase in blood flow[40]. In the cheek pouch, this inhibition is exerted against a variety of mediators, including bradykinin, histamine and LTs[125]. Interestingly, in contrast to the effect in rabbit skin, isoprenaline suppresses oedema responses induced by histamine and in reversed passive Arthus reactions in guinea-pig skin[127]. The underlying mechanism probably involves β-agonist stimulation of venular endothelial cell adenyl cyclase and an increase in cytoplasmic cyclic AMP concentration. In support of such a mechanism, phosphodiesterase inhibitors, such as theophylline, have also been shown to attenuate venular permeability in the hamster cheek pouch[125].

Another class of drugs, corticosteroids, may act at several levels to inhibit inflammatory reactions. Steroids induce the synthesis of lipocortin[128,129] which inhibits phospholipase activity and thus reduces the availability of free arachidonic acid for conversion to vasodilator PGs. Steroids can therefore act in a similar manner to NSAIDs to suppress inflammation by reducing microvascular blood flow. It has also been suggested that some of the anti-inflammatory properties of steroids are due to inhibition of venular permeability[125,130]. Thus, methylprednisolone can inhibit oedema formation induced by co-infusion of bradykinin and PGE_2 in the dog forelimb[40], and another steroid, dexamethasone, has been shown to suppress leakage in the hamster cheek pouch microcirculation[125] and in the mouse footpad[130]. In rabbit skin, pretreatment of sites with betamethasone[131] results in suppression of oedema formation induced by intradermal injection of a combination of C5a and PGE_2. Whether the latter observation involves an action of the steroid on PMN leukocytes or on the venular endothelium remains to be established.

The PMN leukocyte is another target for the modulation of acute inflammatory responses. It has already been described when considering interactions with complement, how an intravenous infusion of PGI_2 can modulate C5a-induced oedema formation, presumably by an inhibitory action on circulating leukocytes. Recently, it has become apparent that certain NSAIDs, particularly ibuprofen, can inhibit PMN leukocyte responses by a mechanism independent of cyclo-oxygenase inhibition[132]. Thus, ibuprofen has been reported to inhibit leukocyte aggregation, locomotion, enzyme release and the oxygen burst in vitro and in vivo[132-134]. In contrast, another NSAID, aspirin, does not appear to possess similar activities[132]. In the rabbit, ibuprofen inhibits FMLP-induced PMN leukocyte accumulation in the eye[134], and experiments in skin suggest that ibuprofen can inhibit the interaction between the PMN leukocyte and venular endothelial cell which leads to chemoattractant-induced increases in vascular permeability[135,136] (Hellewell, Yarwood and Williams, unpublished). Figure 3.6 shows a typical internally-controlled experiment in rabbit skin. Mixtures of FMLP/PGE_2, FMLP/AA, bradykinin/PGE_2 and bradykinin/AA were injected intradermally and the

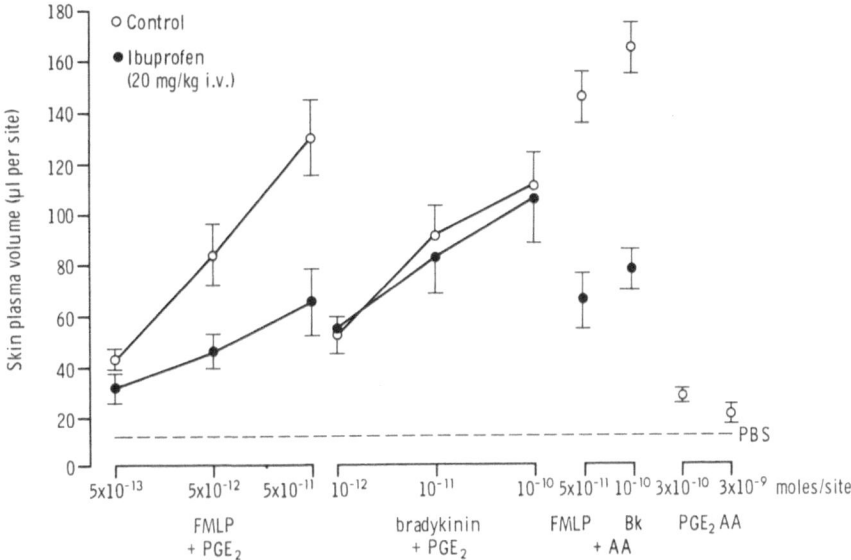

Figure 3.6 Oedema formation in rabbit skin induced by mixtures of FMLP + PGE₂, FMLP + AA, bradykinin + PGE₂ and bradykinin + AA to show the cyclo-oxygenase-dependent and independent effect of intravenous ibuprofen (20 mg kg⁻¹). The experiment was internally controlled. Test agents were given intradermally after intravenous isotope and the reaction allowed to proceed for 30 min. Ibuprofen was then administered and 10 min later, remaining skin sites were injected with the same combination of test agents. Thirty minutes later the animal was killed. Results are means ± SEM of 6 replicate injections per treatment

reactions allowed to proceed for 30 min. Ibuprofen (20 mg kg⁻¹) was then given intravenously and 10 min later remaining skin sites were injected with the same combination of agents. The animals were killed 30 min later and oedema responses assessed. As expected, responses to FMLP/AA and bradykinin/AA were reduced by systemic treatment with ibuprofen. Responses to bradykinin/PGE₂ were not affected by ibuprofen, however, and plasma leakage induced by FMLP/PGE₂ was markedly suppressed. Ibuprofen also reduces vascular permeability responses induced by intradermal injection of C5a and LTB₄ but not the response induced by histamine[136]. These observations may relate to those showing that ibuprofen can suppress the accumulation of PMN leukocytes in experimentally-induced myocardial infarction and thereby reduce infarct size[132].

CONCLUSIONS

From the many observations reported in this chapter, it is clear that interaction between mediators is an important consideration in determining the outcome of an inflammatory reaction. For example, PGs, by decreasing arteriolar tone, may enhance plasma exudation and cell accumulation induced by mediators of increased vascular permeability. In contrast, LTs, by increasing arteriolar tone, may reduce oedema formation. The importance of mediator interactions will undoubtedly vary in different vascular beds: in the peritoneal cavity, where basal blood flow appears to be high compared with skin, inhibition of PG formation has little effect on plasma exudation in our models. However, it is likely that in such circumstances, if vasoconstrictor substances (e.g. LTC_4) are released, they may dramatically influence the magnitude of the inflammatory response. These observations may help to explain why NSAIDs are sometimes very weak or inactive in suppressing inflammatory oedema.

It is also apparent that the site of mediator release is an important consideration in determining the outcome of mediator interaction. The examples quoted in this chapter refer to the observation that PGs may have opposing actions on PMN leukocyte-dependent oedema formation depending on the route of administration or site of generation. Thus, in an inflammatory lesion induced by, for example, a local bacterial invasion, extravascular PGs, by acting on arterioles, can increase the supply of plasma protein and phagocytic cells to the inflammatory site. In contrast, if endothelial cells are stimulated by some mechanism to release PGs, then the local intravascular PG concentration may achieve sufficient concentrations to suppress PMN leukocyte function and hence reduce oedema formation. A knowledge of mediator interactions in the microvasculature and their contribution to inflammation will provide a framework on which to base the design of specific drugs, not only those directed against particular mediators, but also those against the important cellular components, leukocytes and the venular endothelium.

ACKNOWLEDGEMENTS

We would like to thank the Medical Research Council for supporting some of the work described in this chapter. We also thank Elsie Prestige for typing this chapter.

REFERENCES

1. Goldblatt, M.W. (1935). Properties of human seminal plasma. *J. Physiol.*, **84**, 208–218
2. Clegg, P.C., Hall, W.J. and Pickles, V.R. (1966). The action of ketonic prostaglandins on the guinea-pig myometrium. *J. Physiol.*, **183**, 123–144
3. Coceani, F. and Wolfe, L.S. (1966). On the action of prostaglandin E_1 and prostaglandins from brain on the isolated rat stomach. *Can. J. Physiol. Pharmacol.*, **44**, 933–950
4. Khairallah, P.A., Page, I.H. and Turker, R.K. (1967). Some properties of prostaglandin E_1 action on muscle. *Arch. Int. Phramacodyn.*, **169**, 328–341
5. Willis, A.L. (1969). Parallel assay of prostaglandin-like activity in rat inflammatory exudate by means of cascade superfusion. *J. Pharm. Pharmacol.*, **1**, 126–128
6. Horton, E.W. (1963). Action of prostaglandin E_1 on tissues which respond to bradykinin. *Nature* (London), **200**, 892–893
7. Kaley, G. and Weiner, R. (1971). Prostaglandin E_1: A potential mediator of the inflammatory response. *Ann. N.Y. Acad. Sci.*, **180**, 338–350
8. Crunkhorn, P. and Willis, A.L. (1971). Cutaneous reactions to intradermal prostaglandins. *Br. J. Pharmacol.*, **41**, 49–56

9. Vane, J.R. (1971). Inhibition of prostaglandin synthesis as a mechanism of action for aspirin-like drugs. *Nature (London)*, **231**, 232–235
10. Smith, J.B. and Willis, A.L. (1971). Aspirin selectively inhibits prostaglandin production in human platelets. *Nature (London)*, **231**, 235–237
11. Ferreira, S.H., Moncada, S. and Vane, J.R. (1971). Indomethacin and aspirin abolish prostaglandin release from the spleen. *Nature (London)*, **231**, 237–239
12. Williams, T.J. and Morley, J. (1973). Prostaglandins as potentiators of increased vascular permeability in inflammation. *Nature (London)*, **246**, 215–217
13. Williams, T.J. (1976). The pro-inflammatory activity of E-, A-, D- and F-type prostaglandins and analogues 16,16-dimethyl-PGE$_2$ and (15S)-15-methyl-PGE$_2$ in rabbit skin: the relationship between potentiation of plasma exudation and local blood flow changes. *Br. J. Pharmacol.*, **56**, 341–342P
14. Higgs, G.A., Salmon, J.A. and Spayne, J.A. (1981). The inflammatory effects of hydroperoxy and hydroxy acid products of arachidonate lipoxygenase in rabbit skin. *Br. J. Pharmacol.*, **74**, 429–433
15. Solomon, L.M., Juhlin, L. and Kirschenbaum, M.B. (1968). Prostaglandins on cutaneous vasculature. *J. Invest. Dermatol.*, **51**, 280–282
16. Michaelson, G. (1970). Effects of antihistamines, acetylsalicyclic acid and prednisone on cutaneous reactions to kallikrein and prostaglandin E$_1$. *Acta Dermatol. Venereol. Stockholm*, **30**, 31–36
17. Ferreira, S.H. (1972). Prostaglandins, aspirin-like drugs and analgesia. *Nature (London)*, **240**, 200–203
18. Greaves, M.W. and McDonald-Gibson, W. (1973). Itch: role of prostaglandins. *Br. Med. J.*, **3**, 608–609
19. Ferreira, S.H. (1985). Prostaglandin hyperalgesia and the control of inflammatory pain. In Bonta, I.L., Bray, M.A. and Parnham, M.J. (eds.) *Handbook of Inflammation, Volume 5: The Pharmacology of Inflammation*, pp. 107–116. (Amsterdam: Elsevier)
20. Ferreira, S.H., Nakamura, M. and Castro, M.S.A. (1978). The hyperalgesic effects of prostacyclin and prostaglandin E$_2$. *Prostaglandins*, **16**, 31–39
21. Nakano, J. and McMurdy, J.R. (1967). Cardiovascular effects of prostaglandin E$_1$. *J. Pharm. Exp. Ther.*, **156**, 538–547
22. Messina, E.J., Weiner, R. and Kaley, G. (1976). Prostaglandins and local circulatory control. *Fed. Proc.*, **35**, 2367–2375
23. Peck, M.J. and Williams, T.J. (1978). Prostacyclin (PGI$_2$) potentiates bradykinin-induced plasma exudation in rabbit skin. *Br. J. Pharmacol.*, **62**, 464–465P
24. Higgs, E.A., Moncada, S. and Vane, J.R. (1978). Inflammatory effects of prostacyclin (PGI$_2$) and 6-oxo-PGF$_{12}$ in the rat paw. *Prostaglandins*, **16**, 153–162
25. Williams, T.J. and Peck, M.J. (1977). Role of prostaglandin-mediated vasodilatation in inflammation. *Nature (London)*, **270**, 530–532
26. Moncada, S., Ferreira, S.H. and Vane, J.R. (1973). Prostaglandins, aspirin-like drugs and the oedema of inflammation. *Nature (London)*, **246**, 217–219
27. Williams, T.J. (1979). Prostaglandin E$_2$, prostaglandin I$_2$ and the vascular changes in inflammation. *Br. J. Pharmacol.*, **65**, 517–524
28. Williams, T.J. (1977). Chemical mediators of vascular responses in inflammation: a two mediator hypothesis. *Br. J. Pharmacol.*, **61**, 447–448P
29. Majno, G., Schoefl, G.I. and Palade, G. (1961). Studies on inflammation. II. The site of action of histamine and serotonin on the vascular tree; a topographic study. *J. Biophys. Biochem. Cytol.*, **11**, 607–626
30. Thomas, G. and West, G.B. (1974). Prostaglandins, kinins and inflammation in the rat. *Br. J. Pharmacol.*, **50**, 231–235
31. Lewis, A.J., Nelson, D.J. and Sugrue, M.F. (1975). On the ability of prostaglandin E$_1$ and arachidonic acid to modulate experimentally induced oedema in the rat paw. *Br. J. Pharmacol.*, **55**, 51–56
32. Johnston, M.G., Hay, J.B. and Movat, H.Z. (1976). The modulation of enhanced vascular permeability by prostaglandins through alterations in blood flow. *Agents Actions*, **6**, 705–711
33. Basran, G.S., Morley, J., Paul, W. and Turner-Warwick, M. (1982). Evidence in man of synergistic interaction between putative mediators of acute inflammation and asthma. *Lancet*, **1**, 935–937

34. Chahl, L.A. (1976). Interactions of bradykinin, prostaglandin E_1 5-hydroxytryptamine, histamine and adenosine-5'-triphosphate on the dye leakage response in rat skin. *J. Pharm. Pharmacol.*, **28**, 753–757

35. Williams, T.J. (1982). Vasoactive intestinal polypeptide is more potent that prostaglandin E_2 as a vasodilator and oedema potentiator in rabbit skin. *Br. J. Pharmacol.*, **77**, 505–509

36. Brain, S.D. and Williams, T.J. (1985). Inflammatory oedema induced by synergism between calcitonin gene-related peptide (CGRP) and mediators of increased vascular permeability. *Br. J. Pharmacol.*, **86**, 855–860

37. Williams, T.J., Jose, P.J., Forrest, L. H., Smaje, L.H. and Clough, G.F. (1984). Inflammatory oedema induced by synergism between prostaglandins and C5a: the importance of the interaction between neutrophils and venular endothelial cells. In Courtice, G.C., Garlick, D.G. and Perry, M.A. (eds.) *Progress in Microcirculation Research II.* pp. 439–448. (Sydney: Committee in Postgraduate Medical Education, University of NSW)

38. Forrest, M.J., Jose, P.J. and Williams, T.J. (1985). The role of the complement-derived polypeptide C5a in inflammatory reactions. In Higgs, G.A. and Williams, T.J. (eds.) *Inflammatory Mediators.* pp. 99–115. (Basingstoke: Macmillan)

39. Amelang, E. Prasad, C.M., Raymond, R.M. and Grega, G.J. (1981). Interactions among inflammatory mediators on oedema formation in the canine forelimb. *Circ. Res.*, **49**, 298–306

40. Prasad, C.M., Adamski, S.W., Svensjo, E. and Grega, G.J. (1982). Pharmacological modification of the oedema produced by combined infusions of prostaglandin E_1 and bradykinin in canine forelimbs. *J. Pharmacol Exp. Ther.*, **220**, 293–298

41. Eakins, K.E., Higgs, G.A., Moncada, S., Salmon, J.A. and Spayne, J.A. (1980). The effects of arachidonate lipoxygenase products on plasma exudation in rabbit skin. *J. Physiol.*, **307**, 71P

42. Zurier, R.B. and Quagliata, F. (1971). Effect of prostaglandin E_1 on adjuvant arthritis. *Nature (London)*, **234**, 304–305

43. Glenn, E.M. and Rohloff, J. (1972). Antiarthritic and antiinflammatory effects of certain prostaglandins. *Proc. Soc. Exp. Biol. Med.*, **139**, 290–294

44. DiPasquale, G., Rassaert, C., Richter, R., Welaj, P. and Tripp, L. (1973). Influence of prostaglandins (PG) E_2 and F_{2x} on the inflammatory process. *Prostaglandins*, **3**, 741–757

45. Fantone, J.C., Kunkel, S.L., Ward, P.A. and Zurier, R.B. (1980). Suppression by prostaglandin E_1 of vascular permeability by vasoactive inflammatory mediators. *J. Immunol.*, **125**, 2591–2596

46. Rampart, M. and Williams, T.J. (1986). Polymorphonuclear leukocyte-dependent plasma leakage in the rabbit skin is enhanced or inhibited by prostacyclin, depending on the route of administration. *Am. J. Pathol.*, **124**, 66–73

47. Benveniste, J., Henson, P.M. and Cochrane, C.G. (1972). Leukocyte-dependent histamine release from rabbit platelets. The role of IgE, basophils and a platelet-activating factor. *J. Exp. Med.*, **136**, 1356–1377

48. Pinckard, R.N., McManus, L.M. and Hanahan, D.J. (1982). Chemistry and biology of acetylglyceryl ether phosphorylcholine (platelet-activating factor). In Weissmann, G. (ed.) *Advances in Inflammation Research, Volume 4.* pp. 147–180. (New York: Raven Press)

49. Page, C.P., Archer, C.B. and Morley, J. (1985). Properties of PAF-acether appropriate to a mediator of inflammation. In Higgs, G.A. and Williams, T.J. (eds.) *Inflammatory Mediators.* pp. 57–64. (Basingstoke: Macmillan)

50. Vargaftig, B.B. and Ferreira, S.H. (1981). Blockade of the inflammatory effects of platelet-activating factor by cyclooxygenase inhibitors. *Braz. J. Med. Res.*, **14**, 187–189

51. Wedmore, C.V. and Williams, T.J. (1981). Platelet-activating factor (PAF), a secretory product of polymorphonuclear leukocytes, increases vascular permeability in rabbit skin. *Br. J. Pharmacol.*, **74**, 916–917P

52. Morley, J., Page, C.P. and Paul, W. (1983). Inflammatory actions of platelet-activating factor (Paf-acether) in guinea-pig skin. *Br. J. Pharmacol.*, **80**, 503–509

53. Hwang, S-B. Li, C-L., Lam, M-H and Shen, T-Y. (1985). Characterization of cutaneous vascular permeability induced by platelet-activating factor in guinea pigs and rats and its inhibition by a platelet-activating factor receptor antagonist. *Lab. Invest.*, **52**, 617–630

54. McGivern, D.V. and Basran, G.S. (1984). Synergism between platelet-activating factor (PAF-acether) and prostaglandin E_2 in man. *Eur. J. Pharmacol.*, **102**, 183–185

55. Humphrey, D.M., McManus, L.M., Satouchi, K., Hanahan, D.J. and Pinckard, R.N. (1982). Vasoactive properties of acetyl glyceryl ether phosphorylcholine and analogues. *Lab. Invest.*, **46**, 422–427

56. Hellewell, P.G. and Williams, T.J. (1986). A specific antagonist of platelet-activating factor suppresses oedema formation in an Arthus reaction but not oedema induced by leukocyte chemoattractants in rabbit skin. *J. Immunol.*, **137**, 302–307

57. Humphrey, D.M., Hanahan, D.J. and Pinckard, R.N. (1982). Induction of leukocytic infiltration in rabbit skin by acetyl glyceryl ether phosphorylcholine. *Lab. Invest.*, **47**, 227–234

58. Page, W., Page, C.P., Cunningham, F.M. and Morley, J. (1985). The plasma protein extravasation response to PAF-acether is independent of platelet accumulation. *Agents Actions*, **15**, 80–82

59. Bjork, J. and Smedegard, G. (1983). Acute microvascular effects of PAF-acether as studied by intravital microscopy. *Eur. J. Pharmacol.*, **96**, 87–94

60. Worthen, G.S., Gumbay, S., Larsen, G.L. and Henson, P.M. (1983). Prostaglandin E_2 enhances platelet-activating factor-induced lung neutrophil migration, but not vascular permeability. *Am. Rev. Respir. Dis.*, **127**, A57

61. Worthen, G.S. and Henson, P.M. (1983). Mechanisms of acute lung injury. *Clin. Lab. Med.*, **3**, 601–617

62. Williams, T.J. and Jose, P.J. (1981). Mediation of increased vascular permeability after complement activation; histamine-independent action of rabbit C5a. *J. Exp. Med.*, **153**, 136–153

63. Williams, T.J. (1978). A proposed mediator of increased vascular permeability in acute inflammation in the rabbit. *J. Physiol.*, **281**, 44–45P

64. Jose, P.J., Peck, M.J., Robinson, C. and Williams, T.J. (1978). Characterization of a histamine-independent vascular permeability-increasing factor generated on exposure of rabbit plasma to zymosan. *J. Physiol.*, **281**, 13–14P

65. Jose, P.J., Forrest, M.J. and Williams, T.J. (1983). Detection of the complement fragment C5a in inflammatory exudates from the rabbit peritoneal cavity using radioimmunoassay. *J. Exp. Med.*, **158**, 2177–2182

66. Hugli, T.E. and Muller-Eberhard, H.J. (1978). Anaphylatoxins: C3a and C5a. *Adv. Immunol.*, **26**, 1–55

67. Jose, P.J., Forrest, M.J. and Williams, T.J. (1981). Human C5a des Arg increases vascular permeability. *J. Immunol.*, **127**, 1276–1280

68. Wedmore, C.V. and Williams, T.J. (1981). Control of vascular permeability by polymorphonuclear leukocytes in inflammation. *Nature (London)*, **289**, 646–650

69. Camussi, G., Tetta, C., Bussolino, F., Caligaris Capplo, F. Coda, R., Masera, C. and Segoloni, G. (1981). Mediators of immune-complex-induced aggregation of polymorphonuclear neutrophils. II. Platelet-activating factor as the effector substance of immune-induced aggregation. *Int. Arch. Allergy Appl. Immunol.*, **64**, 25–41

70. Hellewell, P.G. and Williams, T.J. (1985). Inhibition of allergic inflammation by PAF antagonists in the rabbit. *Br. J. Pharmacol.*, **86**, 572P

71. Hellewell, P.G. and Williams, T.J. (1985). Suppression of inflammatory oedema in rabbit skin by two PAF antagonists 48740 RP and L-652731. *Prostaglandins*, **30**, 713

72. Forrest, M.J., Peck, M.J. and Williams, T.J. (1981). Is increased vascular permeability induced by C5a dependent on the generation of lipoxygenase products? *Br. J. Pharmacol.*, **74**, 921–922P

73. Schiffmann, E., Corcoran, B.A. and Wahl, S.A. (1975). N-formylmethionyl peptide as chemoattractants for leucocytes. *Proc. Natl. Acad. Sci. USA*, **72**, 1059–1062

74. Showell, H.J., Freer, R.J., Zigmond, S.H., Schiffmann, E., Aswanikumar, S., Corcoran, B. and Becker, E.L. (1976). The structure-activity relations of synthetic peptides as chemotactic factors and inducers of lysosomal enzyme secretion for neutrophils. *J. Exp. Med.*, **143**, 1154–1169

75. Marasco, W.A., Phan, S.H., Krutzsch, H., Showell, H.J., Feltner, D.E., Nairn, R., Becker, E.L. and Ward, P.A. (1984). Purification and identification of formyl-methionyl-leucyl-phenylalanine as the major peptide neutrophil chemotactic factor produced by *Escherichia coli. J. Biol. Chem.*, **259**, 5430–5439

76. Hellewell, P.G., Wedmore, C.V. and Williams, T.J. (1985). Inflammatory oedema induced by bacterial N-formyl peptides. In Higgs, G.A. and Williams, T.J. (eds.) *Inflammatory Mediators*. pp. 237–238. (Basingstoke: Macmillan)

77. Kunkel, S.L., Thrall, R.S., Kunkel, R.G., McCormick, J.R., Ward, P.A. and Zurier, R.B. (1979). Suppression of immune complex vasculitis in rats by prostaglandin. *J. Clin. Invest.*, **64**, 1525–1529

78. Jugdutt, B.I., Hutchings, G.M., Bulkley, B.J., Pit, B. and Becker, L.C. (1979). Effect of indomethacin on collateral blood flow and infarct size in the conscious dog. *Circulation*, **59**, 734–743

79. Issekutz, A.C. and Movat, H.Z. (1980). The *in vivo* quantitation and kinetics of rabbit neutrophil leukocyte accumulation in the skin in response to chemotactic agents and *Escherichia coli*. *Lab. Invest.*, **42**, 310–317

80. Van Epps, D.E., Wiik, A., Garcia, M.L. and Williams, R.C. (1978). Enhancement of human neutrophil migration by prostaglandin E_2. *Cell. Immunol.*, **37**, 142–150

81. Issekutz, A.C. (1981). Effect of vasoactive agents on polymorphonuclear leukocyte emigration *in vivo*. *Lab. Invest.*, **45**, 234–240

82. Issekutz, A.C. and Movat, H.Z. (1982). The effect of vasodilator prostaglandins on polymorphonuclear leukocyte infiltration and vascular injury. *Am. J. Pathol.*, **107**, 300–309

83. Shaw, J.O., Henson, P.M., Henson, J. and Webster, R.O. (1980). Lung inflammation induced by complement-derived chemotactic fragments in the alveolus. *Lab. Invest.*, **42**, 547–558

84. Larsen, G.L., McCarthy, K., Webster, R.O., Henson, J. and Henson, P.M. (1980). A differential effect of C5a and C5a des Arg in the induction of pulmonary inflammation. *Am. J. Pathol.*, **100**, 179–192

85. Craddock, P.R., Fehr, J., Brigham, K.L., Kronenberg, R.S. and Jacob, H.S. (1977). Complement and leukocyte-mediated pulmonary dysfunction in hemodialysis. *N. Engl. J. Med.*, **296**, 769–774

86. Hammerschmidt, D.E., Weaver, L.J., Hudson, L.D., Craddock, P.R. and Jacob, H.S. (1980). Association of complement activation and elevated plasma-C5a with adult respiratory distress syndrome. *Lancet*, **1**, 947–949

87. Till, G.O., Johnson, K.J., Kunkel, R. and Ward, P.A. (1982). Intravascular activation of complement and acute lung injury. Dependency on neutrophils and toxic oxygen metabolites. *J. Clin. Invest.*, **69**, 1126–1135

88. Henson, P.M., Larsen, G.L., Webster, R.O., Mitchell, B.C., Goins, A.J. and Henson, J.E. (1982). Pulmonary microvascular alterations and injury induced by complement fragments: synergistic effects of complement activation, neutrophil sequestration, and prostaglandins. *Ann. NY Acad. Sci.*, **384**, 287–300

89. Larsen, G.L., Webster, R.O., Worthen, G.S., Gumbay, R.S. and Henson, P.M. (1985). Additive effect of intravascular complement activation and brief episodes of hypoxia in producing increased permeability in the rabbit lung. *J. Clin. Invest.*, **75**, 902–910

90. Said, S.I., Yoshida, T., Kitamura, S. and Vreim, C. (1974). Pulmonary alveolar hypoxia: release of prostaglandins and other humoral mediators. *Science*, **185**, 1181–1183

91. Fehr, J., Dahinden, C. and Russi, R. (1984). Formylated chemotactic peptides can mimic the secondary provoking endotoxin injection in the generalized Schwartzman reaction. *J. Infect. Dis.*, **150**, 160–161

92. Worthen, G.S., Haslett, C., Smedly, L.A., Rees, A.J., Gumbay, R.S., Henson, J.E. and Henson, P.M. (1986). Lung vascular injury induced by chemotactic factors: enhancement by bacterial endotoxins. *Fed. Proc.*, **45**, 7–12

93. Kellaway, C.H. and Trethewie, E.R. (1940). The liberation of a slow-reacting smooth muscle-stimulating substance in anaphylaxis. *Q. J. Exp. Physiol.*, **30**, 121–145

94. Brocklehurst, W.E. (1960). The release of histamine and formation of a slow-reacting substance (SRS-A) during anaphylactic shock. *J. Physiol.*, **151**, 416–435

95. Austen, K.F. and Lewis, R.A. (1984). Historical and continuing perspectives on the biology of the leukotrienes. In Chakrin, L.W. and Bailey, D.M. (eds.) *The Leukotrienes. Chemistry and Biology*. pp. 1–12. (London: Academic Press)

96. Brocklehurst, W.E. (1967). *3rd International Symposium on Vasoactive Polypeptides; Bradykinin and Related Kinins*. pp. 189–191. (Oxford: Pergamon Press)

97. Williams, T.J. and Piper, P.J. (1980). The action of chemically pure SRS-A on the microcirculation *in vivo*. *Prostaglandins*, **19**, 779–789

98. Drazen, J.M., Austen, K.F., Lewis, R.A., Clark, D.A., Goto, G., Marfat, A. and Cory, E.J. (1980). Comparative airway and vascular activities of leukotrienes C-1 and D *in vivo* and *in vitro*. *Proc. Natl. Acad. Sci. USA*, **77**, 4354–4358

99. Peck, M.J., Piper, P.J. and Williams, T.J. (1981). The effect of leukotrienes C_4 and D_4 on the microvasculature of guinea-pig skin. *Prostaglandins*, **21**, 315–321

100. Dahlén, S.-E., Björk, J., Hedqvist, P., Arfors, K.-E., Hammarström, S., Lindgren, J.A. and Samuelsson, B. (1981). Leukotrienes promote plasma leakage and leukocyte adhesion in postcapillary venules: *In vivo* effects with relevance to the acute inflammatory response. *Proc. Natl. Acad. Sci. USA*, **78**, 3887–3891

101. Ueno, A., Tanaka, K., Katori, M., Hayashi, M. and Arai, Y. (1981). Species differences in increased vascular permeability by synthetic leukotrienes C_4 and D_4. *Prostaglandins*, **21**, 637–648

102. Camp, R.D.R., Coutts, A.A., Greaves, M.W., Kay, A.B. and Walport, M.J. (1983). Responses of human skin to intradermal injection of leukotrienes C_4, D_4 and B_4. *Br. J. Pharmacol.*, **80**, 497–502

103 Soter, N.A., Lewis, R.A., Corey, E.J. and Austen, K.F. (1983). Local effects of synthetic leukotrienes (LTC_4, LTD_4, LTE_4 and LTB_4) in human skin. *J. Invest. Dermatol.*, **80**, 115–119

104. Ford-Hutchinson, A.W., Bray, M.A., Doig, M.V., Shipley, M.E. and Smith, M.J.H. (1980). Leukotriene B, a potent chemokinetic and aggregating substance released from polymorphonuclear leucocytes. *Nature (London)*, **286**, 264–265

105. Bray, M.A., Ford-Hutchinson, A.W. and Smith, M.J.H. (1981). Leukotriene B_4: an inflammatory mediator *in vivo*. *Prostaglandins*, **22**, 213–222

106. Movat, H.Z., Rettl, C., Burrowes, C.E. and Johnston, M.G. (1984). The *in vivo* effect of leukotriene B_4 on polymorphonuclear leukocytes and the microcirculation. *Am. J. Pathol.*, **115**, 233–244

107. Lewis, R.A., Geotzl, E.J., Drazen, J.M., Soter, J.A., Austen, K.F. and Corey, E.J. (1981). Functional characterization of synthetic leukotriene B and its stereochemical isomers. *J. Exp. Med.*, **154**, 1243–1248

108. Björk, J., Hedqvist, P. and Arfors, K-E. (1982). Increase in vascular permeability induced by leukotriene B_4 and the role of polymorphonuclear leukocytes. *Inflammation*, **6**, 189–200

109. Lindbom, L., Hedqvist, P., Dahlén, S-E., Lindgren, J.A. and Arfors, K-E. (1982). Leukotriene B_4 induces extravasation and migration of polymorphonuclear leukocytes *in vivo*. *Acta Physiol. Scand.*, **116**, 105–108

110. Bray, M.A., Cunningham, F.M., Ford-Hutchinson, A.W. and Smith, M.J.H. (1981). Leukotriene B_4: A mediator of vascular permeability. *Br. J. Pharmacol.*, **72**, 483–486

111. Levine, J.D., Lau, W., Kwait, G. and Goetzl, E.J. (1984). Leukotriene B_4 produced hyperalgesia that is dependent on polymorphonuclear leukocytes. *Science*, **225**, 743–745

112. Bisgaard, H. and Kristensen, J.K. (1985). Leukotriene B_4 produces hyperalgesia in humans. *Prostaglandins*, **30**, 791–797

113. Williams, T.J., Hellewell, P.G. and Jose, P.J. (1986). Inflammatory mechanisms in the Arthus reaction. *Agents Actions*, **19**, 66–72

114. Issekutz, A.C. and Bhimji, S. (1982). Effect of nonsteroidal anti-inflammatory agents on immune complex and chemotactic factor-induced inflammation. *Immunopharmacology*, **4**, 253–266

115. Butler, K. and Lewis, G.P. (1976). The effect of anti-inflammatory compounds on the biochemical changes in the Arthus reaction. *J. Pathol.*, **119**, 175–182

116. Chang, Y.-H. and Otterness, I.G. (1981). Effects of pharmacologic agents on the reversed passive Arthus reaction in the rat. *Eur. J. Pharmacol.*, **69**, 155–164

117. Bailey P.J. and Strum, A. (1983). Immune complexes and inflammation. A study of the activity of anti-inflammatory drugs in the reverse passive Arthus reaction in the rat. *Biochem. Pharmacol.*, **32**, 475–481

118. Ferreira, S.H. (1976). Prostaglandins and immunological trauma. In Lewis, G.P. (ed.) *The Role of Prostaglandins in Inflammation*. pp. 75–87. (Bern: Hans Huber)

119. Cochrane, C.G. and Janoff, A. (1974). The Arthus reaction: a model of neutrophil and complement-mediated injury. In Zweifach, B.W., Grant, L. and McCluskey, R.T. (eds.) *The Inflammatory Process*. Vol. III, pp. 85–162. (New York: Academic Press)

120. Jose, P.J., Forrest, M.J. and Williams, T.J. (1985). Generation of C5a and prostacyclin (PGI_2) in an inflammatory response to zymosan and a reverse passive Arthus-type reaction in the peritoneal cavity of the rabbit. *Agents Actions*, **16**, 39–41

121. Issekutz, A.C. and Szpejda, M. (1986). Evidence that platelet-activating factor may mediate some acute inflammatory responses: studies with the platelet-activating factor antagonist, CV3988. *Lab. Invest.*, **54**, 275–281

122. Deacon, R.W., Melden, M.K., Saunders, R.N. and Handley, D.A. (1986). PAF involvement in dermal extravasation in the reverse passive Arthus reaction. *Fed. Proc.*, **45**, 995

123. Hwang, S.B., Lam, M.H., Biftu, T., Beattie, T.R. and Shen, T.Y. (1985). *Trans*-2,5-bis-(3,4,5-trimethoxyphenyl) tetrahydrofuran. An orally active specific and competitive receptor antagonist of platelet-activating factor. *J. Biol. Chem.*, **260**, 15639–15645

124. Desquand, S., Lefort, J., Deregnaucourt, J., Sedivy P., Lagente, V., Randon, J. and Vargaftig, B.B. (1985). Inhibition by the PAF acether antagonist 48740 RP of the bronchopulmonary effects of PAF-acether. *Int. J. Immunopharmacol.*, **3**, 383

125. Persson, C.G.A. and Svensjo, E. (1985). Vascular responses and their suppression: drugs interfering with venular permeability. In Bonta, I.L. Bray, M.A. and Parnham, M.J. (eds.) *Handbook of Inflammation, Volume 5: The Pharmacology of Inflammation*. pp. 61–82. (Amsterdam: Elsevier)

126. Svensjo, E., Persson, C.G.A. and Rutili, G. (1977). Inhibition of bradykinin induced macromolecular leakage from postcapillary venules by a β_2-adrenoceptor stimulant, terbutaline. *Acta Physiol. Scand.*, **101**, 504–506

127. Kenaway, S.A., Lewis, G.P. and Williams, T.J. (1978). The effects of α- and β-adrenoceptor agonists on inflammatory exudation in rabbit and guinea-pig skin. *Br. J. Pharmacol.*, **64**, 447–448P

128. Flower, R.J. and Blackwell, G.L. (1979). Anti-inflammatory steroids induce biosynthesis of a phospholipase A_2 inhibitor which prevents prostaglandin generation. *Nature (London)*. **278**, 456–459

129. Hirata, F., Schiffmann, E., Venkatasubramanian, K., Salomon, D. and Axelrod, J. (1980). A phospholipase A_2 inhibitory protein in rabbit neutrophils induced by glucocorticoids. *Proc. Natl. Acad. Sci. USA*, **55**, 2533–2536

130. Tsurufuji, S., Sugio, K. and Takemasa, F. (1979). The role of glucocorticoid receptor and gene expression in the anti-inflammatory action of dexamethasone. *Nature (London)*, **280**, 408–410

131. Clough, G. and Williams, T.J. (1985). The inhibitory effect of a corticosteroid on plasma leakage induced by C5a in rabbit skin. In Higgs, G.A. and Williams, T.J. (eds.) *Inflammatory Mediators*. pp. 236–237. (Basingstoke: MacMillan)

132. Flynn, P.J., Becker, W.K., Vercellotti, G.M., Weisdorf, D.J., Craddock, P.R.,Hammerschmidt, D.E., Helehel, R. and Jacob, H.S. (1984). Ibuprofen inhibits granulocyte responses to inflammatory mediators: A proposed mechanism for reduction of experimental myocardial infarct size. *Inflammation*, **8**, 33–44

133. Kaplan, B.K., Edelson, H.S., Korchak, H.M., Given, W.P., Abrahamson, S. and Weissmann, G. (1984). Effects of non-steroidal anti-inflammatory agents on human neutrophil functions *in vitro* and *in vivo*. *Biochem. Pharmacol.*, **33**, 371–378

134. Shimanuki, T., Nakamura, R.M. and Dizerega, G.S. (1985). Modulation of leukotaxis by ibuprofen. *Inflammation*, **9**, 285–295

135. Rampart, M., Hellewell, P.G. and Williams, T.J. (1985). Inhibition by ibuprofen of polymorphonuclear leukocyte-dependent plasma leakage in rabbit skin. *Naunyn Schmiedeberg's Arch. Pharmacol.*, **330**, R53

136. Rampart, M. and Williams, T.J. (1986). Suppression of inflammatory oedema by ibuprofen involving a mechanism independent of cyclooxygenase inhibition. *Biochem. Pharmacol.*, **35**, 581–586

4
Eicosanoids in Immune Regulation

T. J. ROGERS

INTRODUCTION

The analysis of the role of the products of the lipoxygenase (LO) pathway of arachidonic acid metabolisn in the immune system has consumed a great deal of attention recently. It is clear that the biochemical events involved in the metabolism of arachidonic acid are still not fully defined, and it is reasonable to assume that our appreciation of the role of LO products in various biological responses is far from complete. Until the present time, studies have been conducted either with purified LO products or with certain 'specific' inhibitors of LO activity. Our ability to identify, and purify, additional LO products and inhibitors will certainly assist in the understanding of the role of this pathway in the immune response. Our understanding of the precise immune cell target of the effect of these LO products is still evolving, as is our information concerning the biochemical events which mediate their effects. Finally, we are still in the process of dissecting the cellular and molecular nature of immune responses; thus, information derived from experiments conducted with LO products and inhibitors must be evaluated with the understanding that the mechanism of any effect may be uncertain until a later time.

In this chapter, I will attempt to review the studies which have been carried out in an attempt to elucidate the roles of the LO pathway in the immune response. Because of the obvious relationship between the LO pathway and the cyclo-oxygenase (CO) pathway, I will also include a brief review of certain recent studies on the role of prostaglandin synthesis in the function of the cells of the immune system.

OVERVIEW OF THE IMMUNE SYSTEM

The first step in an immune response is the contact between antigen and an accessory cell (such as the monocyte/macrophage or a granulocyte). These cells are responsible for the processing of antigen, and presenting antigen to

67

the various lymphoid cells capable of responding to determinants present on that particular antigen. The monocyte/macrophage lineage also secretes a group of mediators (or monokines), the most important of which is termed interleukin 1 (IL-1).

The accessory cells present antigen to both regulatory lymphocytes and effector lymphocytes. The differentiation of both B-cells and effector T-cells is dependent on the activity of T-helper cells. The T-helper cells also release a variety of mediators (or lymphokines), the most important of which is termed interleukin 2 (IL-2). IL-2 is required for the differentiation and growth of both immature B-cells and T-cytotoxic cells in order to generate antibody-forming plasma cells and mature killer cells, respectively. Suppressor T-cells are capable of exerting their effect on a variety of cell types. These cells secrete a group of suppressor factors which may inhibit the activity of T-helper cells, effector T-cells, or B-cells directly.

Among the various T-cells with effector function is the T-cytotoxic cell. This cell is involved in tumour or allograft rejection. In addition, some T-cells are responsible for the phenomenon of delayed-type hypersensitivity. As a part of this process, these T-cells secrete a group of factors which influence the chemotaxis and migration of accessory cells. Also, there are factors which activate macrophages and induce these accessory cells to increase their capacity for killing infectious agents. Among these macrophage-activating factors is γ-interferon. It is interesting that in this way, the accessory cells can play an important role in both the afferent and efferent arms of the immune response.

A variety of assay systems have been devised to test for the immunocompetence of the various cells of the immune system. Some of these assays are direct. For example, it is possible to test the ability of B-cells to respond and produce antibody both *in vivo* and *in vitro*. It is also possible to test the generation of T-cytotoxic cell activity directly. These direct tests are complicated by the fact that, as I described above, there are several immune cell types involved in both the antibody and cytotoxic cell response. A given drug or compound which influences the antibody response could act on accessory cells, T-helper cells or B-cells. However, although it is more difficult, it is possible to manipulate the immune system (primarily *in vitro*) in such a way that the precise cellular target for the effects of a drug can be assigned.

A variety of indirect assay systems have been employed in order to test for the competence of both B-cells and T-cells. The most common is the use of certain lectins, such as phytohaemmaglutinin (PHA) or concanavalin A (Con A), which stimulate the proliferation (or mitogenesis) of most T-cells. There are also B-cell-specific mitogens, the most common of which is bacterial lipopolysaccharide (LPS) (or endotoxin). The rationale for these agents is that they can substitute for the antigen in the generation of lymphocyte proliferation, and a specific lymphocyte type can be evaluated separate from the other types. It should be pointed out, however, that while the assay with mitogens is technically straightforward, the results can be complicated by the fact that even these mitogenic responses require the function of accessory cells. Therefore, the effect of a given compound on the response to PHA may be due to effects on either accessory cells or T-cells or both.

The use of these proliferative responses to mitogens is currently quite popular. It should be pointed out that it is also possible to induce lymphocyte proliferation by antigenic stimulation. This is usually carried out in what is termed a mixed-lymphocyte reaction (MLR). In this assay, lymphocytes from two histoincompatible donors are mixed together *in vitro*, and the cells from donor A recognize the foreign histocompatibility antigens present on the cells from donor B and respond against them. The same is true in this case for the cells from donor B. The result is a proliferative response. The advantage of the MLR is that it is more biologically relevant than the highly artificial response to the mitogens.

It should be clear that the immune system is highly dynamic, and it is often very difficult to identify the precise cellular, or molecular, mechanism for the effect of any particular compound on this system. It is necessary to evaluate results in the context of what is known about the nature of a particular assay technique. As the research in the area of arachidonic acid metabolism and the immune response is reviewed, it is necessary to appreciate the complexity which exists on both a cellular and molecular level.

ACCESSORY CELL FUNCTION

The accessory cells have a significant role in the association between arachidonic acid metabolism and the immune system. The accessory cells are potent sources of essentially all the known arachidonic acid metabolites. It is well known that macrophages release products of both LO and CO pathways following activation, but the production and release of particular products may vary depending on the nature of the stimulation of the accessory cells. Certain lectins, the calcium ionophore A23187, IgE immune complexes, and particulate antigens are among the list of reagents which induce LO product release from the various accessory cells[1-9]. Studies carried out with macrophages indicate that arachidonic acid metabolism may differ in activated and non-activated macrophages. Resident macrophages release significantly higher levels of both hydroxyeicosatetraenoic acids (HETEs) and leukotriene C_4 (LTC$_4$) in response to inflammatory stimuli *in vitro* than do activated macrophages[10]. It appears, however, that several different stages of activation may exist for the macrophage, and the production of the various arachidonic acid metabolites may vary for each stage.

It has now been shown that the products of the LO pathway are capable of exerting significant effects on accessory cell function. A number of LO products[9-11], including products of both 5-LO and 12-LO, are capable of eliciting neutrophil chemotactic activity. It appears that leukotriene B_4 (LTB$_4$) is particularly potent in this regard[12]. It is conceivable that these products may influence a number of immune responses *in vivo*, including hypersensitivity reactions.

These results suggest that the accessory cells may utilize the LO products as a means of autoregulation. Recent reports with the macrophage product IL-1 tend to bear out this interpretation. Monokines generated from LPS-stimulated macrophages have been shown[13] to significantly enhance the production of LTB_4 and LTC_4. The identity of the monokine(s) actually responsible for this effect has not been defined, although it has been shown that IL-1 has the ability to stimulate phospholipase activity[14,15].

The relationship between the LO activity and IL-1 has been taken a step further by investigators[16] who have shown that LTB_4, and to a lesser extent LTD_4, has the capacity of augmenting the production of IL-1 by human peripheral blood monocytes at concentrations as low as $10^{-8}\,mol\,L^{-1}$. It was also found that the production of IL-1 in response to macrophage stimulation with LPS was augmented by the addition of exogenous LTB_4. The addition of the CO inhibitor, indomethacin, to these monocytes did not inhibit the augmentation of IL-1 production, indicating that the effect of the addition of LTB_4 is not due to a feedback shift in arachidonic acid metabolism to the CO pathway. These results confirm other recent studies[17] in which it was found that agents that block LO activity also inhibit the production of IL-1 in response to macrophage stimulation. Taken together, these studies suggest that LO activity, and possibly the synthesis of LTB_4 specifically, is required for the normal production of IL-1.

Little is known about the relationship between the products of the LO pathway and other monokines. The role of LO products in the processing and presentation of antigen is also uncertain. These subjects are likely to be the focus of much research in the near future.

ANTIBODY-MEDIATED IMMUNITY

It is surprising that very little is known about the role of the LO pathway in the synthesis of antibody by B-lymphocytes. The subject of CO activity and the generation of antibody has received the attention of numerous investigators. As additional LO inhibitors and sources of purified LO products become available, a great deal of additional information is likely to become available in this area.

Among the few studies performed with LO products is a study in which the effect of LTE_4 has been tested to determine the effect on the antibody response of murine splenocytes in vitro[18]. It was found that significant suppression of the primary antibody response could be detected with levels as low as $10^{-7}\,mol\,L^{-1}$. Suppression of the proliferative response to LPS was observed at levels as low as $10^{-8}\,mol\,L^{-1}$. The same investigators observed suppression of the proliferative response to PHA with both LTE_4 and LTD_4 as low as $10^{-12}\,mol\,L^{-1}$. The effects of LO products on T-cell function will be discussed in a later section; however, it appears that the LO pathway may have a more significant influence on T-cell function than on B-cell activity.

In general, the products of the CO pathway have been found to inhibit the primary antibody response to both T-dependent and T-independent antigens[19-22]. On the other hand, this has not been the experience of many investigators who have examined secondary antibody responses. For example, secondary responses to sheep erythrocytes, keyhole limpet haemocyanin, bovine serum albumin, human gamma globulin, and dinitrophenol-*ascaris* are all enhanced[23-27] by E-series prostaglandins (PGE).

The effects of agents which block CO activity have generally supported a suppressive role for the prostaglandins in the antibody response. The primary antibody response is enhanced in the presence of indomethacin[21,22,28]. It appears, however, that the degree of enhancement is dependent on the antigen dose and the basal level of the immune response[21,22]. On the other hand, the secondary response to sheep erythrocytes has been shown to be suppressed by indomethacin[24]. The reason for the dichotomy in the effect of the prostaglandins or CO inhibitors on the primary and secondary responses is not clear. It must be appreciated that the cellular and molecular bases for primary and for secondary antibody responses differ greatly. There may be a process, or processes, which manifests sensitivity to the CO products in one case and not the other.

Because the accessory cells within the immune system serve as a major source of arachidonic acid metabolism, it can easily be seen that these cells may play a significant role in the regulation of B-cell responses. However, relative to other regulatory influences, such as the T-helper and T-suppressor cells, the arachidonic acid metabolites probably play a secondary role in the overall regulation of the antibody response.

CELL-MEDIATED IMMUNITY: EFFECTOR-CELL FUNCTION

Investigations of the effect of LO products on effector T-cell function have been primarily directed toward the MLR, T-cytotoxic cell activity, and natural killer (NK) cells. The results of one study indicate that agents which inhibit CO activity (indomethacin; aspirin; octadeca-9,12-diynoic acid; and d,l-6-chloro-α-methylcarbazole-2-acetic acid) all augment the MLR and T-cytotoxic cell activity[29]. On the other hand, agents which inhibit LO activity, such as nordihydroguaiaretic acid (NDGA) and 5,8,11,14-eicosatetraynoic acid (ETYA), suppress these cellular responses. Finally, agents which block thromboxane synthesis (imidazole and 1-methylimidazole) also inhibit the development of these cellular responses. This study is somewhat difficult to interpret since relatively high concentrations of the LO blockers $(6 \times 10^{-6}\,\mathrm{mol\,L^{-1}})$ were necessary in order to observe an inhibitory effect on the MLR or T-cytotoxic cell activity. These results suggest, however, that the LO and CO products may have opposite effects on these cellular immune responses. This is consistent with other studies which have shown that CO inhibitors enhance MLR and T-cytotoxic cell activity[28,30–32].

The precise CO or LO products which play a role in regulating these cellular responses are not entirely clear. Several reports suggest that PGE may inhibit both the MLR and the activity of T-cytotoxic cells[30–36]. A role for prostacyclin has also been suggested[29]. Little is known about the direct effects of LO products on these cellular responses. One exception is a study in which mice were treated in vivo with 15-hydroxyeicosatetraenoic acid (15-HETE) where the results showed that the MLR responsiveness was inhibited[37].

A number of studies have been directed toward an analysis of the role of LO activity in the function of NK cells. These studies show that agents which inhibit LO activity, such as NDGA, ETYA, BW755C, and quercetin, all inhibit

71

NK activity[38-40]. Indomethacin was shown to have no effect on this inhibition, suggesting that the effect of these LO blockers was not simply to 'shunt' the arachidonic acid metabolism through the CO pathway[38]. In fact, indomethacin has been shown to enhance the activity of NK cells[41,42], and PGE has an inhibitory effect on these cells[41-45]. A number of LO products have been tested to detect enhancing activity in the NK cell assay. Results show that both 5-hydroperoxyeicosatetraenoic acid (5-HPETE) and LTB$_4$ increase NK activity[40,46]. Significantly less, or no, activity was detected with 15-HPETE, 15-HETE, or 5-HETE. Interestingly, the addition of 5-HPETE to cultures of NDGA-treated NK cells significantly restored lytic activity, suggesting that the demand for LO activity could be almost entirely reconstituted by products of the 5-LO pathway alone.

Results of very recent studies show that the novel eicosanoids, lipoxin A and lipoxin B, proposed to be the products of 15-lipoxygenation followed by 5-lipoxygenation, both inhibit NK cell activity[47,48]. This points out an important dichotomy in the role of the LO pathway in the function of these immune cells. The 5-LO products, 5-HPETE and LTB$_4$, enhance the activity of NK cells, whereas the lipoxins, also products in part of 5-LO, have an opposing effect. Hopefully, the explanation for this paradox will be forthcoming over the next few years.

A number of investigators have attempted to determine the role of LO products on the proliferative response to various T-cell mitogens. Agents which block LO activity, such as NDGA, resulted in an inhibition of the T-cell response to PHA[49]. At the same time, however, in general, the results suggest that LO products are inhibitory for the same response. For example, 15-HPETE and 15-HETE exhibit significant suppressive activity for T-cell responses to mitogens[50-52]. This result with 15-HETE may be due to the established ability of 15-HETE to inhibit both 5-LO and 12-LO activity[53,54].

At concentrations as low as 10^{-12} mol L^{-1}, both LTD$_4$ and LTE$_4$ have been reported to inhibit the response of murine splenocytes to PHA[18]. On the other hand, studies with human lymphocytes showed that LTB$_4$, but not LTC$_4$, LTD$_4$ or LTE$_4$, inhibits the response to the T-cell mitogen PHA[55]. The explanation for these differences in results is unclear at present. More recent reports indicate that the effect of LTB$_4$ is directed toward the helper/inducer cell subpopulation of human T-cells[56,57]. These studies show that the response of OKT4$^+$ cells (helper/inducer) to PHA is inhibited, whereas the response of OKT8$^+$ cells (suppressor/cytotoxic) is enhanced by LTB$_4$. The enhancing effect on the suppressor/cytotoxic cell subpopulation could be observed[56] at levels of LTB$_4$ as low as 10^{-12} mol L^{-1}, while the inhibition of the helper/inducer cells was observed at levels as low as 10^{-8} mol L^{-1}.

CELL-MEDIATED IMMUNITY: REGULATORY CELL FUNCTION

Among the most significant functions of the T-helper cell population is the production of IL-2. Recent results[58] show that inhibitors of LO activity, caffeic acid and AA-861, inhibit the production of IL-2 in response to the T-cell mitogen Con A. The effect seems to be limited to the actual production of this lymphokine and not to the reactivity of lymphocytes to this mediator. The results show that these drugs do not inhibit the response to IL-2 once it has been generated. The identity of the LO product(s) responsible for this effect is not currently known.

In a similar fashion, it has been shown that butylated hydroxyanisole, an antioxidant inhibitor of LO activity, suppresses the production of the lymphokine γ-interferon[59]. Furthermore, LTB_4, LTC_4, and LTD_4 are able to replace the requirement for helper cells or IL-2 in the generation of the interferon. It was also observed that the effect of the LO-inhibitor could be reversed by the addition of LTC_4. These studies suggest a significant role for products of the LO pathway for the production of interferon.

Little is known about the role of LO products in the production or activity of other helper factors. Given the very interesting results with γ-interferon, one would expect that additional information concerning the relationship between LO activity and helper cell function will be available in the very near future.

Two very interesting sets of experiments concerning LO products and the function of suppressor cells have recently been reported. In the first case[60,61], LTB_4 was found to induce suppressor cell activity in human peripheral blood cells in $vitro$ at levels as low as 10^{-14} mol L^{-1}. Experiments showed that the suppressor cell activity was exhibited by an $OKT8^+$ T-cell population, although, if the cells were fractionated prior to activation with LTB_4, both $OKT4^+$ and $OKT8^+$ cells developed suppressive capacity. The precise role for this LO product in suppressor cell induction remains uncertain.

A second set of experiments[62,63] has been reported which show that the LO product 15-HETE is capable of inducing murine suppressor cell activity in $vivo$ at levels as low as $10^{-8}-10^{-9}$ mol L^{-1}. The suppressor cells in this case are Lyt 2^+ T-cells, which is consistent with the general suppressor cell phenotype in mice. The mechanism of suppression by these HETE-stimulated cells is unclear; however, it appears that products of both the 5-LO and 15-LO pathways are capable of exerting measurable regulatory cell activity.

It is well established that PGE is capable of inducing suppressor cell activity in both murine and human systems[64-66]. The mechanism of suppression by the PGE-stimulated cells, at least in the case of the murine system, appears to involve the production of a group of suppressor factors[67-73]. Among these factors is a leukotriene-like substance which is apparently responsible for a portion of the suppressive activity[73].

The relevance of the suppressor cells just reviewed to the general regulatory events which take place as a part of normal immune responses is uncertain. Perhaps it would be more relevant to determine the requirement, or the role, of arachidonic acid metabolites in the function of antigen-induced suppressor cells. A number of investigations have been carried out using both antigen- and mitogen-induced suppressor T-cells. The results of several laboratories have suggested that agents which block CO activity either have no effect on suppressor cell function, or augment the suppressive activity[74-79]. On the other hand, the results from our laboratory[80,81] and others[66,82,83] indicate that CO inhibitors prevent the development of suppressor cell activity. The basis for the disagreement concerning the role of CO activity and suppressor cell function has recently been reviewed[84], and probably relates to the great variation in the methods used both to induce the suppressor cells and to alter CO activity.

Our experiments have focussed on the use of staphylococcal enterotoxin B (SEB), an agent which induces potent T-suppressor cell activity. Our experiments show that the CO inhibitors, indomethacin and ETYA, when added within the first 4–6 h of SEB stimulation, prevent the development of suppressor cell function. The LO inhibitor NDGA has no effect on the activity of these cells, and neither do the thromboxane synthase inhibitors, imidazole or pyrogallol. These results suggest that, at least for these suppressor cells, the products of the CO pathway are required for activity, while the products of LO activity have no detectable role.

The nature of the requirement for CO activity in this system has not been investigated but recent reports suggest that PGE may play a significant role in the function of certain suppressor cells which regulate delayed-type hypersensitivity[85]. The results show that these cells act by releasing a suppressor factor. In the presence of indomethacin, the suppressor factor is produced by these cells but is inactive. The addition of exogenous PGE reconstitutes suppressive activity to the factor, indicating that PGE plays a role in the delivery of the suppressive signal in this system.

CONCLUSIONS

It is clear that products of the LO pathway play a role in accessory cell function, the function of effector B- and T-cells, and the function of regulatory T-cells. Two questions remain at this time. How significant is the role the LO products play in these immune processes? Answers to this question will come only after a considerable increase in the number of studies that have been performed with more highly purified LO products (using physiological concentrations) or with highly specific (and well-controlled) inhibitors of the various arachidonic acid pathways. At this time, it would appear that the LO pathway does play a significant role in regulating certain aspects of the immune system. However, it is likely that the influence of these metabolites is less than absolute.

If we accept the proposition that the LO pathway does influence the immune system, the second question relates to the future goals of this line of research. How can we manipulate the complex pathways of arachidonic acid metabolism in order to adjust the immune response in a desired fashion? It may be possible selectively to modulate a particular part of the LO pathways, for example, in order to amplify an immune response which is too weak. Alternatively, it may be possible to manipulate LO activity, or employ a specific metabolite, in order to reduce an undesirable immune response. The latter would be desirable in patients with autoimmune diseases. In any case, the goal of future research will at least serve to illuminate the complexity of both the immune system and arachidonic acid metabolism.

ACKNOWLEDGEMENTS

The excellent editorial assistance of Gregory Harvey is greatly appreciated. Dr Rogers is funded by grants RR 05417 and AI 19045 from the National Institutes of Health.

REFERENCES

1. Razin, E. (1985). Activation of the 5-lipoxygenase pathway in E-mast cells by peanut agglutinin. *J. Immunol.*, **134**, 1142–1145
2. Rigaud, M., Durand, J. and Breton, J.C. (1979). Transformation of arachidonic acid into 12-hydroxy-5,8,10,14-eicosatetraenoic acid by mouse peritoneal macrophages. *Biochim. Biophys. Acta*, **573**, 408–412
3. Yecies, L.D., Wedner, H.J. and Parker, C.W. (1979). Slow reacting substance (SRS) from ionophore A23187-stimulated human leukemic basophils. I. Evidence for a precursor role of arachidonic acid and initial purification. *J. Immunol.*, **123**, 2814–2816
4. Rankin, J.A., Hitchcock, M., Merrill, W.W., Huang, S.S., Brashler, J.R., Bach, M.K. and Askenase, P.W. (1984). IgE immune complexes induce immediate and prolonged release of leukotriene C_4 (LTC_4) from rat alveolar macrophages. *J. Immunol.*, **132**, 1993–1999
5. Rouzer, C.A., Scott, W.A., Cohn, Z.A., Blackburn, P. and Manning, J.M. (1980). Mouse peritoneal macrophages release leukotriene C in response to phagocytic stimulus. *Proc. Natl. Acad. Sci. USA*, **77**, 4928–4932
6. Williams, J.D., Czop, J.K. and Austen, K.F. (1984). Release of leukotrienes by human monocytes on stimulation of their phagocytic receptor for particulate activators. *J. Immunol.*, **132**, 3034–3040
7. Williams, J.D., Lee, T.H., Lewis, R.A. and Austen, K.F. (1985). Intracellular retention of the 5-lipoxygenase pathway product, leukotriene B_4, by human neutrophils activated with unopsonized zymosan. *J. Immunol.*, **134**, 2624–2630
8. Scott, W.A., Pawlowski, N.A., Andreach, M. and Cohn, Z.A. (1982). Resting macrophages produce distinct metabolites from exogenous arachidonic acid. *J. Exp. Med.*, **155**, 535–547
9. Scott, W.A., Pawlowski, N.A., Murray, H.W. Andreach, M., Zrike, J. and Cohn, Z.A. (1982). Regulation of arachidonic acid metabolism by macrophage activation. *J. Exp. Med.*, **155**, 1148–1160
10. Goetzl, E.J., Hill, H.R. and Gorman, R.R. (1980). Unique aspects of the modulation of human neutrophil function by 12-L-hydroperoxy-5,8,10,14-eicosatetraenoic acid. *Prostaglandins*, **19**, 71–85
11. Ford-Hutchinson, A.W., Bray, M.A., Doig, M.V., Shipley, M.E. and Smith, M.J. (1980). Leukotriene B_4, a potent chemokinetic and aggregating substance released from polymorphonuclear leukocytes. *Nature (London)*, **286**, 264–265
12. Dahinden, C.A., Clancy, R.M. and Hugli, T.E. (1984). Stereospecificity of leukotriene B_4 and structure-function relationships for chemotaxis of human neutrophils. *J. Immunol.*, **133**, 1477–1482
13. Dessein, A.J., Lee, T.H., Elsas, P., Ravalese, J., III, Silberstein, D., David, J.R., Austen, K.F. and Lewis, R.A. (1986). Enhancement by monokines of leukotriene generation by human eosinophils and neutrophils stimulated with calcium ionophore A23187. *J. Immunol.*, **136**, 3829–3838
14. Chang, J., Gilman, S.C. and Lewis, A.J. (1986). Interleukin 1 activates phospholipase A_2 in rabbit chondrocytes: a possible signal for IL 1 action. *J. Immunol.*, **136**, 1283–1287
15. Levine, L. and Xiao, D-M. (1985). The stimulations of arachidonic acid metabolism by recombinant murine interleukin 1 and tumor promoters or 1-oleoyl-2-acetyl-glycerol are synergistic. *J. Immunol.*, **135**, 3430–3433
16. Rola-Pleszczynski, M. and Lemaire, I. (1985). Leukotrienes augment interleukin 1 production by human monocytes. *J. Immunol.*, **135**, 3958–3961
17. Dinarello, C.A., Bishai, I., Rosenwasser, L.J. and Coceano, F. (1984). The influence of lipoxygenase inhibitors on the in vitro production of human leukocytic pyrogen and lymphocyte activating factor (interleukin-1). *Int. J. Immunopharmacol.*, **6**, 43–48

18. Webb, D.R., Nowowiejski, I., Healy, C. and Rogers, T.J. (1982). Immunosuppressive properties of leukotriene D_4 and E_4 in vitro. Biochem. Biophys. Res. Commun., **104**, 1617–1622

19. Melmon, K.L., Weinstein, Y., Shearer, G.M. and Bourne, H.R. (1975). Leukocyte separation on the basis of their receptors for biogenic amines and prostaglandins: relation of the receptor to antibody formation. In Braun, W., Lichtenstein, L. and Parker, C.W. (eds.) cAMP, Cell Growth and the Immune Response. pp. 114–134. (New York: Springer-Verlag)

20. Plescia, O.J., Smith, A.H. and Grinwich, K. (1975). Subversion of immune systems by tumor cells and role of prostaglandins. Proc. Natl. Acad. Sci. USA, **72**, 1848–1851

21. Webb, D.R. and Nowowiejski, I. (1977). The role of prostaglandins in the control of the primary 19S immune response to SRBC. Cell. Immunol., **33**, 1–10

22. Zimecki, M. and Webb, D.R. (1976). The regulation of the immune response to T-independent antigens by prostaglandins and B cells. J. Immunol., **117**, 2158–2164

23. Loose, L.D. and DiLuzio, N.R. (1973). Effect of prostaglandin E_1 on cellular and humoral immune responses. J. Reticuloendothel. Soc., **13**, 70–77

24. Wieder, K.J. and Webb, D.R. (1981). The effect of prostaglandin metabolism on immunoglobulin and antibody production in naive and educated whole spleen cells. Prostaglandl. Med., **7**, 79–90

25. Cook, R.G., Stavistky, A.B. and Harold, W.W. (1978). Regulation of the in vitro anamnestic antibody response by cyclic AMP. II. Antigen-dependent enhancement by exogenous prostaglandins of the E series. Cell. Immunul., **40**, 128–140

26. Gerblich, A.A. and Stavitsky, A.B. (1979). Regulation of the in vitro anamnestic antibody response by cyclic AMP. IV. Evidence for participation of prostaglandins of the E series in the early events. Cell. Immunol., **48**, 318–328

27. Kishimoto, T. and Ishizaka, K. (1976). Regulation of the antibody response in vitro. X. Biphasic effect of cyclic AMP on the secondary anti-hapten antibody response to anti-immunoglobulin and enhancing soluble factor. J. Immunol., **116**, 534–541

28. Webb, D.R. and Osheroff, P.L. (1976). Antigen stimulation of prostaglandin synthesis and control of immune responses. Proc. Natl. Acad. Sci. USA, **73**, 1300–1304

29. Leung, K.H., Ehrke, M.J. and Mihich, E. (1982). Modulation of the development of cell-mediated immunity: possible role of the products of the cyclo-oxygenase and the lipoxygenase pathways of arachidonic acid metabolism. Int. J. Immunopharmacol., **4**, 195–204

30. Darrow, T.L. and Tomar, R.H. (1980). Prostaglandin-mediated regulation of the mixed lymphocyte culture and generation of cytotoxic cells. Cell. Immunol., **56**, 172–183

31. Leung, K.H. and Mihich, E. (1980). Prostaglandin modulation of development of cell-mediated immunity in culture. Nature (London), **288**, 597–600

32. Ting, C-C. and Hargrove, M.E. (1983). Activation of natural killer-derived cytotoxic T lymphocytes. I. Regulation by macrophage and prostaglandins. J. Immunol., **131**, 1734–1741

33. Henney, C.S., Bourne, H.R. and Lichtenstein, L.M. (1972). The role of cyclic 3',5'-adenosine monophosphate in the specific cytolytic activity of lymphocytes. J. Immunol., **108**, 1526–1534

34. Strom, T.B., Carpenter, C.B., Garovoy, M.R., Austen, K.F., Merrill, J.P. and Kaliner, M. (1973). The modulating influence of cyclic nucleotides upon lymphocyte-mediated cytotoxicity. J. Exp. Med., **138**, 381–391

35. Hale, A.H., Evans, D.L. and Daniel, L.W. (1982). Effect of prostaglandins on elicitation of anti-viral cytolytic activity. Immunol. Lett., **4**, 171–174

36. Metzger, Z., Hoffeld, J.T. and Oppenheim,J.J. (1980). Macrophage-mediated suppression. I. Evidence for participation of both hydrogen peroxide and prostaglandins in suppression of murine lymphocyte proliferation. J. Immunol., **124**, 983–988

37. Mexmain, S., Gualde, N., Aldigier, J.C., Motta, C., Chable-Rabinovitch, H. and Rigaud, M. (1984). Specific binding of 15 HETE to lymphocytes. Effects on the fluidity of plasmatic membranes. Prostagl. Leukotriene Med., **13**, 93–97

38. Seaman, W.E. (1983). Human natural killer cell activity is reversibly inhibited by antagonists of lipoxygenation. J. Immunol., **131**, 2953–2957

39. Carine, K. and Hudig, D. (1984). Assessment of a role of phospholipase A_2 and arachidonic acid metabolism in human lymphocyte natural cytotoxicity. Cell. Immunol., **87**, 270–283

40. Bray, R.A. and Brahmi, Z. (1986). Role of lipoxygenation in human natural killer cell activation. *J. Immunol.*, **136**, 1783–1790
41. Droller, M.J., Perlmann, P. and Schneider, M.U. (1978). Enhancement of natural and antibody-dependent lymphocyte cytotoxicity by drugs which inhibit prostaglandin production by tumor target cells. *Cell. Immunol.*, **36**, 154–164
42. Tracey, D.E. and Adkinson, N.F. (1980). Prostaglandin synthesis inhibitors potentiate the BCG-induced augmentation of natural killer cell activity. *J. Immunol.*, **125**, 136–141
43. Droller, M.J., Schneider, M.U. and Perlmann, P. (1978). A possible role of prostaglandins in the inhibition of natural and antibody-dependent cell-mediated cytotoxicity against tumor cells. *Cell. Immunol.*, **39**, 165–177
44. Brunda, M.J., Herberman, R.B. and Holden, H.T. (1980). Inhibition of murine natural killer cell activity by prostaglandins. *J. Immunol.*, **124**, 2682–2687
45. Goto, T., Herberman, R.B., Maluish, A. and Strong, D.M. (1983). Cyclic AMP as a mediator of prostaglandin E-induced suppression of human natural killer cell activity. *J. Immunol.*, **130**, 1350–1355
46. Rola-Pleszczynski, M., Gagnon, L. and Sirois, P. (1983). Leukotriene B$_4$ augments human natural cytotoxic cell activity. *Biochem. Biophys. Res. Commun.*, **113**, 531–537
47. Ramstedt, U., Ng, J., Wigzell, H., Serhan, C.N. and Samuelsson, B. (1985). Action of novel eicosanoids lipoxin A and B on human natural killer cell cytotoxicity: effects on intracellular cAMP and target cell binding. *J. Immunol.*, **135**, 3434–3438
48. Serhan, C.N., Fahlstadius, P., Dahlén, S-E., Hamberg, M. and Samuelsson, B. (1985). Biosynthesis and biological activities of lipoxins. In Hayaishi, O. and Yamamoto, S. (eds.) *Advances in Prostaglandin, Thromboxane and Leukotriene Research.* Vol. 15, pp. 163–166. (New York: Raven Press)
49. Kelly, J.P., Johnson, M.C. and Parker, C.W. (1979). Effect of inhibitors of arachidonic acid metabolism on mitogenesis in human lymphocytes: possible role of thromboxanes and products of the lipoxygenase pathway. *J. Immunol.*, **122**, 1563–1571
50. Bailey, J.M., Bryant, R.W., Low, C.E., Pupillo, M.B. and Vanderhoek, J.Y. (1982). Regulation of T-lymphocyte mitogenesis by the leukocyte product 15-hydroxy-eicosatetraenoic acid (15-HETE). *Cell. Immunol.*, **67**, 112–120
51. Gualde, N., Chable-Rabinovitch, H., Motta, C., Durand, J., Beneytout, J.L. and Rigaud, M. (1983). Hydroperoxyeicosatetraenoic acids: potent inhibitors of lymphocyte responses. *Biochim. Biophys. Acta*, **750**, 429–433
52. Low, C-E., Pupillo, M.B., Bryant, R.W. and Bailey, J.M. (1984). Inhibition of phytohemagglutinin-induced lymphocyte mitogenesis by lipoxygenase metabolites of arachidonic acid: structure-activity relationships. *J. Lipid Res.*, **25**, 1090–1095
53. Vanderhoek, J.Y., Bryant, R.W. and Bailey, J.M. (1980). 15-Hydroxy-5,8,11,13-eicosatetraenoic acid: a potent and selective inhibitor of platelet lipoxygenase. *J. Biol. Chem.*, **255**, 5996–5998
54. Vanderhoek, J.Y., Bryant, J.W. and Bailey, J.M. (1980). Inhibition of leukotriene biosynthesis by the leukocyte product 15-hydroxy-5,8,11,13-eicosatetraenoic acid. *J. Biol. Chem.*, **255**, 10064–10066
55. Payan, D.G. and Goetzl, E.J. (1983). Specific suppression of human T lymphocyte function by leukotriene B$_4$. *J. Immunol.*, **131**, 551–553
56. Payan, D.G., Missirian-Bastian, A. and Goetzl, E.J. (1984). Human T-lymphocyte subset specificity of the regulatory effects of leukotriene B$_4$. *Proc. Natl. Acad. Sci. USA*, **81**, 3501–3505
57. Gualde, N., Atluru, D. and Goodwin, J.S. (1985). Effect of lipoxygenase metabolites of arachidonic acid on proliferation of human T cells and T cell subsets. *J. Immunol.*, **134**, 1125–1129
58. Kato, K. and Murota, S. (1985). Lipoxygenase specific inhibitors inhibit murine lymphocyte reactivity to Con A by reducing IL-2 production and its action. *Prostaglandl. Leukotriene Med.*, **18**, 39–52
59. Johnson, H.M. and Torres, B.A. (1984). Leukotrienes: positive signals for regulation of γ-interferon production. *J. Immunol.*, **132**, 413–416
60. Rola-Pleszczynski, M., Borgeat, P. and Sirois, P. (1982). Leukotriene B$_4$ induces human suppressor lymphocytes. *Biochem. Biophys. Res. Commun.*, **108**, 1531–1537
61. Rola-Pleszczynski, M. (1985). Differential effects of leukotriene B$_4$ on T4$^+$ and T8$^+$ lymphocyte phenotype and immunoregulatory functions. *J. Immunol.*, **135**, 1357–1360

77

62. Mexmain, S., Cook, J., Aldigier, J-C., Gualde, N. and Rigaud, M. (1985). Thymocyte cyclic AMP and cyclic GMP response to treatment with metabolites issued from the lipoxygenase pathway. *J. Immunol.*, **135**, 1361–1365
63. Aldigier, J.C., Gualde, N., Mexmain, S., Chable-Ravinovitch, H., Ratinaud, M.H. and Rigaud, M. (1984). Immunosuppression induced *in vivo* by 15-hydroxyeicosatetraenoic acid (15HETE). *Prostaglandl. Leukotriene Med.*, **13**, 99–106
64. Webb, D.R. and Nowowiejski, I. (1981). Mitogen-induced changes in lymphocyte prostaglandin levels: a signal for the induction of suppressor cell activity. *Cell. Immunol.*, **41**, 72–85
65. Fulton, A.M. and Levy, J.G. (1981). The induction of nonspecific T suppressor lymphocytes by prostaglandin E₁. *Cell. Immunol.*, **59**, 54–60
66. Fischer, A., Durandy, A. and Griscelli, C. (1981). Role of prostaglandin E₂ in the induction of nonspecific T lymphocyte suppressor activity. *J. Immunol.*, **126**, 1452–1455
67. Rogers, T.J., Nowowiejski, I. and Webb, D.R. (1980). Partial characterization of a prostaglandin-induced suppressor factor. *Cell. Immunol.*, **50**, 82–93
68. Webb, D.R., Wieder, K., Rogers, T.J. and Nowowiejski, I. (1980). Activation of mouse splenic suppressor cells by endogenous prostaglandin. In de Weck, A., Kristensen, F. and Landy, M. (eds.) *Biochemical Characterization of Lymphokines.* pp. 499–501. (New York: Academic Press)
69. Webb, D.R., Rogers, T.J. and Nowowiejski, I. (1979). Endogenous prostaglandin synthesis and the control of lymphocyte function. *Ann. NY Acad. Sci.*, **332**, 262–270
70. Rogers, T.J., Campbell, L., Calhoun, K., Nowowiejski, I. and Webb, D.R. (1982). Suppression of B-cell and T-cell responses by the prostaglandin-induced T-cell-derived suppressor (PITS). I. Analysis of the PITS_II factor. *Cell. Immunol.*, **66**, 269–276
71. Rogers, T.J., DeHaven, J.I., Donnelly, R.P. and Lamb, B. (1984). Suppression of B-cell and T-cell responses by the prostaglandin-induced T-cell-derived suppressor (PITS). II. Resolution of multiple PITS_II factors. *Cell. Immunol.*, **87**, 703–707
72. Rogers, T.J., DeHaven, J.I. and Donnelly, R.P. (1985). Suppression of B-cell and T-cell responses by the prostaglandin-induced T-cell-derived suppressors (PITS). III. Production of PITS_II factors from T-cell hybridomas. *Int. J. Immunopharmacol.*, **7**, 153–156
73. Webb, D.R., Wieder, K.J., Rogers, T.J., Healy, C.T. and Nowowiejski-Wieder, I. (1985). Chemical identification of a prostaglandin-induced T suppressor (PITS). *Lymphokine Res.*, **4**, 139–149
74. Kemp, J., Louie, D., Mattingly, J., Bennett, J., Higuchi, C., Pretell, J., Horowitz, M. and Gershon, R. (1980). Suppressor cells in vitro: differential effects of indomethacin and related compounds. *J. Immunopharmacol.*, **2**, 471–489
75. Goodwin, J.S. (1980). Modulation of concanavalin-A-induced suppressor cell activation by prostaglandin E₂. *Cell. Immunol.*, **49**, 421–425
76. Skoldstam, L., Zoschke, D. and Messner, R. (1982). Contrasting effects of prostaglandin E₂ and indomethacin in modulating Con A-induced human lymphocyte proliferation and suppressor cell development. *Clin. Immunol. Immunopathol.*, **25**, 32–42
77. Soppi, E., Eskola, J. and Ruuskanen, O. (1982). Effects of indomethacin on lymphocyte proliferation, suppressor cell function, and leukocyte migration inhibitor factor (LMIF) production. *Immunopharmacology*, **4**, 235–242
78. Badger, A.M., Griswold, D.E. and Walz, D.T. (1982). Augmentation of concanavalin A-induced immunosuppression by indomethacin. *Immunopharmacology*, **4**, 149–162
79. Leung, K.H., Ehrke, M.J. and Mihich, E. (1983). Modification by biological products of the generation of suppressor cells in culture. *Immunopharmacology*, **5**, 221–237
80. Donnelly, R.P. and Rogers, T.J. (1985). Inhibitors of prostaglandin synthesis block the induction of Staphylococcal enterotoxin B-activated T-suppressor cells. *Cell. Immunol.*, **81**, 61–70
81. Rogers, C.M., Rogers, T.J. and Gilman, S.C. (1985). Effects of WY-18,251 (3-(p-chlorophenylthiazolo[3,2-a]benzimadazole-2-acetic acid), levamisole and indomethacin in the generation of murine T suppressor cells *in vitro*. *J. Immunopharmacol.*, **7**, 479–488
82. Orme, I.M. and Shand, F.L. (1981). Inhibitors of prostaglandin synthetase block the generation of suppressor T cells induced by concanavalin A. *Int. J. Immunopharmacol.*, **3**, 15–19
83. Orme, I.M. and Shand, F.L. (1982). Concanavalin A-induced alteration of surface marker expression on murine T cells. *Int. J. Immunopharmacol.*, **4**, 137–142

84. Rogers, T.J. (1985). The role of arachidonic acid metabolites in the function of murine suppressor cells. In Goodwin, J.S. (ed.) *Prostaglandins and Immunity*. pp. 79–97. (Boston: Martinus Nijhoff Publishing)

85. Kato, K. and Askenase, P.W. (1984). Reconstitution of an inactive antigen-specific T cell suppressor factor by incubation of the factor with prostaglandins. *J. Immunol.*, **133**, 2025–2031

5
Current Concepts on the Role of Eicosanoids in the Pathogenesis of Bronchial Asthma

C. ROBINSON

INTRODUCTION

The exact global prevalence of bronchial asthma is hard to determine due to difficulties in providing an acceptable definition of the disease. Typically, asthma encompasses a broad spectrum of clinical features. Traditionally, reversible airflow obstruction has been used as a physiological index of asthma but, in extreme cases, this reversibility is sometimes hard to establish. Conversely, in latent asthma there may be asymptomatic periods in which patients require little or no medication. These and other diagnostic problems undoubtedly result in the underdiagnosis of the disease. In this chapter, the inflammatory events underlying the three major pathophysiological elements of asthma will be considered: the early asthmatic reaction, the late reaction and bronchial hyper-reactivity. Although the initiating event in allergic asthma is sensitization to a specific allergen, most asthma encountered in the clinic, i.e. where sensitization has already taken place, is set against an established background of bronchial hyper-reactivity. This is also true of the subjects who participate in studies designed to investigate the cellular and molecular basis of asthma. It is likely that the bronchial hyper-reactivity results from a genetic predisposition for its expression together with the physical events which are thought to trigger it. Thus, by its nature, most of the information about the events causing bronchial hyper-reactivity is indirect and often based on studies in animal models. This will be described in the first part of this chapter.

AIRWAYS INFLAMMATION AND BRONCHIAL HYPER-REACTIVITY

The pathological correlates of asthma include mucosal oedema, mucus hypersecretion, epithelial damage and a marked infiltration of the airways with eosinophil, and, to a lesser extent, neutrophil leukocytes[1-4]. It has become increasingly recognized that a key event linking the observed pathological changes with the pharmacological characteristic of enhanced non-specific bronchial reactivity to a wide spectrum of bronchoconstrictor agents could be the recruitment and activation of inflammatory cells for mediator release[5-7]. Bronchial hyper-reactivity is manifest as chest tightness, cough and wheezing evoked by exposure to cold air and noxious stimuli and is often associated with an exaggerated diurnal rhythm in airway calibre. Although a small proportion of the normal population may exhibit features of bronchial hyper-reactivity as indicated by bronchial provocation testing, it is a more common feature of asthma. Among such inflammatory mediators which may be involved in the pathogenesis of bronchial hyper-reactivity are those lipids derived by the oxidative metabolism of arachidonic acid.

A wide variety of hypotheses have been preferred to account for the pathogenesis of hyper-reactivity. Although such hypotheses can explain the altered airways sensitivity, e.g. by smooth muscle hypertrophy or by a change in the numbers or sensitivity of pharmacological receptors[8-10], these phenomena are not the initiating factors in hyper-reactivity. Furthermore, the variation in the degree of hyper-reactivity induced by changing the exposure to environmental allergens, noxious stimuli or by alterations in pharmacological treatment suggests that external factors, as well as genetic predisposition, all contribute to the condition. Much work has focused upon the possible loss of an inhibitory β_2-adrenoceptor regulatory mechanism[9,10]. However, although such receptors are found in abundance in human airways, few are inervated by adrenergic fibres[11,12]. Similarly, alterations in the pulmonary non-adrenergic non-cholinergic inhibitory nervous system with its putative transmitter vasoactive intestinal peptide, and the substance P-dependent non-cholinergic excitatory nerves, could account for a component of bronchial hyper-reactivity[13-15]. The possible activation of neuronal reflexes from afferent C fibres or irritant receptors in the epithelium may represent a common pathway linking neuronal and inflammatory mediator hypotheses of the pathogenesis of bronchial hyper-reactivity.

Focal disruption of the airway surface epithelium and its tight junctions by inflammatory mediators released from activated inflammatory cells, osmotic forces or physicochemical trauma may expose or modify the firing threshold of sensory afferent receptors which might be directly rendered hypersensitive by inflammatory mediators. In this respect, bronchial hyper-reactivity may be likened to the events which initiate prostaglandin-induced hyperalgesia in the skin[16]. It is noteworthy in relation to the pathophysiology of asthma that eosinophil-derived mediators may affect all of these factors. For example, leukotrienes (LT) C_4 and D_4, which can be released from eosinophils by physiological stimuli[17,18], are potent inflammatory mediators and, additionally, can enhance chloride ion secretion in canine tracheal epithelium[19]. Furthermore, the eosinophil-derived major basic protein is cytotoxic in the airways epithelium and thus results in specific physicochemical trauma. A number of studies have addressed the changes which occur following exposure to the noxious stimuli which produce bronchial hyper-reactivity[20-22]. Exposure to atmospheres containing 3 ppm of ozone can induce enhanced responsiveness to bronchoconstrictor stimuli[20,23] and this has been used widely as a model of some of the events which occur in asthma. The mechanism by which ozone initiates this response is not known, but may involve physical damage to the epithelium resulting in the oxidation of membrane lipids[24,25]. Pathological examination of the airways after ozone exposure reveals an influx of neutrophils into the epithelium and subepithelium. Bronchoalveolar lavage (BAL) of dogs exposed to ozone also demonstrates an increase in the number of neutrophils and epithelial cells recovered[26] albeit the dog being an exquisitely sensitive species in terms of triggering neutrophil infiltration. That these changes are intimately associated with the acquisition of bronchial hyper-reactivity is further suggested by the fact that in ozone-treated dogs which do not become hyper-responsive the number of neutrophils recovered by BAL is normal[27].

Several other lines of evidence implicate the neutrophil in the acquisition of bronchial hyper-reactivity following ozone exposure in the dog. Hydroxyurea-induced neutropaenia results in a smaller degree of hyper-responsiveness after ozone exposure when such animals are compared with dogs treated with ozone alone[28]. Furthermore, BW755C, an inhibitor of cyclo-oxygenase and the 5- and 12-lipoxygenase pathways of human polymorphonuclear leukocytes[29-32], provides protection against the bronchial hyper-reactivity induced by ozone and reduces the inflammatory cell infiltrate[33]. Pharmacological dissection of these events with indomethacin[34] and the thromboxane synthase inhibitor, OKY 046, has further revealed that thromboxane A_2 (TxA_2) generation following the infiltration of the airways with neutrophils is crucial to the acquisition of bronchial hyper-responsiveness after ozone or antigen[35,36]. These observations suggest that for hyper-reactivity to occur in this animal model, neutrophils must be activated to migrate into the airway epithelium[37], and it is noteworthy that the time courses of cellular infiltration and the onset of hyper-reactivity are remarkably similar[27]. A corollary of this hypothesis is that the epithelium itself must play an important role in the recruitment of neutrophils into the airway, or that chemoattractant mediators released from cells resident within the airway lumen, e.g. macrophages, are freely permeant across the epithelium. On purely physicochemical grounds, it would be surprising if the latter were true, and, in the rat at least, there is evidence of selective permeability of lipid mediators[38].

Relatively few investigations of mediator release from the airway epithelium have been performed. In rats and rabbits, tracheal epithelial cells have little capacity to metabolize exogenous arachidonic acid[39]. Isolated canine airway epithelial cells challenged with arachidonic acid synthesize and release 15-HETE and LTB_4 as their major products, together with smaller quantities of other HETEs and LTC_4[40]. When administered by inhalation to dogs, LTB_4 elicits both a reversible augmentation of bronchial reactivity by a TxA_2-dependent mechanism and a concomitant infiltration of neutrophils into the airways[37]. Together, these data make a plausible model for a mediator-driven inflammatory cell influx precipitating enhanced bronchial reactivity. However, experiments have been performed in isolated epithelial cells dispersed from human trachea obtained *post mortem*, which show a profile of products different from that of canine cells. After arachidonic acid challenge, the major product

82

identified by gas chromatography–mass spectrometry was 15-HETE, together with smaller amounts of two 8,15-diHETEs and two 8,15-leukotrienes. Other products detected from human trachea were a 14,15-diHETE, 8-HETE, 12-HETE and 5-HETE, but there was an absence of LTB_4 or its diastereomers[41]. However, the stimulus used in the human tracheal studies was a direct non-physiological challenge with exogenous arachidonic acid and thus the wider significance of these results must be viewed cautiously. It is interesting to note parenthetically that 15-lipoxygenase activity is only unmasked in human neutrophils following cell damage and cytolysis elicited by challenge with a large concentration of arachidonic acid[42]. Additionally, the absence of LTB_4 generation in human tracheal epithelium warns of species differences which have been the bane of asthma research. This is highlighted in ozone-treated guinea pigs where, in contrast to the canine model, neutropaenia does not inhibit the acquisition of bronchial hyper-reactivity, and in which the influx of neutrophils into the airways is slower than the onset of bronchial hyper-reactivity[43]. Thus, if lipid mediator release from the epithelium is an important event in the pathogenesis of hyper-reactivity, we are left with a number of questions: (1) do human airway epithelial cells release other eicosanoids upon challenge with more relevant stimuli; and (2) if 15-HETE is the principal eicosanoid released from these cells, what is its pathophysiological function?

In human polymorphonuclear (PMN) leukocytes, 15-HETE is a weak chemokinetic agent[44,45] compared with platelet activating factor, PAF-acether. On isolated airway smooth muscle, it is a weak spasmogen, although it potentiates histamine-induced contractions of human isolated bronchi[46]. In addition, it can exert a modulatory role on the lipoxygenase activity of other cell types[47–49]. It is also noteworthy that in the dog where 15-HETE is also a major epithelium-derived eicosanoid, it is a potent agonist for tracheal mucus secretion, inflammatory cell infiltration and respiratory fluid loss *in vivo*[50]. The latter action is specific for 15-HETE and is not found with either 5-HETE or 15-HPETE, but its inhibition by indomethacin suggests that a component of the response may be mediated indirectly. This observation deserves further attention in view of the release of 15-HETE from human trachea. The relatively low potency of 15-HETE in PMN migration compared with LTB_4 suggests that it is unlikely to drive an influx of inflammatory cells into the airway. One report has suggested that 8(S),15(S)-dihydroxy-5(Z),9(E),11(Z),13(E)-eicosatetraenoic acid, prepared by incubation of arachidonic acid with soybean lipoxygenase or generated by A23187-dependent stimulation of human PMN leukocytes, is almost equipotent with LTB_4 for human PMN chemokinesis[44]. Subsequent work with chemically synthesized 8,5-diHETEs of known absolute configuration has contradicted these findings[51], although it is possible that other stereoisomers are active. Thus, the 8,15-diHETEs formed by human tracheal epithelial cells are unlikely to account for the inflammatory cell infiltration of the airway epithelium.

If the search for exactly which mediator(s) drive the inflammatory cell influx in the airways of human asthma at the biochemical level has been unrewarding so far, pharmacological studies have implicated a range of putative mediators in the induction of hyper-responsiveness in both man and experimental animals. Some of these studies are summarized in Table 5.1.

Table 5.1 Lipid mediators promoting enhanced reactivity to other agonists

Potentiating agent	Agonists potentiated	Test system	Reference
SRS-A	Histamine	Guinea-pig ileum*	220
LTC_4,LTD_4	Histamine	Guinea-pig trachea*	221
LTE_4	Histamine	Guinea-pig trachea*	222
PGD_2	Histamine methacholine	Asthmatic subjects	52
LTC_4	Fog	Asthmatic subjects	223
LTD_4	Histamine $PGF_{2\alpha}$	Normal subjects	224
PAF	Methacholine	Normal subjects	217
PGI_2	PGD_2	Rhesus monkey	138
LTB_4	Acetylcholine	Guinea pig	225
LTB_4	Acetylcholine potassium chloride	Guinea-pig trachea*	225

*denotes *in vitro* preparation

Many *in vivo* studies of this type have employed the technique of initial challenge with a subthreshold concentration of one agonist. Although inhalation of a subconstrictor concentration of one agonist may produce no measurable effect on airway calibre *per se* it is likely to exert some functional effect on bronchial airway smooth muscle. Subconstrictor concentrations of agonists influence the length–tension relationships of bronchial smooth muscle and this can alter the constrictor threshold of a subsequently administered agonist irrespective of its pharmacological nature. This physiological interaction could lead to a displacement of the concentration response curve to the left which would be unrelated to true pharmacological synergism. This may account for a synergistic interaction that has been reported between histamine and PGD_2 in one study[52], while another report has demonstrated only an additive interaction when employing a technique which does not involve the subconstrictor dose problem[53]. Such interactions may also be influenced by an inhibitory mediator(s) released from the airways epithelium, the release of which may be susceptible to the cellular damage seen in asthma[54].

THE EARLY ASTHMATIC REACTION

When a patient with allergic asthma is challenged by bronchial provocation with specific allergen, a bronchoconstrictor response is evoked and this reaches a maximum 10–30 min after challenge[55]. For many years, mast cells have been implicated as the major cell type initiating this response which is frequently used as a clinical model of one component of the disease[56,57].

In normal human lung, mast cells comprise 0.01–0.1% of the nucleated cell population and are found in the alveoli and airways[58–61]. They contain a wide variety of mediators which are believed to exert their effects directly on target cells within the lung or which may recruit other cells to amplify and attenuate the response[56]. An important preformed product of the secretory granule is histamine which is capable of causing contraction of airway smooth muscle, vasodilatation and augmented vasopermeability. In addition, mast cell granules also contain a variety of neutral proteases and exoglycosidases. Mast cells are activated by the immunoglobulin-dependent cross-linkage of membrane IgE Fc receptors which initiates a series of complex biochemical changes within the cell. (For reviews, see references 56,62 and 63). The influx of calcium ions consequent upon cell activation, results in swelling of the secretory granules and their translocation towards the plasma membrane. Fusion of the perigranular and cytoplasmic membranes exposes the granule matrix to the extracellular environment, where liberation of preformed mediators occurs by ion exchange[64].

Support for mast cell activation in the early asthmatic reactions is provided by the demonstration that, in patients with mild asthma, the plasma concentrations of the preformed mediators histamine and high-molecular weight neutrophil chemotactic factor (HMW–NCF) increase after allergen provocation, and that this increase precedes the onset of maximum bronchoconstriction[65]. Pharmacological evidence also supports a role for the mast cell in this component of the disease. Pretreatment of patients with the mast cell stabilizing drug, sodium cromoglycate, or the β_2-adrenoceptor agonist, salbutamol, inhibits both the onset of bronchoconstriction and the changes in plasma histamine and HMW-NCF concentrations[65]. Both of these drugs inhibit histamine release from human lung mast cells, but, at therapeutic concentrations, are without significant activity against histamine release from basophils[66]. Furthermore, the powerful histamine H_1-receptor antagonists, astemizole and terfenadine, both produce significant inhibition of the initial phase of bronchoconstriction during the early asthmatic response to allergen[55].

In addition to storing preformed mediators, mast cells are also capable of synthesizing mediators on a *de novo* basis. Immunological activation of human dispersed pulmonary mast cells by cross-linkage of IgE results in the generation of large quantities of PGD_2 (40–100 ng/10^6 cells) which proceeds in parallel with the release of histamine[67,68]. Highly purified human pulmonary mast cells also release[68] small amounts of thromboxane TxB_2 and 6-oxo-$PGF_{1\alpha}$. In studies with mast cells prelabelled with tritiated arachidonic acid, the most abundant lipoxygenase product released by IgE-dependent activation is leukotriene LTC_4 (20–25 ng/10^6 cells) together with smaller quantities of LTB_4 and 5-HETE[69]. Leukotriene D_4 was not detected in these experiments, suggesting that the conversion of LTC_4 to other sulphidopeptide leukotrienes occurs in cells other than mast cells. Early experiments employing mast cells enriched by density flotation on metrizamide gradients led to the view that an accessory cell was required for the optimum production of SRS-A leukotrienes by mast cells[70,71]. More recent work with cells of higher purity obtained by countercurrent centrifugal elutriation and isopyknic centrifugation on discontinuous gradients of Percoll has argued against this[72]. However, it would be surprising if mast cells were the only cells within the lung capable of generating LTC_4, as alveolar macrophages are also known to generate LTC_4 and LTD_4 upon IgE-dependent activation[73,74].

The complexity of lipid mediator release following a specific stimulus, such as cross-linkage of IgE, is illustrated by a comparison of the release of cyclooxygenase products from passively sensitized human lung cells enriched to different degrees with mast cells. When challenged with anti-IgE, proteolyt-ically dispersed cells, enriched to contain 1–10% mast cells, release PGD_2 (22–56%), TxB_2 (37–66%), 6-oxo-$PGF_{1\alpha}$ (< 1–2%), PGE_2 (4–6%) and $PGF_{2\alpha}$ (3–5%), together with substantial amounts of histamine[67]. This profile contrasts with antigen challenge of bronchial or subpleural parenchymal fragments where 6-oxo-$PGF_{1\alpha}$ (an index of prostacyclin release) is a major product[75] together with PGD_2. This difference is most likely to be due to the loss of pulmonary vascular endothelial cells during proteolytic digestion. Further enrichment of mast cells, up to 90% purity, reveals that PGD_2 is the major cyclo-oxygenase product of these cells[68,69,76], but fractions containing few or no mast cells also respond to IgE-dependent activation[67] with the release of TxB_2 and smaller quantities of 6-oxo-$PGF_{1\alpha}$, PGE_2 and $PGF_{2\alpha}$. This suggests that other cells release eicosanoids in response to IgE-dependent activation or through the action of substances released from mast cells, such as the oligopeptide prostaglandin generating factor of anaphylaxis, PGF-A[77,78]. Cells which are known to possess Fc receptors for IgE, albeit of a lower affinity than the mast cell receptors, include macrophages[79], B- and T-lymphocytes[80], monocytes[81], eosinophils[82] and platelets[83]. In particular, cells of the monocyte-macrophage series are likely to be major contributors to non-mast cell-derived prostanoids because the pattern of their separation on density gradients corresponds most closely with anti-IgE and ionophore A23187-stimulated prostanoid generation[67]. Monocytes and macrophages have the capacity to release a wide spectrum of mediators, including acid hydrolases TxA_2, LTB_4, sulphidopeptide LTs, mono-HETEs and PAF-acether[84]. Furthermore, the anatomical location of alveolar macrophages raises the possibility that these cells may play a contributory role in the early asthmatic response to inhaled allergens.

Which mast cells are activated in the airways?

For mast cells to be centrally involved in the initiation of the allergen dependent early asthmatic response, sufficient cellular activation needs to occur to initiate mediator release. Cells abutting onto the lumen of the airway are therefore likely to be the initial targets for inhaled allergens. However, most of the mast cells within the airways are located between the basement membrane and the epithelium, with few cells in the stratified columnar epithelium exposed to the lumen[60]. Thus, an important question is how do these sub-epithelial mast cells become activated? Disruption of the tight junctions in the airway epithelium is one mechanism to account for this. Boucher and co-workers have shown that antigen-induced bronchoconstriction in *Ascaris*-sensitive monkeys, and histamine-, methacholine- or antigen-induced bronchoconstriction in guinea pigs, results in an increased epithelial permeability to marker molecules such as horseradish peroxidase[85,86]. However, in human asthma, there is not an enhanced epithelial permeability during phases of enhanced bronchial reactivity[87], although the technique used in these human studies may not discriminate between alveolar and bronchial permeability. Furthermore, it may not be unreasonable to assume that in quiescent phases of mild asthma, bronchial epithelial permeability may not be significantly changed from normal. However, permeability could be increased as a result of the antigen-dependent activation of lumenal mast cells or macrophages, and this may then expose subepithelial mast cells, facilitating their IgE-dependent activation.

Histochemical, biochemical, functional and pharmacological evidence has been presented for the existence of at least two subpopulations of rodent mast cells associated either with connective tissue or mucosal surfaces[88]. On the basis of this, it has been widely assumed that mast cells in the airway epithelium may be 'mucosal' mast cells, while subepithelial mast cells may be classified as connective tissue cells. However, although BAL mast cells contain fewer secretory granules and have a higher nuclear to cytoplasmic ratio than mast cells in the parenchyma, the application of the histochemical methods used for rat cells to human lung have failed to provide convincing evidence for such heterogeneity[89]. However, there is evidence for mediator heterogeneity between mast cells obtained by bronchoalveolar lavage (BAL) and those enzymatically dispersed from lung. Mast cells derived by BAL respond to ionophore or IgE-dependent stimulation with the release of histamine in parallel with PGD_2[90]. In contrast to the parenchymal mast cells, where anti-IgE stimulation is twice as effective as A23187 in releasing PGD_2[6,7], the ratio is considerably higher in BAL mast cells (Agius, Robinson and Holgate, unpublished). Further evidence for mediator heterogeneity in these cells is provided by LTC_4 which is released in barely detectable quantities[91] when compared with enzymatically dispersed parenchymal mast cells.

THE LATE ASTHMATIC REACTION

In patients in whom allergen provocation evokes a late asthmatic reaction some 8–16 h after provocation, there is often an associated increase in bronchial responsiveness. Subjects who exhibit only an immediate response do not exhibit this enhanced airways reactivity. Current evidence links the onset of the late reaction with the recruitment and activation of other inflammatory cells, particularly leukocytes[92–95], and with associated changes in circulating levels of mediators[96]. Cellular and molecular aspects of late reactions have been described in detail in Chapter 2 and possible mechanisms of enhanced responsiveness have been dealt with earlier in this chapter. Both high-molecular weight NCF and histamine have been shown to be present in elevated concentrations in plasma during the late reaction[96]. There have been no published accounts of plasma measurements of lipid mediators in late reactions, but, in documented nasal late reactions, PGD_2 is significant because of its absence in nasal washings[97] although histamine, LTC_4 and NCF are all released into lavage fluid[97,98]. This evidence has been interpreted as arguing against the direct participation of mast cells during nasal late reactions, although the release of mediators in the early reaction may be important for activating the cells which participate in the late response. Salbutamol and other β_2-adrenoceptor agonists, which are potent inhibitors of mast cell histamine secretion *in vitro* and the immediate asthmatic reaction to allergen *in vivo*, have little effect on the pathogenesis of the late reaction[99,100], and, chronically, they may even enhance non-specific bronchial responsiveness[101]. In contrast, sodium cromoglycate, a relatively weak inhibitor of histamine release from human pulmonary mast cells, inhibits the early reaction, the late reaction and the acquisition of non-specific hyper-reactivity[99,102]. These observations highlight possible independent mechanisms for cromoglycate and salbutamol suppression of the immediate reaction. This might be by direct inhibition of mast cell mediator release and secondarily either a direct or indirect action leading to an attenuated influx and activation of leukocytes.

Recent studies in asthmatic volunteers undergoing bronchoalveolar lavage 6 h after bronchial provocation with allergen have shown that, in those patients with both early and late responses, there is an increase in the number of neutrophils recovered in BAL. This change is not seen in those patients who show only early responses[103]. Animal models of allergen-induced immediate and late reactions have been developed in rabbits[104] sheep[105], guinea pigs[106] and Basenji greyhounds[107], and these have further linked the late reaction and enhanced non-specific bronchial reactivity to inflammatory cell infiltration. In rabbits sensitized to produce IgE with *Alternaria tenuis*, late reactions are associated with a reduction in the number of circulating neutrophils[104]. There is also a concomitant neutrophil infiltration of the airways and an increase in the number of neutrophils recovered by BAL. The LT antagonist, FPL 55712, and sodium cromoglycate both inhibit the response in the sheep model, suggesting the involvement of inflammatory mediators[108]. In addition, other neutrophil chemotactic agents, e.g. PAF-acether and HMW-NCF, may also be involved.

Although neutrophil and monocyte infiltration is characteristic of asthma, eosinophil infiltration is numerically more dominant in the pathology of the disease. Of course, this does not necessarily indicate that these cells are more important. Blood and sputum eosinophilia are often correlates of asthma[1,109,110], and, in *post mortem* tissue from asthma deaths, eosinophil infiltration is a striking histopathological feature[1-4]. Eosinophil activation is also signalled by the presence in asthmatic airways or sputum of eosinophil major basic protein and cationic protein[111] and the demonstration of elevated levels of eosinophil proteins in the late reaction[92]. This protein is cytotoxic and may be partly responsible for the disruption of the airway epithelium in asthma[112,113]. Exactly what accounts for this influx and activation of eosinophils is not known. Nor is it known whether eosinophil-derived proteins also serve as triggers for lipid mediator release as would seem likely from their mode of action. Although it is tempting to speculate that the eosinophil influx is dependent on the magnitude of the early response, this is not always the case as late reactions following severe early asthmatic responses are not always accompanied by eosinophilia. A wide variety of agents have chemotactic activity for eosinophils *in vitro*, including PAF-acether[114], LTB$_4$[115] and the ECF-A acidic tetrapeptides[116]. It was speculated earlier that the pathogenesis of bronchial hyper-reactivity may be partly controlled by the release of mediators from a damaged bronchial epithelium. The established link and similarities between aspects of hyper-reactivity and late reactions suggests that common mechanisms may account for a part of these disease features.

An attempt to integrate these components on the basis of mediators known to be released from human tracheal epithelial cells does not provide a convincing answer at present. An obvious candidate as a lipid mediator of eosinophil chemotaxis is PAF-acether, although, at present, it is not known whether epithelial cells generate and release this mediator.

The presence of low-affinity Fc receptors for IgE on alveolar macrophages has led to the belief that these cells might also participate in asthma, particularly since the cells are capable of generating a wide range of mediators both *in vitro* and *in vivo*[84]. This view is supported by the observed correlation between the severity of asthma and the activation state of peripheral blood monocytes measured as IgG and complement C3b receptor expression[117]. The activation of macrophages may be intimately linked to the recruitment of other inflammatory cells, particularly eosinophils. For example, in addition to the eosinophil chemoattractants, PAF-acether and LTB_4, macrophages also release a 40 000 dalton protein termed eosinophil activating factor (EAF)[118] which concentration-dependently augments IgG-dependent LTC_4 generation from human eosinophils[119]. Although EAF has yet to be found in asthma, this and other factors may be a part of the mechanisms regulating the infiltration and activation of eosinophils which is so characteristic of asthma pathology. It is also likely that the recruitment and activation of eosinophils may also be regulated by T-lymphocytes, and specific changes in helper (OKT4) and activated (Ia positive) cells have been documented in asthma[120].

PHARMACOLOGICAL EFFECTS OF EICOSANOIDS IN ASTHMA

Prostaglandins

It has long been recognized that prostaglandins are capable of exerting pharmacological effects on the airways of many species[121-124]. The contractile action of $PGF_{2\alpha}$ and relaxant action of PGE_2 on human bronchial smooth muscle led to the proposal that bronchial hyper-reactivity may develop as a fundamental imbalance between these mediators[122]. Prostacyclin could play a useful role in such a hypothesis since it is the most abundant cyclo-oxygenase product of human airway tissue, and, despite having little or no effect on airway calibre in most subjects[125,126], it can protect against bronchoconstriction induced by exercise, water mist, PGD_2 and methacholine[125,127]. At present, there is no rigorous evidence to support or refute the concept of altered arachidonic acid metabolism causing bronchial hyper-reactivity, save observations of small differences in platelet and leukocyte lipoxygenase activity in asthma[128,129]. Furthermore, in ovalbumin-sensitized guinea pigs, repeated challenge with aerosolized ovalbumin induces changes in the profile of prostaglandin synthesis and metabolism in the lung[130].

The effects of prostaglandins on the tone of isolated airways *in vitro* or on experimental animals *in vivo* are largely predictive of their effects on airway calibre in man. By inhalation, $PGF_{2\alpha}$ produces bronchoconstriction in man, whereas PGE_2 usually produces bronchodilatation[131,132]. The greater sensitivity of asthmatic subjects to the bronchoconstrictor effects of $PGF_{2\alpha}$, and the correlation of this to the severity of the disease as indicated by tests of bronchial reactivity[133], is well documented. This is also true with inhaled PGD_2 which, in molar terms, is at least 3 times more potent than $PGF_{2\alpha}$ and 30 times more potent than histamine[134]. A convenient way of expressing data from this type of study is to use the provocation concentration of agonist, or PC value, required to produce a specified percentage fall in baseline airway calibre when measured by a particular technique. In the study by Hardy *et al.*[134], there was a positive correlation between the PC_{35} for specific airways conductance (sGaw) values for histamine and PGD_2 ($r = 0.7$, $p < 0.05$) and histamine and $PGF_{2\alpha}$ ($r = 0.8$, $p < 0.05$), indicating that sensitivity to the PGs is related to a feature of enhanced non-specific airways reactivity. It should be mentioned parenthetically that none of these prostaglandins have appreciable bronchoconstrictor effects when administered by intravenous infusion[135], this probably being due to their rapid local inactivation. It is interesting to note that $9\alpha,11\beta\text{-}PGF_2$, the initial metabolite formed by the 11-keto reductase-dependent metabolism of PGD_2, is itself a potent contractile agonist on human airways *in vitro* or by inhalation in asthmatic, but not normal, subjects *in vivo*[136,137]. These observations have prompted speculation[136] that a component of the bronchoconstrictor effect of PGD_2 may be mediated by its metabolism to $9\alpha,11\beta\text{-}PGF_2$, although formal proof of this hypothesis is awaited. In rhesus monkeys, prostacyclin has been shown to enhance the bronchoconstriction evoked by PGD_2[138], but, in man, provided that it is administered beforehand, prostacyclin attenuates PGD_2-induced broncho spasm[127].

The presence of discrete receptors for prostaglandins on airway smooth muscle, as indicated by experiments on isolated tissue preparations, suggests that the effects of prostanoids on airway calibre may be mediated by direct dynamic effects on bronchial smooth muscle[139]. However, inhalation of nebulized prostaglandins, irrespective of whether they induce bronchodilatation or bronchoconstriction, is often associated with an initial cough response, one of several problems which has restricted the therapeutic use of prostanoids as bronchodilators. Experiments in both animals and man suggest that a variable proportion of the bronchoconstrictor response to inhaled prostanoids is actually mediated by a cholinergic mechanism inhibitable by muscarinic antagonists and cromoglycate[140–145]. This could be due to activation of non-myelinated C-fibres, stimulation of irritant receptors or direct facilitation of postganglionic cholinergic transmission[146]. Activation of such mechanisms may be especially important in exacerbations of asthma where mucosal oedema and epithelial shedding may expose afferent nerve endings to eicosanoids generated by activated cells.

Leukotrienes

Ever since their discovery as SRS-A, the sulphidopeptide leukotrienes have been assumed to be of central importance in asthmatic bronchospasm. This case has been built up because of the poor efficacy of older H_1-receptor antagonists in the pharmacological management of the early asthmatic reaction[55] and the ability of crude lung-derived SRS-A and chemically synthesized LTC_4 and LTD_4 to elicit contraction of both guinea pig and human airways *in vitro*[147–150]. Furthermore, the ability of SRS-A to enhance the histamine-induced contractions of smooth muscle promoted the belief that SRS-A may be involved in the pathogenesis of bronchial hyper-reactivity[151]. As contractile agonists of human airway smooth muscle, they are 200–1000 times more potent than histamine[147,152], although there is considerable species heterogeneity since airways from monkeys, rats, cats and dogs are less sensitive[153,154].

The mechanism of action of leukotrienes on guinea-pig airways and their relative effects in human asthma, have been the subject of considerable controversy (reviewed in reference 155). In anaesthetized guinea pigs, the mechanism of bronchoconstriction elicited by LTC_4, D_4 or E_4 depends upon the route of administration. Intravenously, leukotrienes evoke a slowly onsetting bronchoconstriction of long duration which can be attenuated by indomethacin[156,157]. In contrast, aerosol administration of leukotrienes produces a more transient response which is refractory to indomethacin[157,158].

In man, there is little doubt that inhaled LTC_4, LTD_4 and, less potently, LTE_4 are more active than histamine in eliciting a persisting bronchoconstriction[159–160]. In normal subjects, the leukotrienes are, on a molar basis, 600–9000 times more potent than histamine or methacholine[159–161,163–166], whereas one study reported that, in asthmatic subjects, LTD_4 is only 140 times more potent than histamine[161]. This observation was interpreted as asthmatic subjects not being hyper-responsive to LTD_4 when compared with the normal group, and was explained by the hypothesis that LTD_4 acted on a portion of the respiratory tree where histamine has little or no effect[161]. In contrast, Smith *et al.* have demonstrated that patients with very mild asthma or rhinitis do exhibit an enhanced responsiveness to inhaled LTD_4 when compared with normal subjects[163]. Moreover, in this study LTD_4 exerted an equal effect on specific conductance and maximal expiratory flow measurements and this was interpreted as indicating that LTD_4 acted on both proximal and peripheral airways. It is unlikely that these parameters of airway function reflect such an absolute demarcation of site of action, but such a non-specific profile of activity may be produced artefactually due to very intense peripheral airway constriction. A feature which has emerged from these investigations is that the index of airway calibre used to measure leukotriene-induced bronchoconstriction can be very important in determining the degree of hyper-reactivity of asthmatic patients compared with normal subjects. The most extreme example of this is when partial expiratory flow volumes are used as the index of airway calibre, when the sensitivity of asthmatic and normal groups can appear similar[155,162].

ARE EICOSANOIDS IMPORTANT IN ASTHMA?

Much of the foregoing discussion of the possible involvement of eicosanoids in asthma has concentrated on the evidence for their synthesis, release and biological actions in target tissues. Two further criteria, which must be satisfied to further establish their roles, are (1) measurement of eicosanoid release during exacerbations of the disease *in vivo*, and (2) specific attenuation of their effects by pharmacological agents which inhibit the synthesis of, or antagonize the actions of, individual mediators or groups of mediators.

Mediator release *in vivo*

The precise and accurate measurement of eicosanoids in biological fluids has been a problematic area of eicosanoid research. The high potency of eicosanoids, coupled with their short *in vivo* half-lives, results in the plasma concentrations of parent prostanoids being very low, usually less than $5 \, pg \, ml^{-1}$, when measured by gas chromatography–mass spectrometry[135,167,168]. Measurement of the same prostanoids by radioimmunoassay techniques has often resulted in the detection of spuriously high values (reviewed in references 167,169). Furthermore, the facile artefactual generation of prostaglandins renders them poor analyte molecules. In contrast, and despite other limitations, the measurement of prostaglandin metabolites has proved to be a much more useful technique with which to investigate prostaglandin release. Their longer half-lives *in vivo*, presence in higher concentration and virtual absence of problems of artefactual generation make them useful analytes, even for radioimmunoassay[169]. Despite this, relatively few studies have been performed in asthma in which physiological concentrations of prostaglandins are reported. Gréen, *et al.*[170] demonstrated that allergen challenge of asthmatic subjects resulted in an increase in the plasma concentration of 13,14-dihydro-15-keto-$PGF_{2\alpha}$. The simplest interpretation of these results is that allergen provocation elicits $PGF_{2\alpha}$ release and that this is reflected in the elevated concentration of the metabolite. However, *in vitro*, IgE-dependent activation of human lung results in relatively little release of $PGF_{2\alpha}$ and nor is $PGF_{2\alpha}$ released as a consequence of smooth muscle contraction *in vivo*[171].

One explanation for the elevated concentrations of 13,14-dihydro-15-keto-$PGF_{2\alpha}$ following allergen provocation comes from recent experiments in which the human metabolism of PGD_2 was studied. Prior to this work, an investigation of PGD_2 metabolism in a monkey had suggested that PGD_2 was metabolized by reduction to yield compounds in which the 3-hydroxycyclopentanone ring of PGD_2 had been reduced to the cyclopentane-1,3-diol ring characteristic of F-series prostaglandins. It was widely assumed that the ring stereochemistry of these metabolites was identical to $PGF_{2\alpha}$. However, using a highly specific radioimmunoassay, Hardy *et al.*[171] demonstrated that, in man, inhalation of PGD_2 did not alter the plasma concentration of 13,14-dihydro-15-keto-$PGF_{2\alpha}$, whereas, after inhalation of $PGF_{2\alpha}$, there was a rapid rise in the level of this metabolite (Figure 5.1).

Investigation of the PGD_2 metabolites present in the urine of a patient with systemic mastocytosis[172–174] and in a normal volunteer following infusion of tritiated PGD_2[175] have confirmed that initial 11-keto reduction is a major metabolic route for PGD_2 in man. However, the product of this reaction is $9\alpha,11\beta$-PGF_2 and not $PGF_{2\alpha}$[174–176]. As mentioned earlier, $9\alpha,11\beta$-PGF_2 is

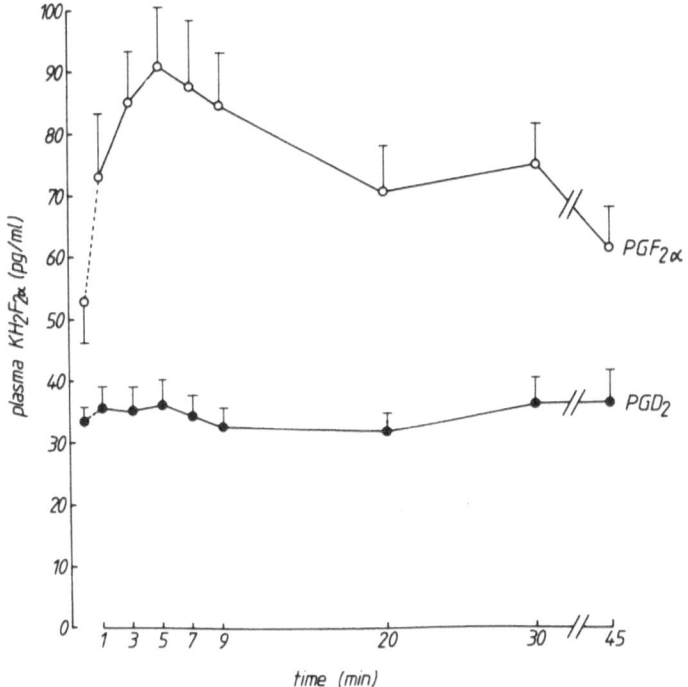

Figure 5.1   Changes in the plasma concentrations of 13,14-dihydro-15-keto-PGF$_{2\alpha}$ (KH$_2$F$_{2\alpha}$) following inhalation of either PGF$_{2a}$ (O) or PGD$_2$ (●) in a group of 14 subjects. Seven of the subjects had mild asthma. There was no difference in response between the asthma and normal groups. Data are presented as mean ± SEM

biologically active and causes contraction of human airways[136,137]. The 9α,11β-epimer of PGF$_2$ has also been detected in human plasma following inhalation or intravenous infusion of [^{3}H$_7$]-PGD$_2$ (Robinson, unpublished). In addition, a major component of the plasma radioactivity following administration by either route was associated with a peak tentatively identified as 13,14-dihydro-15-keto-9α,11β-PGF$_2$ (Figure 5.2). The relatively long biological half-life of this metabolite (10 min) suggests that it may serve as a useful index of the activation of mast cells for newly generated mediator production.

Attention is now being paid to the identification of suitable compounds to serve as indices of leukotriene turnover. In the monkey, tritiated LTB$_4$ is rapidly and extensively degraded, suggesting that no stable metabolite may exist[177]. Only 1–2% of the infused dose was recovered as non-volatile metabolites, and this was mainly 20-hydroxy-LTB$_4$[177]. In man, initial experiments with LTC$_4$ have revealed that most metabolites are excreted in the urine (48%) with a much smaller amount (8%) eliminated in the faeces[178]. As little as 1 h after intravenous injection, 25% of the dose was recovered in the urine and 13% of this material was identified as LTE$_4$[178]. In the rat, the majority of LTC$_4$ metabolites are excreted in the faeces and N-acetyl-LTE$_4$ is an additional

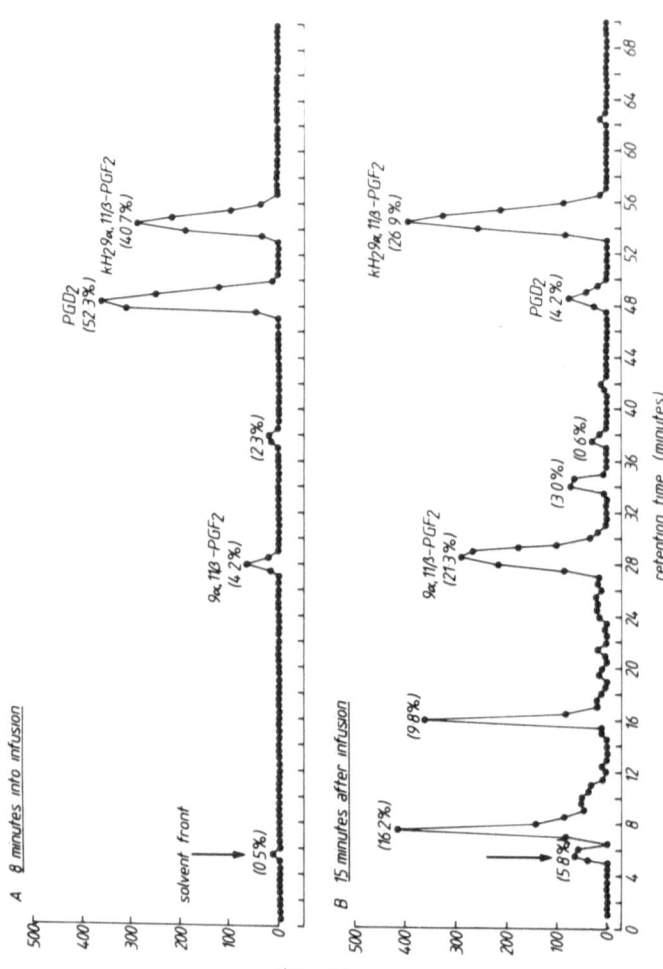

Figure 5.2 Reversed-phase high-performance liquid chromatographic separation of plasma metabolites observed after intravenous infusion of [^{3}H$_4$]-PGD$_2$ into a normal volunteer. The upper panel depicts a sample taken 8 min into the 20 min infusion; the lower panel, a sample taken 15 min after the end of the infusion period

94

metabolite[179,180]. There is now considerable interest in employing LTE_4 as an analyte for the measurement of sulphidopeptide LT turnover, and the recent introduction of a two-step reduction method to facilitate hydrogenation and thioether cleavage may overcome some of the many technical difficulties associated with leukotriene measurement.

Pharmacological manipulation of eicosanoid release and function in asthma

Despite the potent contractile effects of certain prostanoids on airway smooth muscle and their IgE-dependent release from human lung, a role for prostaglandins in asthmatic bronchoconstriction has been largely dismissed on the basis of a small number of clinical studies with cyclo-oxygenase inhibitors. Smith[181] showed that 200 mg indomethacin daily for seven days failed to inhibit the response to antigen measured as FEV_1. However, detailed examination of this data reveals that in five subjects the fall in FEV_1 was smaller after indomethacin, although this was attributed to possible decomposition of the antigen solution[181]. That prostaglandins may be unimportant in asthmatic bronchospasm was supported by a similar lack of protection against exercise challenge[181], although the current view is that newly generated mediators may not be involved in exercise-induced asthma. In a more detailed study, Fish and colleagues[182] studied the effects of indomethacin (200 mg for 4 days) and placebo on the antigen-induced early reaction in both allergic asthmatic and allergic non-asthmatic subjects. Indomethacin enhanced the antigen sensitivity of the non-asthmatic group but no effect was seen on methacholine sensitivity. Indomethacin had no effect in the asthmatic group when responses were measured as FEV_1, but parallel measurements of sGaw indicated a small reduction in the sensitivity to antigen. These and other pharmacological studies[183-186] have failed to clarify whether prostaglandins participate to any extent in exercise- or antigen-induced bronchoconstriction. However, they do not formally exclude a role for prostaglandins in asthmatic bronchoconstriction. For example, no study has yet provided the technically difficult independent evidence that the doses of inhibitor employed actually produced significant inhibition of cyclo-oxygenase activity in airways and lung. Furthermore, most studies have concentrated upon the bronchospasm which occurs within 15 min of antigen provocation and it is possible that newly generated mediators are responsible for a component of the early bronchoconstrictor response which develops after this time.

Recent experiments with the non-steroidal anti-inflammatory drug, flurbiprofen, which is at least 1000 times more potent than aspirin as an inhibitor of cyclo-oxygenase[187], have provided some interesting evidence in support of prostaglandin-mediated allergic bronchoconstriction[57]. Allergen provocation of atopic non-asthmatic subjects was employed as the experimental model and the effects of placebo, the H_1-antagonist, terfenadine (180 mg 3 h prior to challenge), and flurbiprofen (150 mg daily for 3 days) were compared[57]. The antihistamine inhibited the airways response to allergen provocation,

95

confirming that, within the first 15 min of the allergen response, histamine is an important mediator of bronchospasm. Flurbiprofen also had a major effect on allergen-induced bronchoconstriction. However, the activity of this drug differed from that of the antihistamine in that maximum inhibition occurred at 15 min and was sustained for 45 min. As PGD_2 release from mast cells *in vitro* proceeds at a slower rate than that of histamine[67], it is possible that flurbiprofen may act by inhibiting PGD_2 release. When used in combination, the two drugs produced an inhibitory effect which was less than additive. One explanation for these findings is that, in addition to inhibiting PGD_2 formation, flurbiprofen also inhibits the synthesis of a factor(s) which exerts a protective action on the airways. Such factors could include PGE_2 or PGI_2[120,127]. Alternatively, the metabolism of arachidonic acid may have been redirected to the formation of sulphidopeptide LTs[188], or to other lipoxygenase products, such as 5-HETE and 12-HETE, which augment histamine release in rat mast cells[189], elicit neutrophil degranulation[190] and become incorporated into cell membranes in macrophages[191]. However, an increasing number of studies employing isolated human lung cells have provided evidence against the concept of 'shunting' to sulphidopeptide LTs[192,193] although, theoretically, differences in methodology and source of substrate (exogenous or endogenous) could affect the results obtained.

At present, drugs which inhibit the formation of, or block the actions of, leukotrienes are only just becoming available for trial in man. Piriprost (U-60,257) is a pyrrole analogue of prostacyclin and is one compound which inhibits the release of leukotrienes *in vitro*[194,195], although it is without effect on broken-cell preparations. In a double blind placebo controlled study, inhalation of nebulized piriprost (1 mg) failed to offer significant protection against allergen and exercise challenge in patients with allergic asthma[196]. Furthermore, piriprost was without protective effect in subjects with documented late asthmatic reactions[196]. Superficially, this study questions a pivotal role for leukotrienes in allergen- and exercise-induced bronchoconstriction in man, but the same general caveats apply to this study as described earlier for the indomethacin trials.

Intervention in the arachidonic acid cascade at one level might have important consequences for the formation of other metabolites without the redirection of arachidonic acid metabolism. It is possible, therefore, that a clearer idea of the role of leukotrienes may be gained by the use of selective receptor antagonists. A fuller discussion of these compounds is presented in Chapter 8. At the time of writing, only a few of these compounds have undergone evaluation in man. These include 1-[2-hydroxy-3-propyl-4-[4-(1H-tetrazol-5-yl)butoxy]phenyl] ethanone (LY171883) and ($\pm$)-4-[[3-(4-acetyl-3-hydroxy-2-propylphenoxy)propyl]thio]-γ-hydroxy-β-methyl-benzenebutanoic acid (L649,923). Both of these compounds are orally active Ltd_4 antagonists[197,198]. When tested against an allergen-induced asthmatic reaction, L649,923 produced only a very small inhibition of the early respone but was without effect against the late reaction[199]. In contrast, LY171883, which, in sheep sensitive to *Ascaris suum* is a preferential inhibitor of the late reaction[200], also inhibits the late reaction in man and offers some benefit in asthma. However, studies with both of these compounds are only at an early stage and it remains to be established whether these compounds can be used to dissect the putative role of LTD$_4$ in asthma. One compound which may give this answer is 2(S)-hydroxy-3(R)-(2-carboxyethylthio-3-)[2-(8-phenyl-octyl)phenyl] propanoic acid (SK&F104353), an orally active LTD$_4$ antagonist of high selectivity developed by sequential modification of LTD$_4$ itself and the structurally related low-affinity antagonist 2-nor-LTD$_1$. Clinical studies with this compound are eagerly awaited.

A SYNTHESIS OF THE POTENTIAL ROLE OF LIPID MEDIATORS IN ASTHMA

Figure 5.3 shows a schematic overview of some of the cellular events which may be involved in the pathogenesis of early- and late-phase reactions in asthma. Initial exposure to a suitable stimulus, such as allergen, results in primary mediator release. As well as having direct actions on smooth muscle, some of these mediators are responsible for the recruitment of secondary effector cells, such as neutrophils, eosinophils and monocytes/macrophages. The arrival and activation of these cells at the site of provocation in the airway may be responsible for a second wave of inflammation which is manifest as enhanced bronchial reactivity, possibly resulting from epithelial damage, and a further bronchoconstriction. Primary mediator release could act as a tripwire mechanism for the individual, thus explaining why late

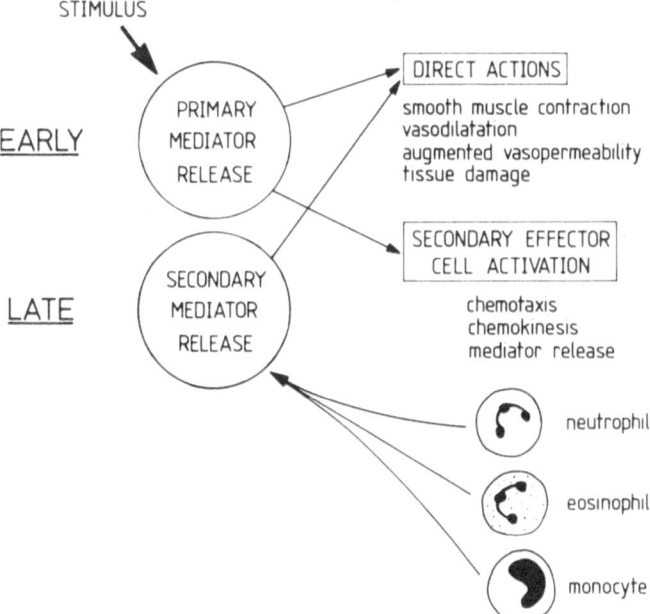

Figure 5.3   A hypothesis for the pathogenesis of early and late phase reactions

97

bronchoconstrictor responses are not seen in all patients following allergen challenge under experimental conditions. If the primary events were sufficiently strong, it is possible that all patients would experience late reactions under these circumstances.

In Figure 5.4 an attempt has been made to identify the cells and putative mediators of some of these events. Initial cellular activation might involve mast cells, macrophages, T-lymphocytes and possibly cells of the epithelium, releasing a complex cocktail of lipid and non-lipid mediators. PAF-acether and interleukin (IL-1) could play potentially important roles in chemotactic responses, provided that they are released from the primary mediator secreting cells. It is known that human pulmonary mast cells may have the capacity to synthesize PAF-acether but little is released extracellularly[201]. Indeed, other PAF-acether-secreting cells, such as neutrophils, release only a small proportion of the PAF-acether they actually synthesize[202]. Interestingly, the same may also be true of IL-1 production by macrophage and epithelial cells. The possible effects of inflammatory cell infiltration into the airways are summarized in Figure 5.5. Desquamation of the bronchial epithelium, resulting from the cytotoxic effects of secretory products derived from activated leukocytes and

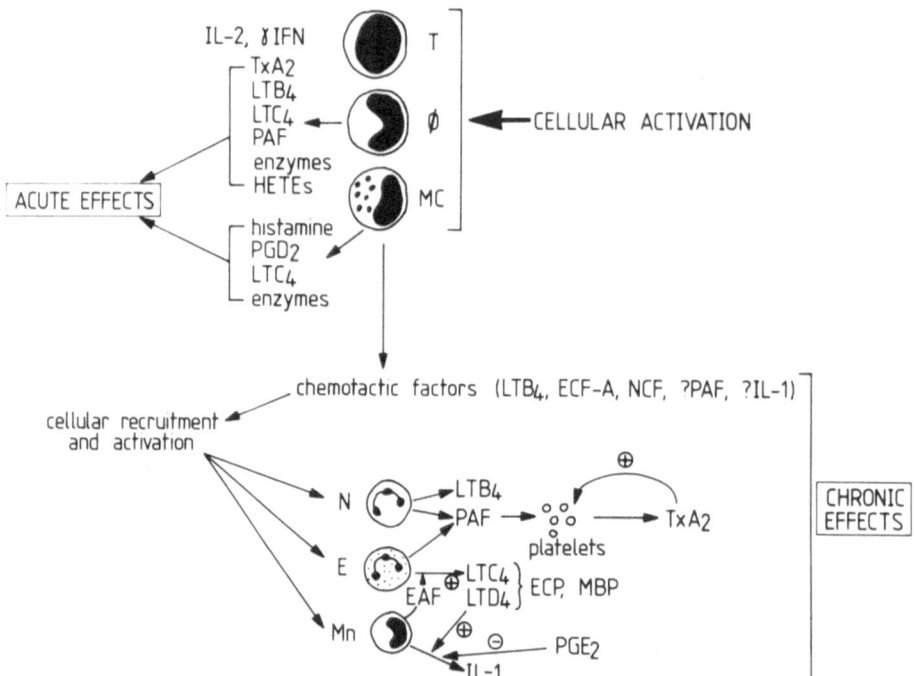

Figure 5.4 A hypothesis for mediator involvement in early and late phase reactions. Abbreviations: T = T-lymphocyte, ϕ = macrophage, MC = mast cell, IL-1,2 = interleukins 1 and 2, N = neutrophil, E = eosinophil, Mn = monocyte, EAF = eosinophil activating factor, ECF-A = eosinophil chemotactic factors, NCF = neutrophil chemotactic factor, ECP = eosinophil cationic protein, MBP = eosinophil major basic protein

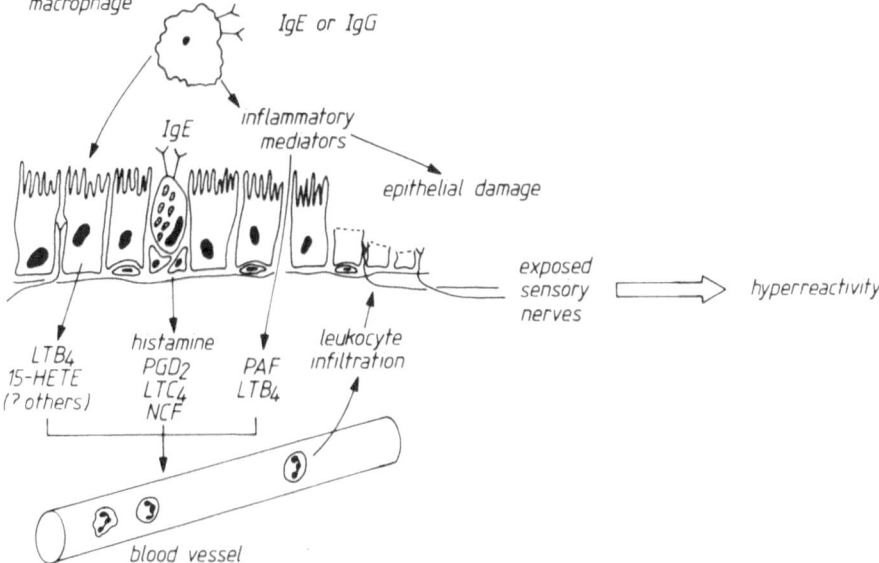

Figure 5.5 A hypothesis for the pathogenesis of airways hyper-reactivity involving inflammatory mediator release from cells within and abutting onto the airway lumen. This results in an influx of leukocytes, causing further inflammation, epithelial desquamation and exposure and heightened sensitivity of sensory nerve endings

the epithelial cells themselves, may result in the exposure of sensory nerves. In a situation analogous to the interaction of mediators on sensory nerves in skin, this would induce a state of hyper-responsiveness to other irritant stimuli and explain the non-specific bronchial hyper-reactivity seen in patients with asthma. In clinical asthma, this component of the disease is likely to be the most dominant feature, representing a subacute inflammatory background against which further bronchial provocations are set.

CONCLUSIONS

This review has attempted to integrate and evaluate the possible roles of eicosanoids into a workable hypothesis for the pathogenesis of allergic asthma. The complexities of the disease are such that it is unreasonable to expect single mediators, or even single models, to account for the great variation in clinical presentation of asthma from patient to patient[203]. This is even more unreasonable when the mechanisms of non-allergic intrinsic asthma and exercise-induced asthma are considered in the same terms as mechanisms proposed from work on allergic asthma[204].

Intensive work on the early events following IgE-dependent challenge both *in vivo* and *in vitro* has made the events underlying the immediate or early asthmatic reaction much clearer. These laboratory models are obviously rather artificial and their relationship to the disease at large may thus be questionable.

Furthermore, the relative importance of mast cells and alveolar macrophages remains to be fully explored. One means of doing this may be to use mediators as probes of specific cellular activation, provided that patients with suitable airways reactivity are chosen. Patients with severe bronchial hyper-reactivity may be inappropriate for such studies because of the small amounts of mediators which are required to produce a given fall in airway calibre[205]. On the basis of current knowledge PGD_2 and its metabolites, $9\alpha,11\beta$-PGF_2 and 13,14-dihydro-15-keto-$9\alpha,11\beta$-PGF_2, may be useful markers for mast cell activation *in situ*. A recent report[206] has documented the release of PGD_2 and 15-HETE into lavage fluid after allergen bronchoprovocation in man and these observations strengthen the view that PGD_2 may be an important mediator of the early asthmatic reaction.

Another feature emerging from work on the sequence of events after the early reaction is the concept that cellular infiltration of the airways is closely associated with both the late asthmatic reaction and the acquisition of bronchial hyper-reactivity. The key to the molecular events which drive these events will offer new therapeutic possibilities. A number of lipid mediators have been identified as mediator candidates on the basis of studies in canine and human airways epithelium. Leukotriene B_4 would initially appear to be an attractive candidate, but, at least in the trachea, this is not supported by studies with human cells. A potential role for 15-HPETE in producing β-receptor desensitization, as proposed in the guinea pig, is an unlikely mechanism in man[207-209]. This also underlines the potential trap of species differences when employing animal models of asthma. Currently, there is a resurgence of interest in the use of the guinea pig as a model of the disease. At one time, this model was very much out of favour: the antibodies mediating the anaphylactic reaction were IgG type[210], lipid mediator production was biased heavily towards the thromboxane pathway[211] and the ozone-induced model of bronchial hyper-reactivity was indomethacin insensitive[212]. A number of IgE-dependent models have now been described[213,214] and it is even possible to study the late reaction, cellular infiltration of the airways and bronchial hyper-reactivity[215]. Furthermore, it is now recognized[216,217] that human lung cells are capable of synthesizing and releasing thromboxane A_2 and so differences in mediator generation may be less apparent. Of course, the ultimate value of any model depends upon its ability to predict events in man and this still remains to be established with these more recent models.

Recent attention has focused on other mediators which may be of potential importance in asthma. Pre-eminent amongst these are PAF-acether and interleukin 1. By analogy with other inflammatory diseases, such as rheumatoid arthritis, interleukin 1 mandates consideration as a putative mediator of the influx of inflammatory cells into the airways. There can be little doubt that, in both animals and man, PAF-acether has pharmacological effects which suggest an important role in inflammatory diseases[218]. In man, it can reproduce bronchial hyper-reactivity to inhaled agonists[219], but it may not be the only mediator capable of doing this. Like the prostaglandins and leukotrienes, the true importance of PAF-acether will not be known until it has been measured in exacerbations of the disease in man.

The importance of inflammatory mediators in asthma has been the subject of great debate among the proponents of various theories of the pathogenesis of the disease, and I am certain that these debates will continue. Good theories and models are of heuristic value, despite the fact that they may have to be extensively modified in the light of new findings. Thus, it is encouraging to see that inflammation and neurogenic theories are coming together to form a plausible, more detailed view of bronchial asthma. I am confident that the next ten years will answer many of the issues which need to be resolved about the likely involvement of inflammatory mediators.

REFERENCES

1. McFadden, E.R. (1984). Pathogenesis of asthma. *J. Allergy Clin. Immunol.*, **73**, 413–424
2. Dunnill, M.S. (1971). The pathology of asthma. In Porter, R. and Birch, J. (eds.) *The Identification of Asthma.* pp. 35–46. (London: Churchill Livingstone)
3. Dunnill, M.S. (1982). *Pulmonary Pathology.* (London: Churchill Livingstone)
4. Hayes, J.A. (1976). The pathology of bronchial asthma. In Weiss, E.B. and Segal, M.S. (eds.) *Bronchial Asthma Mechanisms and Therapeutics.* pp. 347–381. (Boston: Little Brown and Co)
5. Boushey, H.A., Holtzman, M.J., Sheller, R. and Nadel, J.A. (1980). State of the art. Bronchial hyperreactivity. *Am. Rev. Respir. Dis.*, **121**, 389–413
6. Nadel, J.A. (1984). Inflammation and asthma. *J. Allergy Clin. Immunol.*, **73**, 651–653
7. Holtzman, M.J., Fabbri, L.M., O'Byrne, P.M., Gold, B.D., Aizawa, H., Walters, E.H., Alpert, S.E. and Nadel, J.A. (1983). Importance of airway inflammation for hyperresponsiveness induced by ozone. *Am. Rev. Respir. Dis.*, **127**, 686–690
8. Takizawa, T. and Thurlbeck, W.M. (1971). Muscle and mucus gland size in the major bronchi of patients with chronic bronchitis, asthma and asthmatic bronchitis. *Am. Rev. Respir. Dis.*, **104**, 331–336
9. Szentvanyi, A. (1968). The beta-adrenergic theory of atopic abnormality in bronchial asthma. *J. Allergy*, **42**, 203–232
10. Barnes, P.J. (1984). Adrenergic receptors of normal and asthmatic airways. In Zaagsma, J. (ed.) *Receptors and Chronic Obstructive Lung Disease.* pp. 72–79. (Amsterdam: Excerpta Medica)
11. Richardson, J. and Beland, J. (1976). Nonadrenergic inhibitory nervous system in human airways. *J. Appl. Physiol.*, **41**, 764–771
12. Sheppard, M.N., Kurian, S.S., Henzen Longmans, S.C., Michetti F., Cocchia, D., Cole, P., Rush, R.A., Marangos, P.J., Bloom, S.R. and Polak, J.M. (1983). Nerone-specific enolase and S-100: new markers for delineating the innervation of the respiratory tract in man and other mammals. *Thorax*, **38**, 330
13. Barnes, P.J. (1984). The third nervous system in the lung: physiology and clinical perspectives. *Thorax*, **39**, 561–567
14. Barnes, P.J. (1986). Neuropeptides in the airways: functional significance. In: Kay, A.B. (ed.) *Asthma. Clinical Pharmacology and Therapeutic Progress.* pp. 58–72. (Oxford: Blackwell)
15. Barnes, P.J. and Palmer, J.B.D. (1986). Non-adrenergic bronchodilatation. *Bull. Eur. Physiopathol. Respir.*, **22** (Suppl. 7), 153–161
16. Ferreira, S.H., Nakamura, M. and Castro, M.S.A. (1978). The hyperalgesic effects of prostacyclin and prostaglandin E_2. *Prostaglandins*, **16**, 31–39
17. Shaw, R.J., Walsh, G.M., Cromwell, O., Moqbel, R., Spry, C.J.F. and Kay, A.B. (1985). Activated human eosinophils generate SRS-A leukotrienes following IgG-dependent stimulation. *Nature (London)*, **316**, 150–152
18. Bruynzeel, P.L.B., Kok, P.T.M., Hamelink, M.L., Kijne, A.M. and Verhagen, J. (1985). Exclusive leukotriene C_4 synthesis by purified human eosinophils induced by opsonized zymosan. *FEBS Lett.*, **189**, 350–354
19. Leikauf, G.D., Ueki, I.F., Widdicombe, J.H. and Nadel, J.A. (1986). Alteration of chloride secretion across canine tracheal epithelium by lipoxygenase products of arachidonic acid. *Am. J. Physiol.*, **250**, F47–F53

101

20. Golden, J.A., Nadel, J.A. and Boushey, H.A. (1978). Bronchial hyperirritability in healthy subjects after exposure to ozone. *Am. Rev. Respir. Dis.*, **118**, 287–294
21. Laitinen, L.A., Elkin, R.B., Empey, D.W., Jacobs, L., Mills, J., Gold, W.M. and Nadel, J.A. (1976). Changes in bronchial reactivity after administration of live attenuated influenza virus. *Am. Rev. Respir. Dis.*, **113**, 194
22. Islam, M.S., Vastag, E. and Ulmer, W.T. (1972). Sulphur dioxide induced bronchial hyperreactivity against acetylcholine. *Int. Arch. Arbeitsmed.*, **29**, 221–232
23. Holtzman, M.J., Cunningham, J.M., Sheller, J.R., Irsigler, G.B., Nadel, J.A. and Boushey, H.A. (1979). Effect of ozone on bronchial reactivity in atopic and non atopic subjects. *Am. Rev. Respir. Dis.*, **120**, 1059–1067
24. Scheel, L.D., Dobrogorski, O.J., Mountain, J.T. Svirbely, J.L. and Stokinger, H.E. (1959). Physiologic, biochemical, immunologic and pathologic changes following ozone exposure. *J. Appl. Physiol.*, **14**, 67–80
25. Shimasaki, H., Takatori, T., Anderson, W.R., Horten, H.L. and Privett, O.S. (1976). Alteration of lung lipids in ozone exposed rats. *Biochem. Biophys. Res. Commun.*, **68**, 1256–1262
26. Fabbri, L.M., Aizawa, H., Alpert, S.E., Walters, E.H., O'Byrne, P.M., Gold, B.D., Nadel, J.A. and Holtzman, M.J. (1976). Hyperreactivity and changes in cell counts in bronchoalveolar lavage after ozone in dogs. *Am. Rev. Respir. Dis.*, **127**, 224
27. Nadel, J.A. and Holtzman, M.J. (1984). Regulation of airway responsiveness and secretion: role of inflammation. In Kay, A.B., Austen, K.F. and Lichtenstein, L.M. (eds.) *Asthma: Physiology, Immunopharmacology and Treatment. Third International Symposium.* pp. 129–155. (London: Academic Press)
28. O'Byrne, P., Walters, E., Gold, B., Aizawa, H., Fabbri, L., Alpert, S., Nadel, J. and Holtzman, M. (1983). Neutrophil depletion inhibits airway hyperresponsiveness induced by ozone [abstract]. *Physiologist*, **26**, A35
29. Piper, P.J. and Temple, D.M. (1981). The effect of lipoxygenase inhibitors and diethylcarbamazine on the immunological release of slow reacting substance (SRS-A) from guinea-pig chopped lung. *J. Pharm. Pharmacol.*, **33**, 384–386
30. Radmark, O., Malmsten, C. and Samuelsson, B. (1980). The inhibitory effects of BW 755C on arachidonic acid metabolism in human polymorphonuclear leukocytes. *FEBS Lett.*, **110**, 213–215
31. Siegel, M.I., McConnell, R.T., Bonser, R.W. and Cuatrecasas, P. (1981). The production of 5-HETE and leukotriene B₄ in rat neutrophils from carageenan pleural exudates. *Prostaglandins*, **21**, 123–132
32. Higgs, G.A., Flower, R.J. and Vane, J.R. (1979). A new approach to anti-inflammatory drugs. *Biochem. Pharmacol.*, **28**, 1959–1961
33. Fabbri, L.M., Aizawa, H., O'Byrne, P.M., Bethel, R.A., Walters, E.H., Holtzman, M.J. and Nadel, J.A. (1985). An anti-inflammatory drug (BW755C) inhibits airway hyperresponsiveness induced by ozone in dogs. *J. Allergy Clin. Immunol.*, **76**, 162–166
34. O'Byrne, P.M., Walters, E.H., Aizawa, H., Fabbri, L.M., Holtzman, M.J. and Nadel, J.A. (1984). Indomethacin inhibits the hyperresponsiveness but not the neutrophil influx induced by ozone in dogs. *Am. Rev. Respir. Dis.*, **130**, 220–224
35. Aizawa, H., Chung, K.F., Leikauf, G.D. Ueki, I.F., Bethel, R.A., O'Byrne, P.M., Hirose, T. and Nadel, J.A. (1985). Significance of thromboxane generation in ozone induced airway hyperresponsiveness in dogs. *J. Appl. Physiol.*, **59**, 1918–1923
36. Chung, K.F., Aizawa, H., Becker, A.B., Frick, O., Gold, W.M. and Nadel, J.A. (1986). Inhibition of antigen-induced airway hyperresponsiveness by thromboxane synthase inhibitor (OKY-046) in allergic dogs. *Am. Rev. Respir. Dis.*, **134**, 258–261
37. O'Byrne, P.M., Leikauf, G.D., Aizawa, H., Bethel, R.A., Ueki, I.F., Holtzman, M.J. and Nadel, J.A. (1985). Leukotriene B₄ induces airway hyperresponsiveness in dogs. *J. Appl. Physiol.*, **59**, 1941–1946
38. Harper, T.W., Westcott, J.Y., Voelkel, N. and Murphy, R.C. (1984). Metabolism of leukotrienes B₄ and C₄ in isolated perfused rat lung. *J. Biol. Chem.*, **259**, 14437–14440
39. Xu, G.L., Sivarajah, K., Wu, R., Netteshei, P. and Eling, T. (1985). Biosynthesis of prostaglandins by isolated and cultured airway epithelial cells. *Exp. Lung. Res.*, **10**, 101–114
40. Holtzman, M.J., Aizawa, H., Nadel, J.A. and Goetzl, E.J. (1983). Selective generation of leukotriene B₄ by tracheal epithelial cells from dogs. *Biochem. Biophys. Res. Commun.*, **114**, 1071–1076

41. Hunter, J.A., Finkbeiner, W.E., Nadel, J.A., Goetzl, E.J. and Holtzman, M .J. (1985). Predominant generation of 15-lipoxygenase metabolites of arachidonic acid by epithelial cells from human trachea. *Proc. Natl. Acad. Sci. USA*, **82**, 4633–4637

42. McGuire, J., McGee, J., Crittenden, N. and Fitzpatrick, F.A. (1985). Cell damage unmasks 15-lipoxygenase activity in human neutrophils. *J. Biol. Chem.*, **260**, 8316–8319

43. Murlas, C.G. and Roum, J.H. (1985). Sequence of pathologic changes in the airway mucosa of the guinea pig during ozone induced bronchial hyperreactivity. *Am. Rev. Respir. Dis.*, **131**, 314–320

44. Shak, S., Perez, H.D. and Goldstein, I.M. (1983). A novel dioxygenation product of arachidonic acid possesses potent chemotactic activity for human polymorphonuclear leukocytes. *J. Biol. Chem.*, **258**, 14948–14953

45. Turner, S.R. and Tainer, J.A. (1983). Nonchemokinetic neutrophil attractants derived from arachidonic acid. *Cell. Biol. Int. Rep.*, **7**, 843–848

46. Copas, J.L., Borgeat, P. and Gardiner, P.J. (1982). The actions of 5,12- and 15-HETE on tracheobronchial smooth muscle. *Prostagl. Leuk. Med.*, **8**, 105–114

47. Vanderhoek, J.Y., Bryant, R.W. and Bailey, J.M. (1982). Regulation of leukocyte and platelet lipoxygenases by hydroxyeicosanoids. *Biochem. Pharmacol.*, **31**, 3463–3467

48. Maclouf, J., Fruteau de Laclos, B. and Borgeat, P. (1982). Stimulation and leukotriene biosynthesis in human blood leukocytes by platelet derived 12-hydroperoxyeicosatetraenoic acid. *Proc. Natl. Acad. Sci. USA*, **79**, 6042–6046

49. Borgeat, P., Fruteau de Laclos, B. and Maclouf, J. (1983). New concepts in the modulation of leukotriene synthesis. *Biochem. Pharmacol.*, **32**, 381–387

50. Johnson, H.G., McNee, M.L. and Sun, F.F. (1985). 15-Hydroxyeicosatetraenoic acid is a potent inflammatory mediator and agonist of canine tracheal mucus secretion. *Am. Rev. Respir. Dis.*, **131**, 917–922

51. Evans, J., Ford-Hutchinson, A.W., Fitzsimmons, B. and Rokach, J. (1984). Biological activities of isomers of 8,15-dihydroxyeicosatetraenoic acid. *Prostaglandins*, **28**, 435–438

52. Fuller, R.W., Dixon, C.M.S., Dollery, C.T. and Barnes, P.J. (1986). Prostaglandin D$_2$ potentiates airway responsiveness to histamine and methacholine. *Am. Rev. Respir. Dis.*, **133**, 252–254

53. Hardy, C.C., Bradding, P., Robinson, C. and Holgate, S.T. (1986). The combined effects of two pairs of mediators, adenosine with methacholine and prostaglandin D$_2$ with histamine on airway calibre in asthma. *Clin. Sci.*, **71**, 385–392

54. Flavahan, N.A., Aarhus, L.L., Rimele, T.J. and Vanhoutte, P.M. (1985). Respiratory epithelium inhibits bronchial smooth muscle tone. *J. Appl. Physiol.*, **58**, 834–838

55. Holgate, S.T., Emanuel, M.B. and Howarth, P.H. (1985). Astemizole and other H1-antihistamine drug treatment of asthma. *J. Allergy Clin. Immunol.*, **76**, 375–382

56. Robinson, C. and Holgate, S.T. (1985). Mast cell-dependent inflammatory mediators and their putative role in bronchial asthma. *Clin. Sci.*, **68**, 103–112

57. Holgate, S.T., Rafferty, P., Beasley, R., Robinson, C., Hovell, C.J., Curzen, N.P. and Church, M.K. (1987). In vitro and in vivo studies on mast cells of human skin and airways. In Kay, A.B. (ed.) *Allergy and Inflammation.*, pp. 29–52. (London: Academic Press)

58. Jeffery, P. and Corrin, B. (1984). Structural analysis of the upper respiratory tract. In Bienenstock, J. (ed.) *Immunology of the Lung and Upper Respiratory Tract.* pp. 1–27. (New York: McGraw-Hill)

59. Fox, B., Bull, B. and Guz, A. (1981). Mast cells in the human alveolar wall: an electron microscope study. *J. Clin. Pathol.*, **34**, 1333–1342

60. Lamb, D. and Lumsden, A. (1982). Intra-epithelial mast cells in human airway epithelium: evidence for smoking induced changes in their frequency. *Thorax*, **37**, 334–342

61. Guerzon, G.M., Pare, P.D., Michoud, M.C. and Hogg, J.C. (1979). The number and distribution of mast cells in monkey lungs. *Am. Rev. Respir. Dis.*, **119**, 59–66

62. Holgate, S.T. and Church, M.K. (1982). Control of mediator release from mast cells. *Clin. Allergy*, **12** (Suppl.), 5–13

63. Sullivan, T.J. (1981). Diacylglycerol metabolism and the release of mediators from mast cells. In Becker, E.L., Simon, A.S. and Austen, K.F. (eds.) *Biochemistry of the Acute Allergic Reactions.* pp. 229–238. (New York: Alan R. Liss)

64. Wasserman, S.I. (1981). Ion regulation of histamine release from rat serosal mast cells [Abstract]. *Clin. Res.*, **29**, 492A

65. Howarth, P.H., Durham, S.R., Lee, T.H., Kay, A.B., Church, M.K. and Holgate, S.T. (1985). Influence of albuterol, cromolyn sodium and ipratropium bromide on the airway and circulating mediator responses to antigen bronchial provocation in asthma. *Am. Rev. Respir. Dis.*, **132**, 986–992

66. Church, M.K. (1982). The role of basophils in asthma: 1; Sodium cromoglycate on histamine release and content. *Clin. Allergy*, **12**, 223–228

67. Holgate, S.T., Burns, G.B., Robinson, C. and Church, M.K. (1984). Anaphylactic and calcium dependent generation of prostaglandin D_2 (PGD_2), thromboxane B_2 and other cyclooxygenase products of arachidonic acid by dispersed human lung cells and relationship to histamine release. *J. Immunol.*, **133**, 2138–2144

68. Lewis, R.A., Soter, N.A., Diamond, P.T., Austen, K.F., Oates, J.A. and Roberts, L.J. II. (1982). Prostaglandin D_2 generation after activation of rat and human mast cells with anti-IgE. *J. Immunol.*, **129**, 1627–1631

69. Peters, S.P., MacGlashan, D.W., Schulman, E.S., Schleimer, R.P., Hayes, E.C., Rokach, J., Adkinson, N.F. and Lichtenstein, L.M. (1984). Arachidonic acid metabolism in purified human lung mast cells. *J. Immunol.*, **132**, 1972–1979

70. Paterson, N.A.M., Wasserman, S.I., Said, J.W. and Austen, K.F. (1976). Release of chemical mediators from partially purified human lung mast cells. *J. Immunol.*, **117**, 1356–1362

71. Lewis, R.A., Drazen, J.M., Corey, E.J. and Austen, K.F. (1981). Structural and functional characteristics of the leukotriene component of slow reacting substance of anaphylaxis. In Piper, P.J. (ed.) *SRS-A and Leukotrienes*. pp. 101–117. (Chichester: Wiley)

72. MacGlashan, D.W., Schleimer, R.P., Peters, S.P., Schulman, E.S., Adams, G.K., Newball, H.H. and Lichtenstein, L.M. (1982). Generation of leukotrienes by purified human lung mast cells. *J. Clin. Invest.*, **70**, 747–751

73. Rankin, J.A., Hitchcock, M.A., Merrill, W., Bach, M.K., Brashler, J.R. and Askenase, P.W. (1982). IgE-dependent release of LTC_4 from alveolar macrophages. *Nature (London)*, **297**, 329–331

74. Damon, M., Chavis, C., Godard, Ph., Michel, F.B. and Crastes de Paulet, A. (1983). Purification and mass spectrometry identification of leukotriene D_4 synthesized by human alveolar macrophages. *Biochem. Biophys. Res. Commun.*, **111**, 518–524

75. Schulman, E.S., Newball, H.H., Demers, L.M., Fitzpatrick, F.A. and Adkinson, N.F. (1981). Anaphylactic release of thromboxane A_2, prostaglandin D_2 and prostacyclin from human lung parenchyma. *Am. Rev. Respir. Dis.*, **124**, 402–406

76. Schleimer, R.P., Schulman, E.S., MacGlashan, D.W., Peters, S.P., Hayes, E.C., Adams, G.K., Lichtenstein, L.M. and Adkinson, N.F. (1983). Effects of dexamethasone on mediator release from human lung fragments and purified human lung mast cells. *J. Clin. Invest.*, **71**, 1830–1835

77. Steel, L.K. and Kaliner, M.A. (1981). Prostaglandin generating factor of anaphylaxis. Identification and isolation. *J. Biol. Chem.*, **256**, 12692–12698

78. Steel, L.K., Bach, D. and Kaliner, M.A. (1982). Prostaglandin-generating factor of anaphylaxis. II. Characterization of activity. *J. Immunol.*, **129**, 1233–1238

79. Anderson, C.L. and Speigelberg, H.L. (1981). Macrophage receptors for IgE: binding of IgE to specific IgE-Fc receptors on human cell line U937. *J. Immunol.*, **126**, 2470–2473

80. Yodoi, J. and Ishizaka, K. (1979). Lymphocytes bearing Fc receptors for IgE. 1. Presence of human and rat T-lymphocytes with Fc receptors. *J. Immunol.*, **122**, 2577–2583

81. Melewicz, F.M. and Spiegelberg, H.L. (1980). Fc receptors for IgE on a subpopulation of human peripheral blood monocytes. *J. Immunol.*, **125**, 1026–1031

82. Capron, M., Capron, A., Dessaint, J.P., Torpier, G., Gunnar, S., Johansson, O. and Prin, A. (1981). Fc receptors for IgE on human and rat eosinophils. *J. Immunol.*, **126**, 2087–2092

83. Capron, A., Amlisen, J.C., Joseph, M., Auriault, C., Tonnel, A.B. and Caen, J. (1985). New functions for platelets and their pathological implications. *Int. Arch. Allergy Appl. Immunol.*, **77**, 107–114

84. Rankin, J.A. and Askenase, P.W. (1984). The potential role of alveolar macrophages as a source of pathogenic mediators in allergic asthma. In Kay, A.B., Austen, K.F. and Lichtenstein, L.M. (eds.) *Asthma: Physiology, Immunopharmacology and Treatment. Third International Symposium*. pp. 157–171. (London: Academic Press)

85. Boucher, R.C., Pare, P.D., Gilmore, N.J., Moroz, L.A. and Hogg, J.C. (1977). Airway mucosal permeability in the ascaris suum sensitive rhesus monkey. *J. Allergy Clin. Immunol.*, **60**, 134–140

86. Boucher, R.C., Ranga, V., Pare, P.D., Inoue, S., Moroz, L.A. and Hogg, J.C. (1978). Effect of histamine and methacholine on guinea-pig tracheal permeability to HRP. *J. Appl. Physiol.*, **45**, 939–948

87. Elwood R., Kennedy, S., Belzberg, A., Hogg, J.C. and Pare, P.D. (1983). Respiratory mucosal permeability in asthma. *Am. Rev. Respir. Dis.*, **128**, 523–527

88. Metcalfe, D.D. (1983). Effector cell heterogeneity in immediate hypersensitivity reactions. *Clin. Rev. Allergy*, **1**, 311–325

89. Agius, R.M., Howarth, P.H., Robinson, C. and Holgate, S.T. (1986). Human bronchoalveolar mast cells and their mediators. In Kay, A.B. (ed.) *Asthma: Clinical Pharmacology and Therapeutic Progress.* pp. 274–285. (Oxford: Blackwell)

90. Agius, R.M., Robinson, C. and Holgate, S.T. (1985). Release of histamine and newly generated mediators from human bronchoalveolar lavage cells [Abstract]. *Thorax*, **40**, 220

91. Flint, K.C., Hudspith, B.N., Leung, K.B.P., Pearce, F.L., Seiger, K., Hammond, M.D.H., Brostoff, J. and Johnson, N.McI. (1985). IgE-dependent release of leukotriene C_4 and prostaglandin D_2 from human bronchoalveolar cells [Abstract]. *Thorax*, **40**, 716

92. de Monchy, J.G.R., Kauffman, H.F., Venge, P., Koeter, G.H., Jansen, H.M., Sluiter, H.J. and de Vries, K. (1985). Broncho-alveolar eosinophilia during allergen-induced late asthmatic reactions. *Am. Rev. Respir. Dis.*, **131**, 373–376

93. Marsh, W.R. Irvin, C.G., Murphy, K.R., Behrens, L. and Larsen, G.L. (1985). Increases in airway hyperreactivity to histamine and inflammatory cells in bronchoalveolar lavage after the late asthmatic reaction in an animal model. *Am. Rev. Respir. Dis.*, **131**, 875–879

94. Carroll, M. Durham, S.R., Walsh, G.M. and Kay, A.B. (1985). Leukocyte activation in allergen and histamine induced bronchoconstriction. *J. Allergy Clin. Immunol.*, **75**, 290–296

95. Durham, S.R., Carroll M., Walsh, G.M. and Kay, A.B. (1984). Leucocyte activation in allergen-induced late phase asthmatic reactions. *N. Engl. J. Med.*, **311**, 1398–1402

96. Durham, S.R. and Kay, A.B. (1986). Inflammatory cells and mediators in allergen-induced late phase asthmatic reactions. In Kay, A.B. (ed.) *Asthma: Clinical Pharmacology and Therapeutic Progress.* pp. 33–45. (Oxford: Blackwell)

97. Naclerio, R.M., Proud, D., Togias, A.G., Adkinson, N.F., Meyers, D.A., Kagey-Sobotka, A., Plaut, M., Norman, P.S. and Lichtenstein, L.M. (1985). Inflammatory mediators in late antigen-induced rhinitis. *N. Engl. J. Med.*, **313**, 65–70

98. Naclerio, R.M., Meier, H.L., Kagey-Sobotka, A., Adkinson, N.F., Meyers, D.A., Norman, P.S. and Lichtenstein, L.M. (1983). Mediator release after nasal airway challenge with allergen. *Am. Rev. Respir. Dis.*, **128**, 597–602

99. Cockcroft, D.W. and Murdock, K.Y. (1986). Protective effect of inhaled albuterol, cromolyn, beclomethasone and placebo on allergen-induced early asthmatic response (EAR), late asthmatic response (LAR) and allergen-induced increases in bronchial responsiveness to inhaled histamine [Abstract]. *J. Allergy Clin. Immunol.*, **77** (Suppl.), 122

100. Hegardt B., Pauwels, R. and van der Straeten, M. (1981). Inhibitory effect of KWC 2131, terbutaline, and DSCG on the immediate and late allergen-induced bronchoconstriction. *Allergy*, **36**, 115–122

101. Kraan, N., Koeter, G.H., van den Mark, T.W., Sluiter, H.J. and de Vries, K. (1986). Changes in bronchial hyperreactivity induced by 4 week treatment with antiasthmatic drugs in patients with allergic asthma. A comparison between budesonide and terbutaline. *J. Allergy Clin. Immunol.*, **76**, 628–636

102. Lowhagen, O. and Rak, S. (1985). Modification of bronchial hyperreactivity after treatment with sodium cromoglycate during pollen season. *J. Allergy Clin. Immunol.*, **75**, 460–467

103. Kay, A.B., Wardlaw, A.J., Moqbel, R., Buchanan, D.R. and Cromwell, O. (1987). Leukocytes and the asthma process. In Kay, A.B. (ed.) *Allergy and Inflammation.*, pp. 10–28 (London: Academic Press)

104. Larsen, G.L., Shampain, M.P., Marsh, W.R. and Behrens, B.L. (1984). An animal model of the late asthmatic response to antigen challenge. In Kay, A.B., Austen, K.F. and Lichtenstein, L.M. (eds.) *Asthma: Physiology, Immunopharmacology and Treatment. Third International Symposium.* pp. 245–262. (London: Academic Press)

105. Abraham, W.M., Delehunt, J.C., Yerger, L. and Marchetts, B. (1983). Characterization of a late phase pulmonary response following antigen challenge in allergic sheep. *Am. Rev. Respir. Dis.,* **128,** 839–844

106. Church, M.K., Clay, T.P., Holgate, S.T., Hutson, P.A. and Miller, P. (1987). Multiple late phase reactions and cellular correlates in an in vivo guinea-pig model of bronchial asthma [Abstract]. *Br. J. Pharmacol.,* **90** (Proc. Suppl.), 30P

107. Hirshman, C.A. (1985). The Basenji-greyhound dog model of asthma. *Chest,* **87** (Suppl.), 172S–178S

108. Delehunt, J.C., Perruchoud, A.P., Yerger, L., Marchette, B., Stevenson, J.S. and Abraham, W.M. (1984). The role of slow reacting substance of anaphylaxis in the late bronchial response after allergen challenge in allergic sheep. *Am. Rev. Respir. Dis.,* **130,** 748–754

109. Burrows, B., Hasan, F.M. Barbee, R.M., Halonen, M. and Lebowitz, M.D. (1980). Epidemiologic observations on eosinophilia and its relation to respiratory diseases. *Am. Rev. Respir. Dis.,* **122,** 709–719

110. Frigas, E., Loegering, D.A., Solley, G.O., Farrow, G.M. and Gleich, G.J. (1981). Elevated levels of the eosinophil granule major basic protein in the sputum of patients with bronchial asthma. *Mayo Clin. Proc.,* **56,** 345–353

111. Filley, W.V., Holley, K.E., Kephart, G.M. and Gleich, G.J. (1982). Identification by immunofluoresence of eosinophil granule major basic protein in lung tissue of patients with bronchial asthma. *Lancet,* **2,** 11–16

112. Frigas, E., Loegering, D.A. and Gleich, G.J. (1980). Cytotoxic effects of the guinea-pig eosinophil major basic protein on tracheal epithelium. *Lab. Invest.,* **42,** 35–43

113. Gleich, G.J., Frigas, E., Loegering, D.A., Wassom, D.L. and Steinmuller, D. (1979). Cytotoxic properties of the eosinophil major basic protein. *J. Immunol.,* **123,** 2925–2927

114. Wardlaw, A.J. and Kay A.B. (1986). PAF-acether is a potent chemotactic factor for human eosinophils [Abstract]. *J. Allergy Clin. Immunol.,* **77** (Suppl.), 236

115. Nagy, L., Lee, T.H., Goetzl, E.J., Pickett, W. and Kay, A.B. (1982). Complement receptor enhancement and chemotaxis of human neutrophils and eosinophils by leukotrienes and other lipoxygenase products. *Clin. Exp. Immunol.,* **47,** 541–547

116. Kay, A.B., Stechschulte, D.J. and Austen, K.F. (1971). An eosinophil leukocyte chemotactic factor of anaphylaxis. *J. Exp. Med.,* **133,** 602–619

117. Gin, W., Shaw, R.J. and Kay, A.B. (1985). Airways reversibility after prednisolone therapy in chronic asthma is associated with alterations in leukocyte function. *Am. Rev. Respir. Dis.,* **132,** 1199–1203

118. Veith, M.C. and Butterworth, A.E. (1983). Enhancement of human eosinophil mediated killing of Schistosoma mansoni larvae by mononuclear cell products in vitro. *J. Exp. Med.,* **157,** 1828–1843

119. Fitzharris, P., Moqbel, R., Thorne, K.J.I., Richardson, B.A., Butterworth, A.E., Hartnell, A. Cromwell, O. and Kay, A.B. (1986). Monocyte derived eosinophil activating factor (EAF) enhances LTC$_4$ production by human eosinophils [Abstract]. *J. Allergy Clin. Immunol.,* **77,** 235

120. Gerblich, A.A., Campbell, A.E. and Schuyler, M.R. (1984). Changes in T-lymphocyte subpopulations after antigenic bronchial provocation in asthmatics. *N. Engl. J. Med.,* **310,** 1349–1352

121. Robinson, C. and Holgate, S.T. (1986). The synthesis, release and effects of prostaglandins in the lung. In Kay, A.B. (ed.) *Asthma: Clinical Pharmacology and Therapeutic Progress.* pp. 213–225. (Oxford: Blackwell)

122. Horton, E.W. (1969). Hypothesis on physiological roles of prostaglandins. *Physiol. Rev.,* **49,** 122–161

123. Sweatman, W.J.F. and Collier, H.O.J. (1968). Effects of prostaglandins on human bronchial muscle. *Nature (London),* **217,** 69–76

124. Bagli, J. (1984). Prostaglandins and related compounds. In Buckle, D.R. and Smith, H. (eds.) *Development of Anti-asthma Drugs.* pp. 225–260. (London: Butterworths)

125. Bianco, S. Robuschi, B., Ceserani, R., Gandolfi, C. and Kamburoff, P. (1978). Prevention of a specifically induced bronchoconstriction by PGI$_2$ and 20-methyl-PGI$_2$ in asthmatic patients. *Pharmacol. Res. Commun.,* **10,** 657–674

126. Hardy, C.C., Robinson, C., Lewis, R.A., Tattersfield, A.E. and Holgate, S.T. (1985). The airway and cardiovascular responses to inhaled prostaglandin I$_2$ in normal and asthmatic man. *Am. Rev. Respir. Dis.,* **131,** 18–21

127. Hardy, C.C., Robinson, C. Bradding, P. and Holgate, S.T. (1984). Prostacyclin: a functional antagonist of prostaglandin D_2-induced bronchoconstriction [Abstract]. *Thorax*, **39**, 696

128. Yen, S.S. and Morris, H.G. (1981). An imbalance of arachidonic acid metabolism in asthma. *Biochem. Biophys. Res. Commun.*, **103**, 774–779

129. Mita, H., Yui, Y., Taniguchi, N., Yasueda, H. and Shida, T. (1985). Increased activity of 5-lipoxygenase in polymorphonuclear leukocytes from asthmatic patients. *Life Sci.*, **37**, 907–914

130. Boot, J.R. Cockerill, A.F., Dawson, W., Mallen, D.N.B. and Osborne D.J. (1978). Modification of prostaglandin and thromboxane release by immunological sensitization and successive immunological challenge from guinea-pig lung. *Int. Arch. Allergy Appl. Immunol.*, **57**, 159–164

131. Mathé, A.A. and Hedqvist, P. (1975). Effect of prostaglandins $F_{2\alpha}$ and E_2 on airway conductance in healthy subjects and asthmatic patients. *Am. Rev. Respir. Dis.*, **111**, 313–320

132. Smith, A.P., Cuthbert, M.F. and Dunlop, L.S. (1975). Effects of inhaled prostaglandins E_1, E_2 and $F_{2\alpha}$ on the airway resistance of normal and asthmatic man. *Clin. Sci. Mol. Med.*, **48**, 421–430

133. Mathé, A.A., Hedqvist, P., Holmgren, A. and Svanborg, N. (1973). Bronchial hyperreactivity to prostaglandin $F_{2\alpha}$ and histamine in patients with asthma. *Br. Med. J.*, **1**, 193–196

134. Hardy, C.C., Robinson, C., Tattersfield, A.E. and Holgate, S.T. (1984). The bronchoconstrictor effect of inhaled prostaglandin D_2 in normal and asthmatic man. *N. Engl. J. Med.*, **311**, 209–213

135. Heavey, D.J., Lumley, P., Barrow, S.E., Murphy, M.B., Humphrey, P.P.A. and Dollery, C.T. (1984). Effects of intravenous infusions of prostaglandin D_2 in man. *Prostaglandins*, **28**, 755–767

136. Beasley, C.R.W., Robinson, C., Featherstone R.L., Varley, J.G., Hardy, C.C., Church, M.K. and Holgate, S.T. (1987). $9\alpha,11\beta$-Prostaglandin F_2, a novel metabolite of prostaglandin D_2, is a potent contractile agonist of human and guinea pig airways. *J. Clin. Invest.*, **79**, 978–983

137. Robinson, C., Beasley, C.R.W., Varley, J.G. and Holgate, S.T. (1987). The effects of inhaled $9\alpha,11\beta$-prostaglandin F_2 on airway function in man. In Samuelsson, B. Paoletti, R. and Ramwell, P.W. (eds.) *Advances in Prostaglandin, Thromboxane and Leukotriene Research*. Vol. 17B, pp. 1053–1057. (New York: Raven Press)

138. Patterson, R., Harris, K.E. and Greenberger, P.A. (1980). Effect of prostaglandin D_2 and I_2 on the airways of rhesus monkeys. *J. Allergy Clin. Immunol.*, **65**, 269–273

139. Gardiner, P.J. and Collier, H.O.J. (1980). Specific receptors for prostaglandins in the airways. *Prostaglandins*, **19**, 819–841

140. Newball, H.H. and Lenfant, C. (1977). The influence of atropine and cromolyn on human bronchial hyperreactivity to aerosolized prostaglandin $F_{2\alpha}$. *Respir. Physiol.*, **24**, 139–146

141. Wasserman, M.A. (1976). Bronchopulmonary responses to prostaglandin $F_{2\alpha}$, histamine and acetylcholine in the dog. *Eur. J. Pharmacol.*, **32**, 146–155

142. Nakanishi, H., Yoshida, H. and Suzuki, T. (1976). Inhibitory effects of prostaglandins E_1 and E_2 on cholinergic transmission in isolated canine tracheal muscle. *Jpn. J. Pharmacol.*, **26**, 669–674

143. Roberts, A.M., Armstrong, D.J., Coleridge, H.M. and Coleridge, J.C.G. (1981). Paradoxical tracheal contraction produced by bronchodilator prostaglandins PGE_2 and PGI_2. *Fed. Proc.*, **40**, 595

144. Coleridge, H.M. and Coleridge, J.C.G. (1977). Impulse activity in afferent vagal C-fibres with endings in the intrapulmonary airways of dogs. *Respir. Physiol.*, **29**, 125–142

145. Coleridge, H.M., Coleridge, J.C.G., Ginzel, K.H., Baker, D.G., Banzett, R.B. and Morrison, M.A. (1976). Stimulation of irritant receptors and afferent C-fibres in the lungs by prostaglandins. *Nature (London)*, **264**, 451–453

146. Hahn, H.L. (1986). Role of the parasympathetic nervous system and of cholinergic mechanisms in bronchial hyperreactivity. *Bull. Eur. Physiopathol. Respir.*, **22** (Suppl. 7), 112–142

147. Dahlén, S.E., Hedqvist, P., Hammarstrom, S. and Samuelsson, B. (1980). Leukotrienes are potent constrictors of human bronchi. *Nature (London)*, **288**, 484–486

148. Lewis, R.A., Austen, K.F., Drazen, J.M., Clark, D. A. and Corey, E.J. (1980). Slow reacting substance of anaphylaxis: identification of leukotrienes C_1 and D from human and rat sources. *Proc. Natl. Acad. Sci. USA*, **77**, 3710–3714

149. Piper, P.J. (1983). Pharmacology of leukotrienes. *Br. Med. Bull.*, **39**, 255–259
150. Brocklehurst, W.E. (1960). The release of histamine and formation of a slow reacting substance (SRS-A) during anaphylactic shock. *J. Physiol.*, **151**, 416–435
151. Brocklehurst, W.E. (1981). Steps in the dark – an outline history of the study of SRS-A. In Piper, P.J. (ed.) *SRS-A and Leukotrienes*, pp. 7–11. (Chichester: Wiley)
152. Hanna, C.J., Bach, M.K., Pare, P.D. and Schellenberg, R.R. (1981). Slow reacting substances (leukotrienes) contract human airway and pulmonary vascular smooth muscle in vitro. *Nature (London)*, **290**, 343–344
153. Smedegard, G., Hedqvist, P., Dahlén, S.E., Revenas, B., Hammarstrom, S. and Samuelsson, B. (1982). Leukotriene C_4 affects pulmonary and cardiovascular dynamics in the monkey. *Nature (London)*, **295**, 327–329
154. Krell, R.D., Osborn, R., Vickery, L., Falcone, K., O'Donnell, M., Gleason, J., Kinzig, C. and Bryan, D. (1981). Contraction of isolated airway smooth muscle by synthetic leukotrienes C_4 and D_2. *Prostaglandins*, **22**, 387–409
155. Drazen, J.M. (1986). Inhalation challenge with sulphidopeptide leukotrienes in human subjects. *Chest*, **89**, 414–418
156. Piper, P.J. and Samhoun, M.N. (1981). The mechanism of action of leukotrienes C_4 and D_4 in guinea-pig isolated perfused lung and parenchymal strips of guinea-pig, rabbit and rat. *Prostaglandins* **21**, 793–803
157. Hamel, R., Masson, P., Ford-Hutchinson, A.W., Jones, T.R., Brunet, G. and Piechuta, H. (1982). Differing mechanisms of leukotriene D_4 induced bronchoconstriction in guinea pigs following intravenous and aerosol administration. *Prostaglandins*, **24**, 432
158. Weichman, B.M., Muccitelli, R.M., Osborn, R.R., Holden, D.A., Gleason, J.G. and Wasserman, M.A. (1982). In vitro and in vivo mechanisms of leukotriene mediated bronchoconstriction in the guinea-pig. *J. Pharmacol. Exp. Ther.*, **222**, 202–208
159. Weiss, J.W., Drazen, J.M., Coles, N., McFadden, E.R., Lewis, R.A., Weller, P.F., Corey, E.J. and Austen, K.F. (1982). Bronchoconstrictor effects of leukotriene C in humans. *Science*, **216**, 196–198
160. Weiss, J.W., Drazen, J.M., McFadden, E.R., Weller, P.F., Corey, E.J., Lewis, R.A. and Austen, K.F. (1982). Comparative bronchoconstrictor effects of histamine, leukotriene C and leukotriene D in normal human volunteers. *Trans. Assoc. Am. Phys.*, **95**, 30–35
161. Griffin, M., Weiss, J.W., Leitch, A.G., McFadden, E.R., Corey, E.J., Austen, K.F. and Drazen, J.M. (1983). Effects of leukotriene D in the airways in asthma. *N. Engl. J. Med.*, **308**, 436–439
162. Bisgaard, H., Groth, S. and Madsen, F. (1985). Bronchial hyperreactivity to leukotriene D_4 and histamine in exogenous asthma. *Br. Med. J.*, **290**, 1468–1471
163. Smith, L.J., Greenberger, P.A., Patterson, R., Krell, R.D. and Bernstein, P.R. (1985). The effect of inhaled leukotriene D_4 in humans. *Am. Rev. Respir. Dis.*, **131**, 368–372
164. Barnes, N.C., Piper, P.J. and Costello, J.F. (1984). Comparative effects of inhaled leukotriene C_4, leukotriene D_4 and histamine in normal human subjects. *Thorax*, **39**, 500–541
165. Barnes, N.C., Piper, P.J. and Costello, J.F. (1984). Actions of inhaled leukotrienes and their interactions with other allergic mediators. *Prostaglandins*, **28**, 629–631
166. Adelroth, E., Morris, M.M., Hargreave, F.E. and O'Byrne, P.M. (1984). Airway responsiveness to leukotrienes C_4 and D_4 and to methacholine in patients with asthma and normal controls. *N. Engl. J. Med.*, **315**, 480–484
167. Blair, I.A., Barrow, S.E., Waddell, K.A., Lewis, P.J. and Dollery, C.T. (1982). Prostacyclin is not a circulating hormone in man. *Prostaglandins*, **23**, 579–589
168. Barrow, S.E., Heavey, D.J., Ennis, M., Chappell, C.G., Blair, I.A. and Dollery, C.T. (1984). Measurement of prostaglandin D_2 and identification of metabolites in human plasma during intravenous infusion. *Prostaglandins*, **28**, 743–754
169. Granstrom, E. and Kindahl H. (1978). Radioimmunoassay of prostaglandins and thromboxanes. In Frölich, J.C. (ed.) *Advances in Prostaglandin and Thromboxane Research*. Vol. 5, pp. 119–210. (New York: Raven Press)
170. Gréen, K., Hedqvist, P. and Svanborg, N. (1974). Increased plasma levels of 15-keto-13,14-dihydro-prostaglandin $F_{2\alpha}$ after allergen provoked asthma in man. *Lancet*, **2**, 1419–1421
171. Hardy, C.C., Holgate, S.T. and Robinson, C. (1986). Evidence against the formation of 13,14-dihydro-15-keto-prostaglandin $F_{2\alpha}$ following inhalation of prostaglandin D_2 in man. *Br. J. Pharmacol.*, **87**, 563–568

172. Roberts, L.J.II, Sweetman, B.J., Lewis, R.A., Austen, K.F. and Oates, J.A. (1980). Increased production of prostaglandin D_2 in patients with systemic mastocytosis. N. Engl. J. Med. **303**, 1400–1404
173. Oates, J.A., Sweetman, B.J. and Roberts, L.J.II (1984). The release of mediators of the human mast cell: investigations in mastocytosis. In Kay, A.B., Austen, K.F. and Lichtenstein, L.M. (eds.) Asthma: Physiology, Immunopharmacology and Treatment. Third International Symposium. pp. 55–62. (London: Academic Press)
174. Roberts, L.J. II and Sweetman, B.J. (1985). Metabolic fate of endogenously synthesised prostaglandin D_2 in a human female with mastocytosis. Prostaglandins, **30** 383–401
175. Liston, T.E. and Roberts, L.J. II. (1985). Metabolic fate of radiolabelled prostaglandin D_2 in a normal human male volunteer. J. Biol. Chem., **260**, 13172–13180
176. Liston, T.E. and Roberts, L.J. II. (1985). Transformation of prostaglandin D_2 to $9\alpha,11\beta$-15(S)-trihydroxy-prosta-(5Z,13E)-dien-l-oic acid ($9\alpha,11\beta$-prostaglandin F_2): a unique biologically active prostaglandin produced enzymatically in vivo in humans. Proc. Natl. Acad. Sci. USA, **82**, 6030–6034
177. Serafin, W.E., Oates, J.A. and Hubbard, W.C. (1984). Metabolism of leukotriene B_4 in the monkey. Identification of the principal non-volatile metabolite in the urine. Prostaglandins, **27**, 899–911
178. Orning, L., Kaijser L. and Hammarstrom, S. (1985). In vivo metabolism of leukotriene C_4 in man: urinary excretion of leukotriene E_4. Biochem. Biophys. Res. Commun., **130**, 214–220
179. Bernstrom, K. and Hammarstrom, S. (1986). Metabolism of leukotriene E_4 by rat tissues. Formation of N-acetyl-leukotriene E_4. Arch. Biochem. Biophys., **244**, 486–491
180. Orning, L., Norin, E., Gustafsson, B. and Hammarstrom, S. (1986). In vivo metabolism of leukotriene C_4 in germ free and conventional rats: fecal excretion of N-acetyl-leukotriene E_4. J. Biol. Chem., **261**, 766–771
181. Smith, A.P. (1975). Effect of indomethacin in asthma: evidence against a role for prostaglandins in its pathogenesis. Br. J. Clin. Pharmacol. **2**, 307–309
182. Fish, J.E., Ankin, M.G., Adkinson, N.F. and Peterman, V.I. (1981). Indomethacin modification of immediate-type immunologic airway responses in allergic asthmatic and non-asthmatic subjects. Am. Rev. Respir. Dis., **123**, 609–614
183. Hume, M. and Eddy, V. (1977). Treatment of chronic airways obstruction with indomethacin. Scand. J. Respir. Dis., **58**, 284–286
184. Rudolph, M., Grant, B., Saunders, K.B., Brostoff, J., Salt, P.J. and Walker, D.S. (1975). Aspirin in exercise induced asthma. Lancet, **1**, 450
185. Schacter, E.N., Kreisnian, H. and Bouhuys, A. (1978). Prostaglandin synthesis inhibition and exercise bronchospasm. Ann. Int. Med., **89**, 287–288
186. Kordansky, D., Adkinson, N.F., Norman, P.S. and Rosenthal, R.R. (1978). Asthma improved by non-steroidal anti-inflammatory drugs. Ann. Int. Med., **88**, 508–511
187. Crook, D., Collins, A.J. Bacon, P.A. and Chan, R. (1976). Prostaglandin synthetase activity from human rheumatoid synovial microsomes: effect of aspirin-like drug therapy. Ann. Rheum. Dis., **35**, 327–332
188. Walker, J.L. (1973). The regulatory function of prostaglandins in the release of histamine and SRS-A from passively sensitized human lung tissue. In Bernhard, S. (ed.) Advances in the Biosciences. Vol. 9, pp. 235–240. (Oxford: Pergamon Press)
189. Stenson, W.F., Parker, C.W. and Sullivan, T.J. (1980). Augmentation of IgE mediated release of histamine by 5-hydroxyeicosatetraenoic acid and 12-hydroxyeicosatetraenoic acid. Biochem. Biophys. Res. Commun. **96**, 1045–1052
190. Stenson, W.F. and Parker, C.W. (1980). Monohydroxyeicosatetraenoic acids (HETEs) induce degranulation of human neutrophils. J. Immunol., **124**, 2100–2104
191. Stenson, W.F., Nickells, M.W. and Atkinson, J.P. (1983). Esterification of monohydroxy fatty acids into the lipids of a macrophage cell line. Prostaglandins, **26**, 253–264
192. Sautebin L., Vigano, T., Grassi, E., Crivellari, M.T., Galli, G., Berti, F. Mezzetti, M. and Folco, G. (1985). Release of leukotrienes, induced by the Ca^{++} ionophore A23187, from human lung parenchyma in vitro. J. Pharmacol. Exp. Ther., **234**, 217–221
193. Peters, S.P., MacGlashan, D.W., Schleimer, R.P. Hayes, E.C., Adkinson, N.F. and Lichtenstein L.M. (1985). The pharmacological modulation of the release of arachidonic acid metabolites from purified human lung mast cells. Am. Rev. Respir. Dis., **132**, 367–373

194. Bach, M.K., Brashler, J.R., Smith, H.W., Fitzpatrick, F.A., Sun, F.F. and McGuire, J.C. (1982). 6,9-Deepoxy-6,9-(phenylimino)-$\Delta^{6,8}$-prostaglandin I_1 (U-60,257) a new inhibitor of leukotriene C and D synthesis: in vitro studies. *Prostaglandins*, **23**, 759–727

195. Sun, F.F. and McGuire, J.C. (1983). Inhibition of human neutrophil arachidonate 5-lipoxygenase by 6,9-deepoxy-6,9-(phenylimino)-$\Delta^{6,8}$-prostaglandin I_1 (U-60,257). *Prostaglandins*, **26**, 211–221

196. Mann, J.S., Robinson C., Sheridan, A.Q., Clement, P., Bach, M.K. and Holgate, S.T. (1986). Effect of piriprost (U-60,257) a novel leukotriene inhibitor on allergen and exercise induced bronchoconstriction in asthma. *Thorax*, **41**, 746–752

197. Fleisch, J.H., Rinkema, L.E., Haisch, K.D., Swanson-Bean, D., Goodson, T., Ho, P.P.K. and Marshall, W.S. (1985). LY171883, 1-[2-hydroxy-3-propyl-4-[4-(1H-tetrazol-5- yl)butoxy]-phenyl]ethanone, an orally active leukotriene D_4 antagonist. *J. Pharmacol. Exp. Ther.*, **233**, 148–157

198. Barnes, N. Piper, P.J. and Costello, J.F. (1987). Studies of an orally active leukotriene antagonist L649,923 in normal man. In Samuelsson, B., Paoletti, R. and Ramwell, P.W. (eds.) *Prostaglandin, Thromboxane and Leukotriene Research.* Vol. 17B, pp. 1000–1002. (New York: Raven Press)

199. Britton, J.R., Hanley, S.P. and Tattersfield, A.E. (1987). Effect of an oral leukotriene antagonist L649,923 on the response to inhaled antigen in asthma. In Samuelsson, B., Paoletti, R. and Ramwell, P.W. (eds.) *Advances in Prostaglandin, Thromboxane and Leukotriene Research.* Vol. 17B, pp. 1003–1006

200. Abraham, W.M., Wanner, A., Stevenson, J.S. and Chapman, G.A. (1986). The effect of an orally active leukotriene D_4/E_4 antagonist, LY171883, on antigen-induced airway responses in allergic sheep. *Prostaglandins*, **31**, 457–467

201. Schleimer, R.P., McGlashan, D.W., Peters, S.P. Pinckard, R.N., Adkinson, N.F. and Lichtenstein, L.M. (1986). Characterization of inflammatory mediator release from purified human lung mast cells. *Am. Rev. Respir. Dis.*, **133**, 614–617

202. Lynch J.M. and Henson, P.M. (1986). The intracellular retention of newly synthesized platelet-activating factor. *J. Immunol.*, **137**, 2653–2661

203. Robinson, C. and Holgate, S.T. (1985). Do leukotrienes fully account for immediate hypersensitivity. *Ann. Inst. Past. Immunol.*, **136D**, 205–212

204. Lee, T.H., Cromwell, O. Nagakura, T. and Kay, A.B. (1984). Mediators in exercise induced asthma. In Kay, A.B., Austen, K.F. and Lichtenstein, L.M. (eds.) *Asthma: Physiology, Immunopharmacology and Treatment. Third International Symposium.* pp. 276–296. (London: Academic Press)

205. Howarth, P.H., Durham, S.R., Kay, A.B. and Holgate, S.T. (1987). The relationship between mast cell mediator release and bronchial reactivity in allergic asthma. *J. Allergy Clin. Immunol.* In press

206. Murray, J.J., Tonel, A.B., Brash, A.R., Roberts, L.J. II, Gosset, P., Workman, R., Capron, A. and Oates, J.A. (1986). Release of prostaglandin D_2 into human airways during acute antigen challenge. *N. Engl. J. Med.* **315**, 800–804

207. Omini, C., Abbrachio, M.P. Coen, E., Daffonchio, L., Fano, M. and Cattabeni, F. (1984). Involvement of arachidonic acid metabolites in β-adrenoceptor desensitization. *Eur. J. Pharmacol.*, **106**, 601–606

208. Daffoncio, L., Abbrachio, M.P., Hernandez, A., Giani, E. Cattabeni, F. and Omini, C. (1985). Arachidonic acid metabolites induce β-adrenoceptor desensitization in rat lung in vitro. *Prostaglandins*, **30**, 799–809

209. Nijkamp, F.P. and van Oosterhout, A.J.M. (1984). Influence of 15-hydroperoxyarachidonic acid on lung beta-adrenoceptor function and airway reactivity. *Agents Actions*, **15**, 85–86

210. Anderson, P. (1980). Antigen-induced bronchial anaphylaxis in actively sensitized guinea-pigs. Antianaphylactic effects of sodium cromoglycate and aminophylline. *Br. J. Pharmacol.*, **69**, 467–472

211. Robinson, C., Hoult, J.R.S., Waddell, K.A., Blair, I.A. and Dollery, C.T. (1984). Total profiling by GC/NICIMS of the major cyclooxygenase products from antigen and leukotriene-challenged guinea-pig lung. *Biochem. Pharmacol.*, **33**, 395–400

212. Lee, H.K. and Murlas, C. (1985). Ozone-induced bronchial hyperreactivity in guinea-pigs is abolished by BW 755C or FPL 55712 but not by indomethacin. *Am. Rev. Respir. Dis.*, **132**, 1005–1009

213. Andersson, P. (1980). Antigen-induced bronchial anaphylaxis in actively sensitized guinea-pigs. Pattern of response in relation to immunization regimen. *Allergy*, **35**, 65–71

214. Carney, I.F. (1976). IgE-mediated anaphylactic bronchoconstriction in the guinea pig and effect of DSCG. *Int. Arch. Allergy Appl. Immunol.*, **50**, 322–328

215. Hutson, P.A., Church, M.K., Clay, T.P., Miller, P. and Holgate, S.T. Early and late phase bronchoconstriction following allergen challenge of non-anaesthetized guinea pigs: I. The association of disordered airway physiology to leukocyte infiltration. *Am. Rev. Respir. Dis.* In press

216. Dahlén, S.E., Hansson, G., Hedqvist, P., Bjorck, T., Granstrom, E. and Dahlén, B. (1983). Allergen challenge of lung tissue from asthmatics elicits bronchial contraction that correlates with the release of leukotrienes C_4, D_4 and E_4. *Proc. Natl. Acad. Sci. USA*, **80**, 1712–1716

217. Harvey, J., Holgate, S.T., Peters, B.J., Robinson, C. and Walker, J.R. (1985). Oxidative transformations of arachidonic acid in human dispersed lung cells: disparity between utilization of endogenous and exogenous substrate. *Br. J. Pharmacol.*, **86**, 417–426

218. Lynch, J.M., Worthen, G.S. and Henson, P.M. (1984). Platelet-activating factor. In Buckle, D.R. and Smith, H. (eds.) *Development of Anti-asthmatic Drugs*, pp. 73–88. (London: Butterworth)

219. Cuss, F.M., Dixon, C.M.S. and Barnes, P.J. (1986). Effects of inhaled platelet activating factor on pulmonary function and bronchial responsiveness in man. *Lancet*, **2**, 189–192

220. Brocklehurst, W.E. (1962). Slow reacting substance and related compounds. *Prog. Allergy*, **6**, 539–558

221. Creese, B.R. and Bach, M.K. (1983). Hyperreactivity of airways smooth muscle produced in vitro by leukotrienes. *Prostagl. Leuk. Med.*, **11**, 161–169

222. Lee, T., Austen, K.F., Corey, E.J. and Drazen, J.M. (1984). Leukotriene E_4 induced airway hyperresponsiveness of guinea-pig tracheal smooth muscle to histamine and evidence for three separate sulfidopeptide leukotriene receptors. *Proc. Natl. Acad. Sci. USA*, **81**, 4922–4925

223. Bianco, S., Robuschi, M., Vaghi, A., Simone, P., Folco, G., Berti F. and Pasargiklian, M. (1985). Effects of leukotriene C_4 on the bronchial response to ultrasonic mist of distilled water. *Respir. Res.*, **19**, 82–86

224. Barnes, N.C. and Costello, J.F. (1986). Leukotrienes and asthma. In Kay, A.B. (ed.) *Asthma: Clinical Pharmacology and Therapeutic Progress*, pp. 194–204. (Oxford: Blackwell)

225. Thorpe, J.E. and Murlas, C.G. (1986). Leukotriene B_4 potentiates airway muscle responsiveness in vivo and in vitro. *Prostaglandins*, **31**, 899–908

6
The Role of Eicosanoids in Inflammatory Disorders of the Skin

R. D. R. CAMP and F. M. CUNNINGHAM

INTRODUCTION

Inflammatory skin diseases encompass a full spectrum of pathological changes varying from acute urticaria and angio-oedema, in which transient increased vascular permeability and plasma exudation are the main abnormalities, to a wide variety of disorders characterized by chronic inflammatory cell infiltrates. The distinction between acute and chronic inflammatory skin disease is not always clear, as in the case of chronic plaque psoriasis in which lesions may persist for years and yet are infiltrated repeatedly by neutrophils which are classically regarded as acute inflammatory cells.

Inflammatory diseases of the skin are often of obscure cause and are extremely common, psoriasis and atopic eczema together affecting more than 4% of the European population. The most widely used anti-inflammatory drugs are topically applied corticosteroids and oral antihistamines. Although these compounds have an important part to play, their usefulness is often limited by poor therapeutic effectiveness and unwanted side effects, the latter being particularly common with long-term potent topical steroids. It is also noteworthy that non-steroidal anti-inflammatory drugs such as aspirin and indomethacin are of little benefit in the treatment of inflammatory skin disease. Therefore, there appears to be ample scope for the development of new therapeutic modalities.

In defining the role of a compound as a mediator of a particular inflammatory change, the criteria discussed by Dale[1], in relation to the pharmacology of neurotransmitters, should also be satisfied. Thus, in investigating the pathogenetic role of a putative mediator of an inflammatory skin disorder, it is important (a) to recover elevated levels of the compound from the inflamed tissue, (b) to reproduce that aspect of the inflammatory change for which the compound is thought to be responsible by use of appropriate doses of the compound, (c) to demonstrate mechanisms for the formation of the mediator in the inflamed tissue, and (d) to abolish that aspect of the inflammatory reaction for which the compound is thought to be responsible with inhibitors of its formation or selective receptor antagonists. It is significant that three of these four criteria can only be investigated by *in vivo* studies, and the unique accessibility of the skin makes it the only human organ in which comprehensive experiments can be carried out *in vivo* in a controlled and ethical manner. The results of studies concerning the role of eicosanoids in inflammatory skin diseases will be described in the following sections.

THE PRO-INFLAMMATORY PROPERTIES OF EICOSANOIDS IN HUMAN SKIN

Chemical mediators of inflammation may be broadly divided into those compounds attracting inflammatory cells (chemoattractants) and vasoactive agents producing vasodilation and/or increased plasma exudation. The vasoactive and chemotactic properties of eicosanoids have been widely studied in the skin of laboratory animals. Studies in man have inevitably been less detailed but have highlighted apparent species differences.

Vasoactive eicosanoids

Since the discovery that the sulphidopeptide 5-lipoxygenase products, leukotrienes (LT) C_4 and D_4, are components of slow-reacting substance of anaphylaxis, attention has been focused on the vasoactive properties of these compounds. LTC_4 and LTD_4 have been shown to exert vasoconstrictor effects in guinea-pig skin[2], but we have found no visual evidence of vasoconstriction in human skin following intradermal injection of 5–200 ng of each compound, although dose-related erythema and wealing were seen[3]. Others have reported pallor in weals produced by intradermal injection of LTC_4 and D_4 in human subjects and have interpreted this as being due to intrinsic arteriolar constriction[4]. We have found[3] no difference between the pallor in histamine-induced weals and that due to LTC_4 and D_4 and believe that this effect, which is often seen in urticarial weals in clinical disease, is due to extrinsic compression of the vasculature by oedema fluid. This interpretation is supported by results obtained using laser Doppler flowmetry, which demonstrated increased blood flow without evidence of vasoconstriction following both intradermal injection of LTC_4 and LTD_4 in human subjects[5] and topical application of LTD_4 to human nasal mucosa[6]. The apparent lack of vasoconstrictor effects of these sulphidopeptide leukotrienes in human skin perhaps increases their importance as pro-inflammatory agents.

There are also apparent species differences in the response of skin to intradermal injection of prostaglandin (PG) E_2. This eicosanoid is a potent vasodilator but has little direct effect on plasma protein extravasation in guinea-pig or rabbit skin in doses up to 1 μg or 300 ng respectively[7,8]. In human skin, dose-related erythema has been found following intradermal injection of 1–10 ng PGE_2, although there was considerable inter-subject variation[9]. Little swelling was noted at these doses, but, in other studies[10,11], swelling was apparent after injection of higher doses of PGE_2 (e.g. 25 ng). In a more recent study, the ability of 0.5 μg doses of PGE_2 to cause swelling has been confirmed by measurement of human skin fold thickness with calipers[12]. Thus, it appears that PGE_2 is able to cause both vasodilation and exudation in human skin and should not be considered purely as a vasodilator mediator, as suggested by studies in rabbit skin[13]. Nevertheless, the ability of PGE_2 to potentiate the effects of other mediators, a phenomenon which may largely be due to its vasodilator properties and which has been demonstrated in animal and human skin, should not be discounted in considering the importance of this eicosanoid as a mediator of inflammation in the skin[7,8,12,14].

Interest in PGD_2 as a mediator of inflammation has increased recently in view of evidence that it is the major prostaglandin produced by mast cells[15,16]. Prostaglandin D_2 (10–100 ng) produced variable dose-related erythema in human subjects following intradermal injection and caused increased vascular permeability in rat skin[9]. Histamine-induced changes in vascular permeability were also potentiated by PGD_2 in rat skin[9], although no significant enhancement of histamine-induced weal responses by PGD_2 were observed in human skin[17]. The pro-inflammatory effects of prostacyclin (PGI_2), which is a potent systemic vasodilator, have also received little attention in man. In a meeting abstract, PGI_2 was reported to produce erythema on intradermal injection in human subjects and to be less potent than PGE_2, but details of these findings have not been published. However PGI_2 has been shown to produce vasodilation and increased blood flow, without plasma exudation, in rabbit skin[18].

As well as exerting pro-inflammatory effects on the vasculature, PGE_2 and PGI_2 may act as anti-inflammatory agents by virtue of their ability to elevate intracellular levels of cyclic adenosine monophosphate (cAMP) in mast cells and leukocytes through stimulation of adenylate cyclase. The possible consequences of these effects in the skin were reviewed some years ago[19,20]. In addition, it has been postulated that the exacerbation of diseases such as asthma and urticaria by the non-steroidal anti-inflammatory drugs, aspirin and indomethacin, may result from the abolition of such inhibitory effects[21,22]. Recent examples of the anti-inflammatory actions of prostaglandins include the inhibition by PGE_2 and PGI_2 of lymphocyte chemotaxis and interleukin-1 synthesis by macrophages[23,24]. In view of these anti-inflammatory properties, it becomes difficult to establish the overall contribution of the vasoactive prostaglandins to the initiation and maintenance of inflammatory reactions in the skin.

Chemoattractant eicosanoids

The first eicosanoid shown to exert dose-related chemoattractant activity for neutrophils *in vitro* was the lipoxygenase product, 12(S)-hydroxy-5,8,10,14-eicosatetraenoic acid (12(S)-HETE)[25–27]. Although 12-HETE was first recognized as a platelet product[28,29], interest in this compound as a mediator of inflammation has resulted from the detection of large amounts in lesions of the inflammatory and proliferative skin disease, psoriasis[30,31]. The *in vivo* chemoattractant activity of 12-HETE has been studied in guinea-pigs by intraperitoneal injection of 4–8 μg doses which resulted in accumulation of both neutrophils and eosinophils in the peritoneal cavity[32]. In human volunteers, single intradermal injections of 5 and 40 μg racemic 12-HETE, prepared by photo-oxidation of arachidonic acid, produced no visible inflammatory effects during an 8 hour observation period. Intradermal infusion of platelet 12(S)-HETE or racemic 12-HETE (5 μg per hour for 8 hours) produced an erythematous response which was no greater than that seen with control infusions, although histological examination of biopsies showed increased accumulations of mononuclear cells and neutrophils on comparison with control biopsies[33]. Topical application of racemic 12-HETE (2–50 μg) to localized areas of skin, followed by occlusion of the deposits for 6 h, produced dose-related erythematous reactions lasting up to 24 h in human volunteers[33]. Erythema was observed at 6–8 h in all volunteers after application of 20 μg racemic 12-HETE. Biopsies at this time showed accumulations of mononuclear cells and neutrophils in the dermis in all samples, and intraepidermal neutrophil infiltrates in some. Similar findings, with more consistent intraepidermal neutrophil accumulations were seen in 24 h biopsies[33]. A comparison of the inflammatory potency of 12-HETE with that of the other monohydroxy metabolites of arachidonic acid in human skin showed that 12-HETE was the most potent of the positional isomers in producing erythema[34]. It is of interest that 5-HETE, which is 10 times more potent as a chemoattractant *in vitro* than the other monohydroxy products of arachidonic acid, had little pro-inflammatory activity following topical application *in vivo*[26,27,34]. Although microgramme amounts of 12-HETE are required to produce inflammatory changes in human skin, and greatly exceed the doses of leukotriene B$_4$ which would evoke similar responses, such amounts are in the range of those identified in psoriatic skin lesions[30,31].

A recent, unexpected finding, which will be described in a later section, has indicated that 12-HETE, recovered from the surface scale of psoriatic lesions, is stereochemically different from platelet 12(S)-HETE and appears to be the 12(R) epimer[35]. *In vitro* studies have shown that 12(R)-HETE is a more potent neutrophil chemoattractant than 12(S)-HETE, the EC$_{50}$ values for the two compounds being 6 x 10^{-7} mol L^{-1} and 1.2 x 10^{-6} mol L^{-1} respectively. In addition, cells migrated twice as far after maximal stimulation with 12(R)-HETE when compared with the distance moved after maximal stimulation with 12(S)-HETE[36]. The *in vivo* properties of 12(R)-HETE are currently under investigation.

Leukotriene B$_4$ (LTB$_4$, 5(S),12(R)-dihydroxy-6,14-*cis*-8,10-*trans*- eicosatetra-enoic acid) is a potent neutrophil chemoattractant[27,37,38]. Intradermal injections of 50–500 ng LTB$_4$ in human volunteers produced ill-defined inflammatory reactions, and biopsies taken after 4–6 h showed perivascular accumulations of polymorphonuclear leukocytes, which were predominantly neutrophils[3,4]. Topical application of LTB$_4$ (5–500 ng) to normal human skin, followed by occlusion for 6 h, produced localized dose-related erythema and swelling which first appeared 12–24 h after application, reached a maximum at 24–48 h and persisted for about 7 days. Biopsy of sites to which 100 ng LTB$_4$

had been applied revealed large numbers of neutrophils in the dermis and epidermis. The neutrophil infiltrates were maximal at 24 h, forming florid collections within discrete vacuoles in the upper epidermis[39] (Figure 6.1). The ability of LTB$_4$ and 12-HETE to produce these intraepidermal neutrophil microabscesses appears to be of significance since this pattern of epidermal cellular infiltration is, in some respects, similar to that seen in psoriatic skin lesions, from which both LTB$_4$ and 12-HETE have been recovered in biologically active amounts (for details see later sections).

FORMATION OF EICOSANOIDS BY HUMAN SKIN *IN VIVO* AND *IN VITRO*

Eicosanoid formation by skin preparations *in vitro* may not necessarily reflect the *in vivo* state and results are subject to variation according to the incubation conditions used. It has therefore been our practice to identify and measure eicosanoids *in vivo* and to study the *in vitro* formation of relevant compounds, if indicated, in subsequent experiments. Consequently, it has been necessary to develop appropriate *in vivo* sampling methods, as well as assays of sufficient sensitivity and specificity to allow analysis of the small quantities of material obtained from human skin.

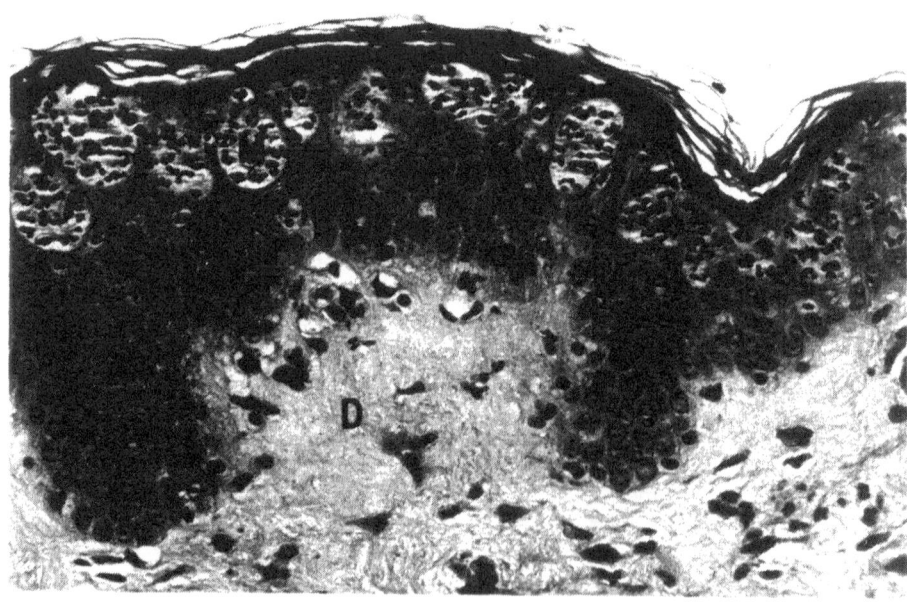

Figure 6.1   Intraepidermal neutrophil microabscesses following topical application of 100 ng LTB$_4$ to human skin. E = epidermis; D = dermis; M = neutrophil microabscess. Magnification x 280

Methods of sampling human skin

A suction blister technique[40] has been widely used to obtain samples from both normal and inflamed skin[41–43]. Perspex cups containing perforated diaphragms are attached to the skin and a negative pressure of about − 200 mmHg applied for 2–3 h, during which time blisters are formed. The blister fluid (100–200 μl or more) can be withdrawn with a syringe and needle, and sampled for mediator content. The technique cannot be used satisfactorily for obtaining exudate from the skin lesions of psoriasis since blisters form less readily and are liable to haemorrhage and rupture. In view of this, a skin chamber technique was developed for sampling the lesions and clinically normal skin of psoriatic patients[44,45]. Abrasions (diameter approximately 2 cm) are produced with a scalpel blade and cylindrical plastic chambers fixed to the abraded sites with cyanoacrylate glue. Sterile physiological solution (1 ml) is placed in each chamber, removed after an appropriate time (usually 30 min in our studies), extracted, purified and assayed. Eicosanoid assays may also be carried out on lipid extracts of surface scale which can be recovered from psoriatic and other scaly lesions by gentle abrasion with a scalpel blade. The results can then be compared with those obtained using scale recovered by abrasion of large areas of normal skin[46]. Useful analyses have also been carried out on extracts of skin slices obtained under local anaesthetic by the use of a keratome[30]. In earlier work a dermal perfusion method was used to identify certain prostaglandins. Sterile physiological solution was introduced into, and drained from, the skin through perforated hypodermic needles placed parallel to each other in the dermis[47,48]. Attempts have also been made to measure prostanoids in venous blood draining an area of inflamed skin such as that of the forearm[49].

Analytical methods used to measure eicosanoid production in skin *in vivo*

The analytical methods used to detect eicosanoid production by human skin include radioimmunoassay (RIA), biological assays and physicochemical techniques, particularly gas chromatography–mass spectrometry (GS–MS). The biological methods include the cascade superfusion technique[50], which has been used to measure PGE_2 in suction blister fluid from human skin[51], and an assay of neutrophil locomotor activity, the agarose microdroplet chemokinesis technique[52]. The latter, used in conjunction with prior chromatographic purification of samples, has been applied successfully to the measurement of chemoattractant eicosanoids[45,46] and is more convenient for the measurement of small quantities of material in large numbers of samples than conventional chemotaxis assays. However, the development of a multiwell microchemotaxis apparatus now appears to provide rapid and sensitive chemotaxis assays if polyvinylpyrrolidone-free polycarbonate membranes and an image analysis system are used[53].

GC–MS methods have been used to quantify a number of eicosanoids in samples from human skin. Compounds measured in our laboratories include arachidonic acid, PGE_2, PGI_2 and a variety of monohydroxy fatty acids.

117

Leukotriene B_4 may be detected in picogramme amounts in samples of human skin by the agarose microdroplet chemokinesis method, but the small quantities present and interference from impurities have prevented routine measurement by GC–MS.

Radioimmunoassay (RIA) for several different eicosanoids are available commercially, but in some instances lack of specificity may be disadvantageous. For example, a commercially available RIA for LTB_4 displays 2% cross-reactivity with 12-HETE, which may be present in suction blister fluid from inflamed human skin in levels[54] which are 100–200 fold higher than those of LTB_4. In extracts of psoriatic scale, the molar ratio of 12-HETE to LTB_4 per unit wet weight of extracted tissue[31,46] may exceed 1000. It therefore appears that measurement of LTB_4 in skin samples with currently available RIA antibodies will only be reliable if adequate purification is carried out prior to assay. The assay of *in vivo* PGD_2 production by RIA, GC–MS, or other methods has proved difficult. Recently, an antiserum against the methyl oxime derivative of PGD_2 has been developed and used in an RIA to detect PGD release into skin chambers during immediate hypersensitivity reactions[55] and into cubital vein blood draining acutely inflamed forearm skin[56]. The PGD_2 methyl oxime is formed by direct derivatization of the aqueous biological sample which may then be assayed without the need for further purification.

Eicosanoid production in model inflammatory reactions of human skin

Some of the initial studies of eicosanoid production in human skin involved measurement of prostaglandins in model inflammatory reactions such as the response to ultraviolet irradiation and to application of tetrahydrofurfuryl nicotinate.

Irradiation of human skin with three times the minimal erythema dose of ultraviolet B (290–320 nm) produces erythema which appears after 4–6 h, reaches a maximum at 24–48 h and thereafter persists for several days. Analysis of suction blister fluid from ultraviolet B irradiated human skin by the cascade superfusion bioassay method revealed PGE_2-like material. The levels of PGE_2-equivalents were significantly greater in inflamed skin when compared with control skin at 6 h after irradiation and reached a maximum at 24 h but returned to control levels by 48 h despite continued intense erythema[51]. More detailed quantitative GC–MS analysis of suction blister fluid recovered at 2,6,18,24 and 48 h after ultraviolet B irradiation confirmed a significant and progressive elevation of PGE_2 occurring in parallel with the appearance of the erythematous reaction and reaching a maximum (49.4 $\pm$ 5.2 ng ml^{-1}, mean $\pm$ SEM, $n = 13$) at 24 h before returning to near control levels (17.1 $\pm$ 0.7 ng ml^{-1}, $n = 47$) at 48 h, in spite of continued intense erythema[41]. Arachidonic acid levels were also elevated at 24 h after ultraviolet B irradiation in the same suction blister samples (785 $\pm$ 57 ng ml^{-1}, $n = 13$, for 24 h post-irradiation samples versus 276 $\pm$ 20 ng ml^{-1}, $n = 47$, for controls). Arachidonic acid was also quantified by GC–MS[41]. Topical or systemic administration of the cyclo-oxygenase inhibitor indomethacin after ultraviolet B irradiation prevented the increase in PGE_2 levels seen in suction blister fluid at 24 h, at the same time as partially reducing the inflammatory reaction[57]. The suppression of ultraviolet B erythema by indomethacin when used in the first 24 h after irradiation has been confirmed by others who have shown[58], in addition, that this drug has no overt anti-inflammatory effect after 24 h, a finding which coincides with the return of PGE_2 to near baseline levels after this time. These results, together with the knowledge that epidermal cells are capable of synthesizing PGE_2 in vitro[59,60], provide firm evidence for a role for this prostaglandin in mediating at least part of the early ultraviolet B reaction (sunburn).

Similar results were obtained with nicotinate ester-induced erythema in human skin. The levels of PGE_2-equivalents (measured by the cascade superfusion technique) were significantly greater in suction blister fluid from inflamed, compared with control, skin and prior administration of aspirin reduced or abolished the inflammatory reaction at the same time as blocking the increase in PGE_2 equivalents[42].

To our knowledge, there is only one report of the measurement of LTB_4 in a model inflammatory reaction in human skin[43]. Suction blister fluid was obtained from areas of acute allergic contact dermatitis (a delayed hypersensitivity reaction) elicited by topical application of antigen (nickel sulphate or potassium dichromate) in specifically allergic volunteers. Samples were extracted, purified by high performance liquid chromatography (HPLC) and appropriate fractions evaporated and assayed by the agarose microdroplet chemokinesis method. Biologically active levels of LTB_4-like material were found in a high proportion of samples from the inflamed, antigen-treated skin (range 100–190 pg LTB_4 equivalents/ml, $n = 10$) but not in samples from vehicle-treated skin. In the same experiments, the levels of 12-HETE, measured by quantitative GC–MS, were not significantly different in allergen and vehicle-treated skin (24.5 ± 5.5 versus 15.3 ± 1.3 ng ml^{-1}, $n = 10$)[43]. A statistically significant elevation of the levels of 12-HETE was found in suction blister fluid from ultraviolet B-irradiated skin (41.5 ± 8.6 ng ml^{-1} for 24 h post-irradiation samples versus 13.7 ± 2.6 ng ml^{-1} for control samples, $n = 6$)[61]. Further evidence for the production of arachidonate lipoxygenase products in human skin has come largely from studies of psoriasis.

Eicosanoid production in inflammatory skin disease

Although PGE_2 appears to play a role in mediating some model inflammatory reactions in human skin, there is, as yet, no firm evidence that this or any other prostaglandin plays a significant pathogenetic role in inflammatory skin diseases, which are almost uniformly unresponsive to, and may be aggravated by, cyclo-oxygenase inhibitors. Increased amounts of PGD_2, a major metabolite of arachidonic acid produced by mast cells, have been detected in venous blood draining areas of cold-induced urticaria[49] although no such increase could be demonstrated in suction blister fluid from cold challenged skin[62]. A major metabolite of PGD_2 has also been identified in increased amounts in the urine of patients with mastocytosis[63], but whether the parent compound accumulates in the skin in sufficient amounts to account for part of the inflammatory reaction seen in this disease is unknown.

Hammarström et al.[30] reported modest increases in the levels of PGE_2 in extracts of keratome slices from psoriatic lesions compared with clinically normal skin (33.1 $\pm$ 5.7 ng g^{-1} versus 23.6 $\pm$ 5.0 ng g^{-1}, $n = 7$, as determined by quantitative GC–MS). In our laboratories, PGE_2 levels have been determined by GC–MS in purified extracts of chamber fluid from abraded lesional and clinically normal psoriatic skin but were not found to be significantly different (9.6 $\pm$ 1.8 ng ml^{-1} lesional versus 7.7 $\pm$ 1.9 ng ml^{-1} clinically normal, $n = 5$)[65]. It therefore appears unlikely that PGE_2 plays an important pro-inflammatory role in psoriasis, a view supported by clinical experience which indicates that drugs such as indomethacin are therapeutically ineffective in, and may even aggravate, this disease[65]. The apparent exacerbation of certain skin diseases by indomethacin[66–68] may be explained by a diversion of the metabolism of arachidonic acid to biologically active lipoxygenase products via indomethacin-insensitive pathways, or by the removal of the inhibitory effects exerted by prostaglandins on certain cellular functions.

Much information concerning the role of arachidonate lipoxygenase products in human inflammatory disease has come from the study of psoriasis. This is a common and often hereditary skin disease characterized by inflammation and epidermal cell proliferation which, together, give rise to the typical chronic, red, scaly skin lesions. The aetiology and pathogenesis of the disease are obscure. Neutrophil infiltrates in the dermis and epidermis are a consistent feature of psoriasis[69] and appear to be an early phenomenon in developing lesions[70]. The pathogenetic importance of locally produced neutrophil chemoattractants has therefore been of interest.

The first report of abnormal arachidonic acid metabolism in psoriasis was by Hammarström et al.[30] who used quantitative GC–MS to show that arachidonic acid (36.3 $\pm$ 16.7 μg g^{-1} versus 1.4 $\pm$ 0.4 μg g^{-1}, $n = 7$) and 12-HETE (4.1 $\pm$ 1.9 μg g^{-1} versus < 0.05 $\pm$ 0.01 μg g^{-1}, $n = 7$) levels were significantly raised in lipid extracts of keratome slices from lesional as opposed to clinically normal skin. Subsequently it was shown that 12-HETE was present in biologically active amounts in extracts of chamber fluid and scale from lesional psoriatic skin. In these experiments, extracts were purified by straight phase HPLC and evaporated fractions assayed by the agarose microdroplet chemokinesis method[31]. Semi-quantitative GC–MS analysis of purified extracts of lesional psoriatic scale has confirmed the presence of large amounts of 12-HETE (730 $\pm$ 300 ng g^{-1} $n = 10$)[71]. GC–MS analysis of chamber fluid has also shown greater release of 12-HETE from abraded lesional as opposed to clinically normal skin (45.9 $\pm$ 4.2 ng ml^{-1} versus 18.5 $\pm$ 5.1 ng ml^{-1}, $n = 5$)[64]. The difference between the amounts of 12-HETE in lesional and uninvolved samples was not as great as that described by Hammarström et al.[30]. This discrepancy may be explained by the sampling methods used. Hammarström et al. assayed extracts of keratome slices, which would include large amounts of scale in the lesional but not uninvolved skin samples. The microgramme amounts of 12-HETE found in the keratomed lesional samples may therefore be derived largely from the scale which is rich in 12-HETE[71] and which may act as a reservoir for lipid compounds. In contrast, the chamber fluid sampling method involves removal of scale during the abrasion procedure and is likely to reflect release of material from the deeper, viable, epidermal layers. Use of the skin chamber sampling method, combined with GC–MS analysis, also confirmed elevated levels of arachidonic acid in lesional versus clinically normal skin ($494 \pm 88 \, \text{ng ml}^{-1}$ versus $154 \pm 38 \, \text{ng ml}^{-1}$, $n = 5$)[64], but again the difference was less than that found when keratome slices were analysed[30].

For some years it was widely assumed that the 12-HETE in lesional psoriatic scale was stereochemically identical to 12(S)-HETE produced by platelets. However, recent work has shown that this is not the case[35]. Lipid extracts of psoriatic scale were purified chromatographically to yield material which produced a single ultraviolet (UV) absorbing peak on straight phase HPLC. This peak co-eluted with racemic 12-HETE prodced by a photo-oxidation technique and with platelet 12(S)-HETE, and displayed the GC–MS characteristics of 12-HETE. However, resolution of the 12-HETE hydroxyl enantiomers 12(R)- and 12(S)-HETE by HPLC of their tert-butyl dimethylsilyl ester dehydroabietyl urethane derivatives, together with co-injection of the derivatives of 12-HETE from platelets or psoriatic scale, showed that platelet 12(S)-HETE could be resolved from psoriatic 12-HETE, which co-eluted with 12(R)-HETE[35]. The potential importance of this unique 12(R) molecule is heightened by the finding that it is more potent than 12(S)-HETE in the agarose microdroplet assay[36] and that it has a higher binding affinity for neutrophil LTB_4 receptors than 12(S)-HETE (J. Evans and A. Ford-Hutchinson, personal communication).

Biologically active amounts of LTB_4 have also been detected in extracts of scale[46] and chamber fluid[45] from abraded psoriatic lesions. In these experiments, lipid extracts were purified by straight and reversed phase HPLC and evaporated fractions assayed by the agarose microdroplet chemokinesis method. Assay of HPLC purified extracts against standard LTB_4 by the chemokinesis method revealed $1.8–8 \, \text{ng} \, LTB_4$ equivalents per gramme of psoriatic lesional scale ($n = 4$, values uncorrected for recovery), whereas LTB_4 was undetectable in scale obtained by abrading large areas of normal skin[46]. Similarly LTB_4 was undetectable in the majority of chamber fluid samples from uninvolved skin, but $68 \pm 15 \, \text{pg ml}^{-1} \, LTB_4$ equivalents ($n = 7$, values uncorrected for recovery) were found in lesional chamber fluid samples[45]. Although LTB_4 was detectable in these samples by a biological assay, as stated earlier, the amounts present were too low and the interference from impurities too great to allow routine assay by GC–MS.

Other monohydroxy metabolites of arachidonic acid have been identified by GC–MS in extracts of chamber fluid and scale from psoriatic lesions, and include 15-HETE, 11-HETE, 9-HETE, 8-HETE and 5-HETE[31,71]. Most of these compounds are chemotactically active, but appeared to be present in amounts which are too low to stimulate neutrophil movement. The 5-lipoxygenase product 5-HETE was present in the lowest amounts of all the mono-HETE compounds measured and proved to be the most difficult compound to assay. It is of interest that the most abundant monohydroxy fatty acid identified in samples from psoriatic lesions is the chemokinetically inactive linoleic acid metabolite, 13-hydroxyoctadecadienoic acid (13-HODD)[31,71]. This compound has the same ω-configuration as 15-HETE which appears to have 5-lipoxygenase inhibiting properties[72]. Subsequently, it was shown that 13-HODD was also capable of inhibiting the release of LTB_4 from ionophore-stimulated human neutrophils, although its IC_{50} value $(32\,\mu mol\,L^{-1})$ in this respect was higher than that of 15-HETE $(6\,\mu mol\,L^{-1})$[73]. Nevertheless, the large amounts of 13-HODD found in psoriatic lesions suggest that it could play a role as a modulator of 5-lipoxygenase activity in skin. It is also of interest that 13-HODD has recently been found to inhibit the adherence of platelets to vascular endothelium[74] suggesting that it may act to maintain vascular patency in inflammatory skin disease.

Further evidence of increased lipoxygenase activity in psoriasis has come from the identification of the vasoactive sulphidopeptide leukotrienes LTC_4 and LTD_4 in lesional extracts. LTC_4 and D_4 immunoreactivity, measured as LTC_4 equivalents, was greater in chamber fluid from abraded lesional as opposed to clinically normal skin. Purification of lesional chamber fluid and scale extracts by HPLC, followed by radioimmunoassay of fractions, confirmed[^] that the immunoreactivity co-eluted with standard LTC_4 and LTD_4. The formation of these vasoactive compounds may contribute to the erythema and increased blood flow[76] seen in psoriatic lesions.

In vitro production of eicosanoids by skin cells

As described in the introduction to this chapter, one of the criteria to be satisfied if a mediator is to be held responsible for an inflammatory reaction, is the identification of a mechanism for the formation of that mediator in the inflamed tissue. With regard to eicosanoids and skin inflammation, this criterion usually demands the demonstration of eicosanoid biosynthesis by preparations of human skin *in vitro*. Such studies have been carried out with either cultured epidermal cells, or cell suspensions, freshly prepared by trypsinization of epidermal slices, and usually consisting of a mixture of keratinocytes, the predominant cell type, and the macrophage-like Langerhans cells.

It appears to be firmly established that epidermal cell preparations are capable of producing prostaglandin E_2 *in vitro*[59,60]. There have also been several reports of the production of arachidonate lipoxygenase products by epidermal cells *in vitro*. The variable results reported may be partly due to differing experimental conditions, but also to questionable analytical methods. In our hands, small, but biologically active, amounts of LTB_4-like material (pg amounts per 10^7 cells) are produced by epidermal cells, in the presence of exogenous arachidonic acid[77]. However, 12-HETE appears to be the major lipoxygenase product of arachidonic acid produced by epidermal cells *in vitro*[77,78], a finding recently confirmed in studies of the metabolism of radioactive arachidonic acid in our laboratory (P.M. Woollard, personal communication). Whether this *in vitro* epidermal cell product is the 12(R)- or th 12(S)-epimer of 12-HETE, described above, remains to be determined. A recent report that 15-HETE is the major lipoxygenase product in keratin-ocytes[79] is not in agreement with *in vivo* findings, at least in psoriasis, in

122

which 12-HETE is produced in significantly greater quantities than 15-HETE[31,71]. Furthermore, high speed supernatants prepared from sonicated keratinocytes were used in the experiments in which 15-HETE was found to be the major lipoxygenase product[79], and there is evidence that sonication may unmask a 15-lipoxygenase which is not active in intact cells[80,81].

THE PATHOGENETIC ROLE OF CHEMOATTRACTANT ARACHIDONATE LIPOXYGENASE PRODUCTS IN PSORIASIS

The recovery of biologically active amounts of LTB$_4$ and 12-HETE from psoriatic lesions, together with the biological effects of these compounds in human skin, and in particular their ability to elicit the formation of intraepidermal neutrophil microabscesses, sugest that LTB$_4$ and 12-HETE may play an important role in the pathogenesis of psoriasis. This view was reinforced by reports that benoxaprofen, a proposed 5-lipoxygenase inhibitor, was therapeutically effective in psoriasis[82,83]. Subsequently, doubt has been cast upon the ability of benoxaprofen to inhibit 5-lipoxygenase in cell-free systems[84] and in inflammatory exudates in rats *in vivo*[85], and the mode of action of benoxaprofen in psoriasis therefore remains open to question.

Attempts were made to elicit psoriatic lesions in the uninvolved skin of volunteer patients by single and multiple topical applications of LTB$_4$. No patient developed psoriatic lesions at any application site. In addition, daily application of 50 ng LTB$_4$ under occlusion to the same skin site for ten days was unexpectedly associated with a decreased inflammatory response in both normal and psoriatic volunteers. This state of decreased responsiveness did not appear to be due to an effect on circulating leukocytes, since it was possible to elicit a full, acute, response to LTB$_4$ in a previously untreated site adjacent to an area in which decreased responsiveness had been elicited. Histological examination of biopsies also showed that there were significantly fewer intraepidermal neutrophils in biopsies of sites of multiple application of LTB$_4$ when compared with sites of single application[86]. This state of localized decreased responsiveness has also been demonstrated in rabbit skin following repeated intradermal injections of LTB$_4$, as well as the complement fragment, C5a, and formyl-methionyl-leucyl-phenylalanine (FMLP)[87,88].

The mechanism underlying this desensitization phenomenon has not been established, but explanations may include tachyphylaxis at the level of interaction between endothelial cells and neutrophils, or the local release of an inhibitor of neutrophil movement. Whatever the explanation, the phenomenon may represent an important mechanism, preventing uncontrolled neutrophil accumulation, particularly in response to such chemoattractants as LTB$_4$ which is produced by neutrophils themselves.

Similar 'tachyphylaxis' and an inability to elicit psoriatic lesions have been observed following repeated applications of racemic 12-HETE and combinations of LTB$_4$ and racemic 12-HETE[89]. These findings have suggested that the production of LTB$_4$ and 12-HETE is unlikely to be a primary event in the pathogenesis of psoriasis, although their formation may be part of a series of phenomena which together culminate in the development of a lesion.

Furthermore, neither compound is specific to psoriasis − production of LTB$_4$ has been demonstrated, for example, in allergic contact dermatitis[43] and atopic dermatitis[90], and 12-HETE in the ultraviolet B reaction[61]. In addition, other neutrophil chemoattractants have been identified in psoriasis, including platelet activating factor[91,92] and an interleukin-1-like compound[93]. The relative importance of the various chemoattractants in psoriasis remains to be established and may ultimately only be determined by the use of specific inhibitors of the formation or effects of these compounds in volunteer patients.

REFERENCES

1. Dale, H.H. (1934). Progress in autopharmacology. A survey of present knowledge of the chemical regulation of certain functions by natural constituents of the tissues. *Bull. Johns Hopkins Hosp.*, **53**, 297−347
2. Peck, M.J., Piper, P.J. and Williams, T.J. (1981). The effects of leukotrienes C$_4$ and D$_4$ on the microvasculature of guinea pig skin. *Prostaglandins*, **21**, 315−321
3. Camp, R.D.R., Coutts, A.A., Greaves, M.W., Kay, A.B. and Walport, M.J. (1983). Responses of human skin to intradermal injection of leukotrienes C$_4$, D$_4$ and B$_4$. *Br. J. Pharmacol.*, **80**, 497−502
4. Soter, N.A., Lewis, R.A., Corey, E.J. and Austen, K.F. (1983). Local effects of synthetic leukotrienes (LTC$_4$, LTD$_4$, LTE$_4$ and LTB$_4$) in human skin. *J. Invest. Dermatol.*, **80**, 115−119
5. Bisgaard, H., Kristensen, J. and Sondergaard, J. (1982). The effect of leukotriene C$_4$ and D$_4$ on cutaneous blood flow in humans. *Prostaglandins*, **23**, 797−801
6. Bisgaard, H., Olsson, P. and Bende, M. (1984). Leukotriene D$_4$ increases nasal blood flow in humans. *Prostaglandins*, **29**, 611−619
7. Williams, T.J. and Morley, J. (1973). Prostaglandins as potentiators of increased vascular permeability in inflammation. *Nature (London)*, **246**, 215−217
8. Williams, T.J. and Peck, M.J. (1977). Role of prostaglandin-mediated vasodilation in inflammation. *Nature (London)*, **270**, 530−532
9. Flower, R.J., Harvey, E.A. and Kingston, W.P. (1976). Inflammatory effects of prostaglandin D$_2$ in rat and human skin. *Br. J. Pharmacol.*, **56**, 229−233
10. Juhlin, L. and Michaelsson, G. (1969). Cutaneous reactions to prostaglandins in healthy subjects and in patients with urticaria and atopic dermatitis. *Acta Derm. Venereol.*, **49**, 251−261
11. Crunkhorn, P. and Willis, A.L. (1971). Cutaneous reactions to intradermal prostaglandins. *Br. J. Pharmacol.*, **41**, 49−56
12. Basran, G.S., Morley, J., Paul, W. and Turner-Warwick, M. (1982). Evidence in man of synergistic interactions between putative mediators of acute inflammation and asthma. *Lancet*, **1**, 935−937
13. Williams, T.J. (1977). Chemical mediators of vascular responses in inflammation: a two mediator hypothesis. *Br. J. Pharmacol.*, **61**, 447−448P
14. Wedmore, C.V. and Williams, T.J. (1981). Control of vascular permeability by polymorphonuclear leucocytes in inflammation. *Nature (London)*, **289**, 646−650
15. Roberts, L.J., Lewis, R.A., Oates, J.A. and Austen, K.F. (1979). Prostaglandin, thromboxane and 12-hydroxy-5,8,10,14-eicosatraenoic acid production by ionophore-stimulated rat serosal mast cells. *Biochim. Biophys. Acta*, **575**, 185−192
16. Lewis, R.A., Soter, N.A., Diamond, P.T., Austen, K.F., Oates, J.A. and Roberts, L.J. (1982). Prostaglandin D$_2$ generation after activation of rat and human mast cells with anti-IgE. *J. Immunol.*, **129**, 1627−1631
17. Barnes, V.F. and Heavey, D.J. (1986). Effect of prostaglandin D$_2$ on histamine-induced weals in human skin. *Br. J. Pharmacol.*, **87**, 357−360
18. Williams, T.J. (1979). Prostaglandin E$_2$, prostaglandin I$_2$ and the vascular changes of inflammation. *Br. J. Pharmacol.*, **65**, 517−524

19. Bonta, I.L. and Parnham, M.J. (1978). Prostaglandins and chronic inflammation. *Biochem. Pharmacol.*, **27** 1611–1623
20. Goodwin, J.S. and Webb, D.R. (1980). Regulation of the immune response by prostaglandins. *Clin. Immunol. Immunopathol.*, **15**, 106–122
21. Asad, S.I., Youlten, L.J.F. and Lessof, M.H. (1985). Specific desensitisation in 'aspirin-sensitive' urticaria. In Champion, R.H., Greaves, M.W., Kobza Black, A. and Pye, R.J. (eds.) *The Urticarias*, pp. 32–38. (London: Churchill Livingstone)
22. Capron, A., Amiesen, J.C., Joseph, M., Auriault, C., Tonner, A.B. and Caen, J. (1985). New functions for platelets and their pathological implications. *Int. Arch. Allergy Appl. Immunol.*, **77**, 107–114
23. van Epps, D.E. (1984). Mediators and modulators of human lymphocyte chemotaxis. *Agents Actions*, **12** (Suppl.), 217–223
24. Kunkel, S.L., Chensue, S.W. and Phan, S.H. (1986). Prostaglandins as endogenous mediators of interleukin 1 production. *J. Immunol.*, **136**, 186–192
25. Turner, S.R., Tainer, J.S. and Lynn, W.S. (1975). Biogenesis of chemotactic molecules by the arachidonic lipoxygenase system of platelets. *Nature (London)*, **257**, 680–681
26. Goetzl, E.J. and Sun, F.F. (1979). Generation of unique monohydroxy-eicosatraenoic acids from arachidonic acid by human neutrophils. *J. Exp. Med.*, **150**, 406–411
27. Palmer, R.M.J., Stepney, R.J., Higgs, G.A. and Eakins, K.E. (1980). Chemokinetic activity of arachidonic acid lipoxygenase products on leucocytes of different species. *Prostaglandins*, **20**, 411–418
28. Hamberg, M. and Samuelsson, B. (1974). Prostaglandin endoperoxides. Novel transformations of arachidonic acid in human platelets. *Proc. Natl. Acad. Sci. USA*, **71**, 3400–3404
29. Nugteren, D.H. (1975). Arachidonate lipoxygenase in blood platelets. *Biochim. Biophys. Acta*, **380**, 299–307
30. Hammarström, S., Hamberg, M., Samuelsson, B., Duell, E.A., Stawski, M. and Voorhees, J.J. (1975). Increased concentrations of nonesterified arachidonic acid, 12L-hydroxyeicosatetraenoic acid, prostaglandin E_2 and prostaglandin F_{2x} in the epidermis of psoriasis. *Proc. Natl. Acad. Sci. USA*, **72**, 5130–5134
31. Camp, R.D.R., Mallet, A.I., Woollard, P.M., Brain, S.D., Kobza Black, A. and Greaves, M.W. (1983). The identification of hydroxy fatty acids in psoriatic skin. *Prostaglandins*, **26**, 431–448
32. Goetzl, E.J., Valone, F.H., Reinhold, V.N. and Gorman, R.R. (1979). Specific inhibition of the polymorphonuclear leukocyte chemotactic response to hydroxy-fatty acid metabolites of arachidonic acid by methyl ester derivatives. *J. Clin. Invest.*, **63**, 1181–1186
33. Dowd, P.M., Kobza Black, A., Woollard, P.M., Camp, R.D. and Greaves, M.W. (1985). Cutaneous responses to 12-hydroxy-5,8,10,14-eicosatetraenoic acid (12-HETE). *J. Invest. Dermatol.*, **84**, 537–541
34. Cunningham, F.M., Woollard, P.M. and Camp, R.D.R. (1985). Proinflammatory properties of unsaturated fatty acids and their monohydroxy metabolites. *Prostaglandins*, **30**, 497–509
35. Woollard, P.M. (1986). Stereochemical difference between 12-hydroxy-5,8,10,14-eicosatetraenoic acid in platelets and psoriatic lesions. *Biochem. Biophys. Res. Commun.*, **136**, 169–176
36. Cunningham, F.M., Greaves, M.W. and Woollard, P.M. (1986). Chemokinetic activity of 12(S) and 12(R) hydroxyeicosatetraenoic acids for human polymorphonuclear leucocytes. *Br. J. Pharmacol.*, **87**, 107P
37. Ford-Hutchinson, A.W., Bray, M.A., Doig, M.V., Shipley, M.E. and Smith, M.J.H. (1980). Leukotriene B_4, a potent chemokinetic and aggregating substance released from polymorphonuclear leucocytes. *Nature (London)*, **286**, 264–265
38. Goetzl, E.J. and Pickett, W.C. (1980). The human PMN leukocyte chemotactic activity of complex hydroxy-eicosatetraenoic acids (HETEs). *J. Immunol.*, **125**, 1789–1791
39. Camp, R., Russell Jones, R., Brain, S., Woollard, P. and Greaves, M. (1984). Production of intraepidermal microabscesses by topical application of leukotriene B_4. *J. Invest. Dermatol.*, **82**, 202–204
40. Kobza Black, A., Greaves, M.W., Hensby, C.N., Plummer, N.A. and Eady, R.A.J. (1977). A new method for recovery of exudate from normal and inflamed human skin. *Clin. Exp. Dermatol.*, **2**, 209–216

41. Black, A.K., Fincham, N., Greaves, M.W. and Hensby, C.N. (1980). Time course changes in levels of arachidonic acid and prostaglandin D_2, E_2, $F_{2\alpha}$ in human skin following ultraviolet B irradiation. *Br. J. Clin. Pharmacol.*, **10**, 453–457

42. Plummer, N.A., Hensby, C.N., Kobza Black, A. and Greaves, M.W. (1977). Prostaglandin activity in sustained inflammation of human skin before and after aspirin. *Clin. Sci. Mol. Med.*, **52**, 615–620

43. Barr, R.M., Brain, S., Camp, R.D.R., Cilliers, J., Greaves, M.W., Mallet, A.I. and Misch, K. (1984). Levels of arachidonic acid and its metabolites in the skin in human allergic and irritant contact dermatitis. *Br. J. Dermatol.*, **111**, 23–28

44. Brain, S.D., Camp, R.D.R., Dowd, P.M., Kobza Black, A., Woollard, P.M., Mallet, A.I. and Greaves, M.W. (1982). Psoriasis and leukotriene B_4. *Lancet*, **2**, 762–763

45. Brain, S., Camp, R., Dowd, P., Kobza Black, A. and Greaves, M.W. (1984). The release of leukotriene B_4-like material in biologically active amounts from the lesional skin of patients with psoriasis. *J. Invest. Dermatol.*, **83**, 70–73

46. Brain, S.D., Camp, R.D.R., Cunningham, F.M., Dowd, P.M., Greaves, M.W. and Kobza Black, A. (1984). Leukotriene B_4-like material in scale of psoriatic lesions. *Br. J. Pharmacol.*, **83**, 313–317

47. Greaves, M.W., Sondergaard, J. and McDonald-Gibson, W. (1971). Recovery of prostaglandins in human cutaneous inflammation. *Br. Med. J.*, **2**, 258–260

48. Greaves, M.W. and Sondergaard, J. (1970). Pharmacological studies in cutaneous inflammation in man using an *in vivo* perfusion method. *Br. J. Dermatol.*, **82** (Suppl. 6), 82–85

49. Heavey, D.J., Kobza Black, A., Barrow, S.E., Chappell, C.G., Greaves, M.W. and Dollery, C.T. (1985). Prostaglandin D_2 and histamine release in cold urticaria. *Br. J. Clin. Pharmacol.* **20**, 270P

50. Vane, J.R. (1964). The use of isolated organs for detecting active substances in the circulating blood. *Br. J. Pharmacol.*, **23**, 360–373

51. Kobza Black, A., Greaves, M.W., Hensby, C.N. and Plummer, N.A. (1978). Increased prostaglandins E_2 and $F_{2\alpha}$ in human skin at 6 and 24 h after ultraviolet B irradiation (290–320 nm). *Br. J. Clin. Pharmacol.*, **5**, 431–436

52. Smith, M.J.H. and Walker, J.R. (1980). The effects of some antirheumatic drugs on an *in vitro* model of human polymorphonuclear leucocyte chemokinesis. *Br. J. Pharmacol.*, **69**, 473–478

53. Harvath, L., Falk, W. and Leonard, E.J. (1980). Rapid quantitation of neutrophil chemotaxis: use of a polyvinylpyrrolidone-free polycarbonate membrane in a multiwell assembly. *J. Immunol. Meth*, **37**, 39–45

54. Greaves, M.W., Barr, R. and Camp, R. (1984). Leukotriene B_4-like immunoreactivity and skin disease. *Lancet*, **2**, 160

55. Barr, R.M., Black, A.K., Francis, D.M., Koro, O., Numata, T. and Greaves, M.W. (1986). Release of prostaglandin D_2 (PGD_2) from human skin *in vivo* during cutaneous anaphylaxis. *Br. J. Pharmacol.* (In press)

56. Barr, R.M., Black, A., Dover, J.S., Francis, D., Greaves, M.W., Kelly, R.W. and Koro, O. (1986). Prostaglandin D_2 release in localised heat urticaria. *Br. J. Pharmacol.*, **87**, 103P

57. Black, A.K., Greaves, M.W., Hensby, C.N., Plummer, N.A. and Warin, A.P. (1978). The effects of indomethacin on arachidonic acid and prostaglandins E_2 and $F_{2\alpha}$ levels in human skin 24 h after u.v.B and u.v.C irradiation. *Br. J. Clin. Pharmacol.*, **6**, 261–266

58. Farr, P.M. and Diffey, B.L. (1985). A quantitative study of the effects of topical indomethacin on cutaneous erythema induced by ultraviolet radiation (UVR). *Br. J. Dermatol.*, **113**, 771–772

59. Jonsson, C-E. and Anggard, E. (1972). Biosynthesis and metabolism of prostaglandin E_2 in human skin. *Scand. J. Clin. Lab. Invest.*, **29**, 289–296

60. Ziboh, V.A. (1973). Biosynthesis of prostaglandin E_2 in human skin: subcellular localisation and inhibition by unsaturated fatty acids and anti-inflammatory drugs. *J. Lipid Res.*, **14**, 377–384

61. Kobza Black, A., Barr, R.M., Wong, E., Brain, S., Greaves, M.W., Dickenson, R., Shroot, B. and Hensby, C.N. (1985). Lipoxygenase products of arachidonic acid in human inflamed skin. *Br. J. Clin. Pharmacol.*, **20**, 185–190

62. Misch, K., Black, A.K., Barr, R.M., Hensby, C.N., Mallet, A.I. and Greaves, M.W. (1982). Histamine and non-histamine pharmacological activity in cold urticaria. *J. Invest. Dermatol.*, **78**, 329

63. Roberts, L.J., Sweetman, B.J., Lewis, R.A., Austen, K.F. and Oates, J.A. (1980). Increased production of prostaglandin D₂ in patients with systemic mastocytosis. *N. Engl. J. Med.*, **303**, 1400–1404

64. Barr, R.M., Wong, E., Mallet, A.I., Olins, L.A. and Greaves, M.W. (1984). The analysis of arachidonic acid metabolites in normal, uninvolved and lesional psoriatic skin. *Prostaglandins*, **28**, 57–65

65. Ellis, N., Fallon, J.D., Heezen, J.L. and Voorhees, J.J. (1983). Topical indomethacin exacerbates lesions of psoriasis. *J. Invest. Dermatol.*, **80**, 362

66. Griffiths, C.E.M., Leonard, J.N. and Fry, L. (1985). Dermatitis herpetiformis exacerbated by indomethacin. *Br. J. Dermatol.*, **112**, 443–445

67. Harrington, C.I. and Messenger, A.G. (1986). Dermatitis herpetiformis. *Br. J. Dermatol.*, **114**, 265–266

68. Katayama, H. and Kawada, A. (1981). Exacerbation of psoriasis induced by indomethacin. *J. Dermatol.*, **8**, 323–327

69. Ragaz, A. and Ackerman, A.B. (1979). Evolution, maturation, and regression of lesions of psoriasis. *Am. J. Dermatopathol.*, **1**, 199–214

70. Chowaniec, O., Jablonska, S., Beutner, E.H., Proniewska, M., Jarzabek-Chorzelska, M. and Rzesa, G. (1981). Earliest clinical and histological changes in psoriasis. *Dermatologica*, **163**, 42–51

71. Woollard, P.M. and Mallet, A.I. (1984). Lipoxygenase products. A novel gas chromatographic–mass spectrometric assay for monohydroxy fatty acids. *J. Chromatogr.*, **306**, 1–21

72. Vanderhoek, J.Y., Bryant, R.W. and Bailey, J.M. (1980). Inhibition of leukotriene biosynthesis by the leukocyte product 15-hydroxy-5,8,11,13-eicosatetraenoic acid. *J. Biol. Chem.*, **255**, 10064–10066

73. Camp, R.D.R. and Fincham, N.J. (1985). Inhibition of ionophore-stimulated leukotriene B₄ production in human leucocytes by monohydroxy fatty acids. *Br. J. Pharmacol.*, **85**, 837–841

74. Buchanan, M.R., Haas, T.A., Lagarde, M. and Guichardant, M. (1985). 13-Hydroxyoctadecadienoic acid is the vessel wall chemorepellant factor LOX. *J. Biol. Chem.*, **260**, 16056–16059

75. Brain, S.D., Camp, R.D.R., Kobza Black, A., Dowd, P.M., Greaves, M.W., Ford-Hutchinson, A.W. and Charleson, S. (1985). Leukotrienes C₄ and D₄ in psoriatic skin lesions. *Prostaglandins*, **29**, 611–619

76. Klemp, P. and Staberg, B. (1983). Cutaneous blood flow in psoriasis. *J. Invest. Dermatol.*, **81**, 503–506

77. Fincham, N., Camp, R. and Leigh, I. (1985). Synthesis of arachidonate lipoxygenase products by epidermal cells. *J. Invest. Dermatol.*, **84**, 447

78. Hammarstrom, S., Lindgren, J.A., Marcelo, C., Duell, E.A., Andersson, T.F. and Voorhees, J.J. (1979). Arachidonic acid transformations in normal and psoriatic skin. *J. Invest. Dermatol.*, **73**, 180–183

79. Burrall, B.A., Wintroub, B.U. and Goetzl, E.J. (1985). Selective expression of 15-lipoxygenase activity by cultured keratinocytes. *Biochem. Biophys. Res. Commun.*, **133**, 208–213

80. Kuhn, H., Ponicke, K., Halle, W., Wiesner, R., Schewe, T. and Forster, W. (1985). Metabolism of [1-¹⁴C]-arachidonic acid by cultured calf aortic endothelial cells: evidence for the presence of a lipoxygenase pathway. *Prostagl. Leuk. Med.*, **17**, 291–303

81. McGuire, J., McGee, J., Crittenden, N. and Fitzpatrick, F. (1985). Cell damage unmasks 15-lipoxygenase activity in human neutrophils. *J. Biol. Chem.*, **260**, 8316–8319

82. Kragballe, K. and Herlin, T. (1983). Benoxaprofen improves psoriasis. *Arch. Dermatol.*, **119**, 548–552

83. Allen, B.R. and Littlewood, S.M. (1982). Benoxaprofen : effect on cutaneous lesions in psoriasis. *Br. Med. J.*, **285**, 1241

84. Masters, D.J., Spruce, K.E., Vickers, V.C. and McMillan, R.M. (1985). Measurement of arachidonate metabolism using cyanopropyl mini-columns: effects of cyclooxygenase and lipoxygenase inhibitors. *Br. J. Pharmacol.*, **84**, 45P

85. Salmon, J.A., Higgs, G.A., Tilling, L., Moncada, S. and Vane, J.R. (1984). Mode of action of benoxaprofen. *Lancet*, **2**, 848

127

86. Wong, E., Camp, R.D. and Greaves, M.W. (1985). The responses of normal and psoriatic skin to single and multiple topical applications of leukotriene B$_4$. *J. Invest. Dermatol.*, **84**, 421–423
87. Colditz, I.G. and Movat, H.Z. (1984). Chemotactic factor-specific desensitization of skin to infiltration by polymorphonuclear leukocytes. *Immunol. Lett.*, **8**, 83–87
88. Colditz, I.G. and Movat, H.Z. (1984). Desensitization of acute inflammatory lesions to chemotaxins and endotoxin. *J. Immunol.*, **133**, 2163–2168
89. Dowd, P.M., Kobza Black, A., Woollard, P.M. and Greaves, M.W. (1986). Cutaneous tolerance and cross-tolerance to 12(R,S)-HETE and LTB$_4$. *Clin. Exp. Dermatol.*, **11**, 199–200
90. Ruzicka, T., Simmet, T., Peskar, B.A. and Ring, J. (1986). Skin levels of arachidonic acid-derived inflammatory mediators and histamine in atopic dermatitis and psoriasis. *J. Invest. Dermatol.*, **86**, 105–108
91. Mallet, A.I., Cunningham, F.M. and Daniel, R. (1984). Rapid isocratic high performance liquid chromatographic purification of platelet activating factor (PAF) and lyso-PAF in human skin. *J. Chromatogr.*, **309**, 160–164
92. Mallet, A.I. and Cunningham, F.M. (1985). Structural identification of platelet activating factor in psoriatic scale. *Biochem. Biophys. Res. Commun.*, **126**, 192–198
93. Camp, R.D.R., Chu, A., Cunningham, F.M., Fincham, N.J., Greaves, M.W. and Morris, J. (1986). Identification of an interleukin-1-like peptide in psoriasis. *Br. J. Pharmacol.*, (In press)

7
The Role of Eicosanoids in Inflammatory Diseases of the Joints

B. HENDERSON

INTRODUCTION

The synovial joint is prey to a variety of diseases including a number of inflammatory lesions. The most serious of these inflammatory diseases is rheumatoid arthritis (RA). This distressing condition is relatively common, affecting about 1% of the population. Because of the severity and incidence of RA, most studies of the role of eicosanoids in inflammatory joint disease have concentrated on this lesion.

SYMPTOMS AND PATHOLOGY OF RHEUMATOID ARTHRITIS

Rheumatoid arthritis is a chronic inflammatory, probably autoimmune, disease, afflicting the peripheral synovial joints in a symmetrical manner. The synovial joints are involved in the following order of frequency: (1) hands, wrists and ankles; (2) shoulders, elbows, hips and knees; and (3) vertebral column. The principal symptoms of disease are pain and swelling in the afflicted joints. Large joints, such as the knee, often contain an effusion. Associated with these symptoms is the progressive destruction of the collagenous structures of the joints: articular cartilage; subchondral bone; ligaments etc. It is this damage to tissues that results in rheumatoid joints becoming crippled.

The structure of a 'typical' synovial joint is shown in Figure 7.1 alongside diagrammatic representations of the histology of the normal and rheumatoid synovial lining. The synovial joint consists of two or more bone ends covered with a resilient layer of articular cartilage. Surrounding these bone ends is a strong fibrous capsule which functions to maintain joint congruity and stability. The inner aspect of the joint capsule is a thin glistening tissue termed the synovial lining. This highly vascularized tissue is believed to keep the joint space free from debris and to facilitate the nutrition of the cartilage

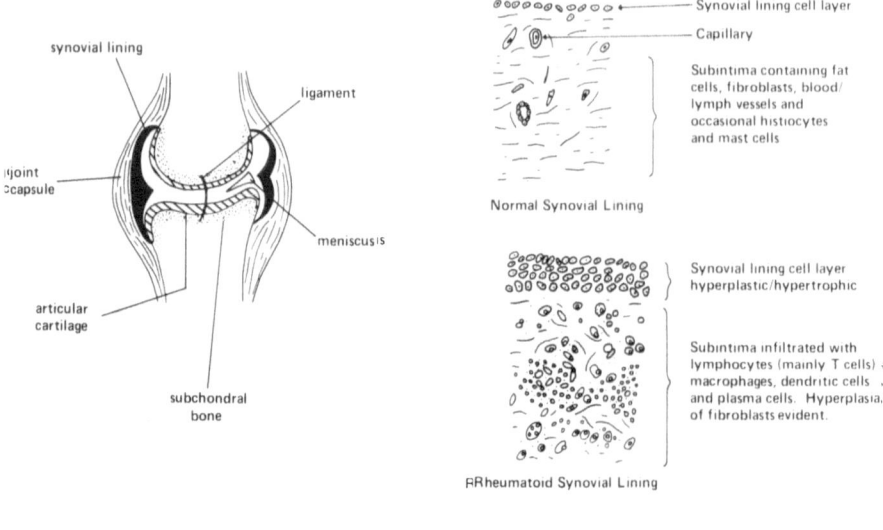

Figure 7.1 Schematic representation of : (A) the structure of the synovial joint and (B) histology of the normal and rheumatoid synovial lining

among other functions[1]. It is this synovial lining which is the target tissue in RA. The normal synovial lining is a pleomorphic connective tissue, characterized by the presence of a layer of cells (composed of macrophages and fibroblast-like cells and collectively called synovial lining cells) at the tissue surface, i.e. adjacent to the joint space. An extensive capillary network is present beneath the synovial lining cell layer (Figure 7.1). In rheumatoid arthritis, the synovial lining is heavily infiltrated with mononuclear cells. The T lymphocyte is the predominant lymphoid cell present in the synovial infiltrate. Immunocytochemical studies using monoclonal antibodies specific for T cell subsets suggest that the majority of these cells are activated helper T cells[2]. The rheumatoid synovial lining also contains large numbers of HLA-DR positive macrophages and the macrophage-like dendritic cells which are now believed to be important in the perpetuation of this lesion[3]. Studies of the distribution of infiltrating cells in the rheumatoid synovial lining have led to the suggestion that this tissue has many of the characteristics of a hyperactive, immunologically-stimulated lymphoid organ[3]. In addition to the increased cellularity of the rheumatoid synovial lining, as a result of cellular infiltration, there is a further increase in tissue cellularity due to hyperplasia of the synovial lining cell, fibroblast and blood vessel cell populations[1]. Few polymorphonuclear leukocytes (PMN) are found in the rheumatoid synovial lining. However, large numbers of these cells are present in the synovial fluid. How these cells manage to get into the synovial effusion without being seen, in any great numbers, in the synovial lining, is unexplained. The presence of infiltrating cells in the RA joint is associated with damage to articular cartilage and bone.

The mechanisms believed to be responsible for this tissue erosion will be discussed.

If pain and swelling in the synovial joints were the only consequences of RA, this disease would not be regarded as particularly serious. Unfortunately, in a sizeable proportion of patients, there is progressive damage to articular cartilage, subchrondral bone and intra-articular ligaments and tendons. Destruction of cartilage and bone occurs in a centripetal fashion, and, as with ligament and tendon damage, is believed to be due to the action of the inflamed synovial lining. The mechanism by which this tissue damage is brought about is still not fully understood and will be discussed in a later section. It should be pointed out at this stage that of the wide range of anti-inflammatory and antirheumatic drugs used in the treatment of RA, only gold compounds appear to have an influence, albeit limited, on the progress of tissue damage[4].

DRUG THERAPY IN RHEUMATOID ARTHRITIS

Salicylic acid was processed from salicin (obtained from the willow tree) in 1860 and was used in the treatment of rheumatic diseases a few years later. The preparation, acetylsalicylic acid, was introduced by Bayer in 1899 under the trade name aspirin and has been used in the treatment of rheumatic diseases, including RA, ever since[5]. A host of explanations were propounded to account for the anti-inflammatory and analgesic actions of aspirin. The discovery that aspirin-like anti-inflammatory drugs are potent and selective inhibitors of prostaglandin biosynthesis led Vane to propose this biochemical intervention as the mode of action[6]. This theory is now generally accepted and the inhibition of the synthesis of PGE_2 and prostacyclin explains the antioedema, antierythema, antipyretic and analgesic properties of aspirin and the newer non-steroidal anti-inflammatory drugs (NSAIDs). Vane's hypothesis implicated the prostaglandins, and, with their subsequent discovery, other cyclo-oxygenase products, as important mediators of the pathology of RA. In the years since this seminal work, much attention has been paid to measuring prostanoids, and more recently, leukotrienes, in synovial fluid and to the study of the production of these mediators by tissues of the normal and inflamed joint.

EICOSANOIDS IN SYNOVIAL FLUID AND THE INFLUENCE OF DRUG THERAPY

If eicosanoids contribute to the pathology of RA, then they should be present at biologically active levels within the joint. As a corollary, administration of NSAIDs should significantly lower these levels in joint tissues. The first studies of prostaglandin levels in rheumatoid patients were reported by Higgs and colleagues[7] and Robinson and Levine[8]. The former group used bioassay to measure prostaglandins and reported a concentration of $18.8 \pm 5.3\ \text{ng ml}^{-1}$ (mean $\pm$ SEM) PGE_2 equivalent in untreated synovial effusions compared

131

with 2.6 ± 0.8 ng ml^{-1} in patients receiving aspirin-like drugs (Table 7.1). In one patient, who volunteered to change from a NSAID to the centrally acting analgesic dextropropoxyphene (which does not inhibit cyclo-oxygenase), the PGE$_2$-equivalent levels in the synovial fluid rose from 6.9 ng ml^{-1} to 14.9 ng ml^{-1} 100 h after cessation of NSAID and fell to 10.7 ng ml^{-1} when treatment recommenced. The rise in prostaglandin levels on cessation of NSAID therapy was not accompanied by any change in the leucocyte count in the synovial fluid. Three patients treated with prednisolone were included in this survey. One of these patients had the highest level of PGE$_2$ recorded in this study and the remaining two had relatively high levels compared with the NSAID-treated group.

Using a radioimmunoassay for PGB (the stable product obtained by treating PGE/PGA with alkali), Robinson and Levine[8] reported qualitatively similar results to Higgs et al.[7]. However, the concentrations of PGB found in the rheumatoid synovial effusions were very much lower (Table 7.1). The difference may, in part, be accounted for by the fact that Robinson and Levine grouped patients with RA, gout, pseudogout or infectious arthritis together. whereas Higgs and co-workers only studied patients with RA.

Subsequent studies have confirmed these initial findings that the treatment of rheumatoid patients with NSAIDs lowers the concentration of PGE$_2$ and of other prostanoids in the synovial fluid (Table 7.1). The limited number of studies in which various prostanoids have been assayed suggests that PGE$_2$ is the major product of cyclo-oxygenase activity in rheumatoid synovial fluid[9-14] (Table 7.2).

Table 7.1 Influence of drugs on PGE$_2$ concentrations in rheumatoid synovial fluid

Concentration of PGE$_2$ in ng ml^{-1}				
Untreated	NSAID treated	Steroid treated	Assay	Reference
18.8 ± 5.3 (11)	2.6 ± 0.8 (11)	24.4 ± 18.8 (3)	Bioassay	7
0.35 (34)	0.086 (18)	—	RIA of PGB	8
8.6 ± 2.7 (5)	0.15 ± 0.04 (9)	—	RIA	9
0.15 ± 0.02 (6)	0.015 ± 0.004 (6)	—	RIA	12
0.11 ± 0.02 (17)	—	0.11 ± 0.02	RIA	12
3.6 ± 3.0 (8)	1.9 ± 0.8 (8)	—	RIA	13

( ) number of patients studied
Results expressed as mean $\pm$ SEM

Table 7.2 Concentration of eicosanoids in rheumatoid synovial fluids

Concentration of eicosanoids in ng ml^{-1}					
PGE$_2$	PGD$_2$	PGF$_{2\alpha}$	6-Keto-PGF$_{1\alpha}$	TxB$_2$	Reference
8.6 ± 2.7	—	1.2 ± 0.3	—	0.7 ± 0.1	9
1.3 ± 0.8	—	0.1 ± 0.07	—	—	11
0.1 ± 0.02	—	0.03 ± 0.004	0.1 ± 0.03	0.13 ± 0.03	12
0.9 ± 0.1	0.16 ± 0.02	0.16 ± 0.02	0.18 ± 0.02	0.19 ± 0.02	14

The reported concentrations of PGE_2 in rheumatoid synovial fluid cover a wide range (0.1−18.8 ng ml^{-1} for fluids from patients not receiving drug therapy). It is not immediately clear what factors are responsible for this variation in the PGE_2 concentrations reported by various groups. Probably the major factor is the treatment of the synovial fluid after withdrawal from the joint. Stimulation of inflammatory cells in the effusion could result either in the release or the breakdown of prostanoids. Other variables, such as the groups of patients selected, the severity of the disease, and the assays used, may also influence the concentrations of eicosanoids measured.

Pharmacokinetic studies[15] of the aspirin-like drug, indoprofen, show that it rapidly enters the synovial cavity and inhibits the production of PGE_2. In contrast, the administration of 6α-methylprednisolone (4− 8 mg/day) for 4 − 8 days had no effect on synovial fluid PGE_2, $PGF_{2\alpha}$ or TxB_2 levels, while indoprofen, given for the same duration, significantly lowered the levels of these prostanoids[12]. Neither of these drugs had any effect on the numbers of leukocytes in the rheumatoid synovial fluid.

Very high levels of LTB_4 (in the order of 150 ng ml^{-1}) have been reported to be present in the synovial fluids of patients with seropositive RA[16]. Even higher levels were found in patients with spondylarthritis (arthritis of the spine). No correlation was found between the concentration of LTB_4 and the number of infiltrating cells in the synovial fluid as might be expected if LTB_4 was functioning as a chemoattractant. A further surprise was the ability to extract more LTB_4 from control than from rheumatoid synovial lining tissue. The method used to quantitate the LTB_4 was UV absorbance which is insensitive. Using the same method, Smith and co-workers could not detect LTB_4 in RA synovial fluid. However, using a sensitive bioassay, it was demonstrated[17] that LTB_4 was present at a mean concentration of 0.3 ng ml^{-1} (0.34 ± 0.14 ng ml^{-1}; mean ± SEM; n = 12). Larger amounts of bioassayable LTB_4 have been found in the synovial fluids of patients with gout[18] (mean concentration 2.7 ng ml^{-1}: range 0.2−7.4).

In antigen-induced arthritis in the rabbit, an experimental lesion closely resembling rheumatoid arthritis, biologically active levels of PGE_2 are present in the synovial fluids of arthritic joints during the acute and chronic stages of disease. In contrast, immunoreactive LTB_4 is only found in any quantity during the acute phase. The pattern of prostanoid production by the arthritic synovial lining from these experimental animals is similar to that found with rheumatoid synovial lining explants[19]. However, the inflamed synovial lining of the rabbit produced[20] only small quantities of LTB_4. These studies will be dealt with in more detail in Chapter 9.

JOINT TISSUES RESPONSIBLE FOR EICOSANOID SYNTHESIS

Prostanoids and LTB_4 are found in the cell-free synovial effusions of patients with rheumatoid arthritis. The likely source of these mediators include: (1) the infiltrating cells in the fluid, (2) the inflamed synovial lining and (3) articular cartilage.

The predominant cells in the rheumatoid synovial fluid infiltrate are PMN leukocytes. PMNs are also the predominant infiltrating cells in many experimental inflammatory exudates such as those induced by implanting carrageenin-soaked sponges in rats. In both the rheumatoid synovial fluid and the sponge exudate, PGE_2 is the major eicosanoid detected. The PMNs in the sponge are not a major source of PGE_2 as levels of this prostanoid are not diminished when PMN accumulation is prevented by colchicine[21]. By inference, it is assumed that the PMNs in rheumatoid synovial effusions are not producing PGE_2. Cells present in rheumatoid synovial effusions have been found to produce small quantities of PGE_2 (range $0.4-1.9 \, ng/10^6$ cells per 24 h, $n = 4$) but it is assumed that this is due to the activity of the macrophages in the fluid[10].

Homogenates and microsomal preparations of normal, osteoarthritic or rheumatoid synovial lining produce PGE_2, $PGF_{2\alpha}$ and small amounts of TxB_2. Rheumatoid tissues are the most active producers of prostanoids[22,23]. Of course, this is likely to be a reflection of the relative cellularity of rheumatoid and non-rheumatoid synovial lining tissue. Homogenates of most tissues will produce prostanoids and this methodology gives little information about the cellular control of eicosanoid metabolism.

Explants of rheumatoid synovial lining[10,24,25], maintained for several days in culture medium containing serum, produced PGE_2 and smaller amounts of $PGF_{2\alpha}$. Rheumatoid synovial lining explants, maintained under similar conditions, produced significantly more PGE_2 than explants of normal synovial lining removed from patients undergoing amputation[26]. Similar results were found when explants were maintained under serum-free conditions although the maximum production of PGE_2 was lower. To determine whether cells isolated from the synovial lining would also show such differences in PGE_2 synthesis, both normal and rheumatoid tissues were enzymatically disaggregated. The adherent cells were then assayed, at various intervals for their production of PGE_2. Rheumatoid adherent cells only produced more PGE_2 during the first few days following isolation. During this time the non-adherent, possibly lymphoid, cells were still present. This suggests that cellular interactions are required for the stimulation of eicosanoid synthesis[26].

Explants of non-rheumatoid (obtained at meniscectomy) or rheumatoid synovial lining have been maintained in serum-free, adult organ maintenance culture for 24 h to investigate the capacity of these tissues to produce a range of prostanoids. The major product, both of the chronically inflamed rheumatoid and the mildly inflamed non-rheumatoid tissues, was PGE_2. The rhematoid synovial lining produced significantly more PGE_2 than the non-rheumatoid tissue (mean of $7.3 \, ng \, mg^{-1}$ tissue compared with $2.5 \, ng \, mg^{-1}$). The rheumatoid tissues also produced more prostacyclin (measured as its stable hydrolysis product, 6-keto-$PGF_{1\alpha}$) but the difference was not statistically significant. However, measurement of thromboxane levels in culture fluids revealed that the rheumatoid tissue produced a mean of 15 times as much of this prostanoid as the control (Figure 7.2). The presence of PGE_2, 6-keto-$PGF_{1\alpha}$ and TxB_2 in extracts of the culture fluid was positively confirmed by gas–liquid chromatography and mass spectrometry[19].

These studies demonstrate that the rheumatoid synovial lining produces large amounts of prostanoids, including thromboxane. It has not been

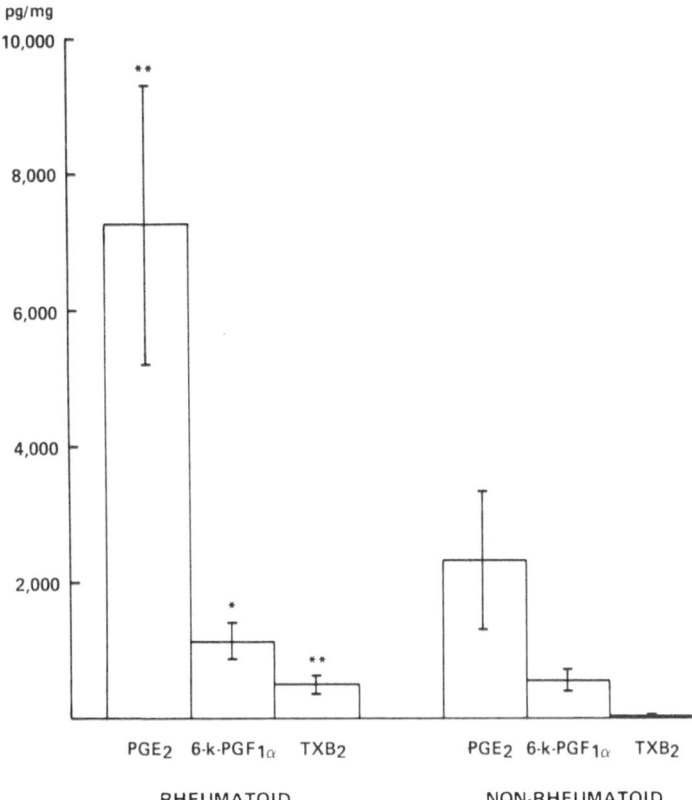

Figure 7.2 Mean concentrations of PGE_2, 6-keto-$PGF_{1\alpha}$ and TxB_2 in the culture media from rheumatoid (n = 9) and non-rheumatoid (n = 6) synovial lining explants. The bars represent $\pm$ SEM. *p < 0.1, **p < 0.05, compared with the non-rheumatoid group. (Reproduced from reference 19, with permission)

established whether the rheumatoid synovial lining can produce 5-lipoxygenase products such as LTB_4.

Rheumatoid synovial lining explants have been used to determine the ability of a range of drugs used in the treatment of RA to inhibit cyclooxygenase activity[25]. As would be expected, all NSAIDs tested inhibited PGE_2 synthesis. The IC_{50} for each NSAID in culture was equivalent to, or less than, the peak free plasma concentration of the drug. The glucocorticoids were potent inhibitors of PGE_2 synthesis with IC_{50} values of 3-30 nmol L^{-1}. Antirheumatic drugs commonly used in the treatment of RA, (hydroxy)-chloroquine, penicillamine, gold sodium thiomalate and azathioprine, were all weak inhibitors of prostaglandin synthesis. Gold and penicillamine have also been shown to have weak anti-inflammatory activity *in vivo* in carrageenin sponge-induced acute inflammation[27].

Chondrocytes, the cellular elements of articular cartilage, produce various prostanoids in culture[28,29]. The rate of production of PGE_2 is similar to that

135

of synovial cells and it is not known if production is increased in RA. However, in view of the hypocellularity of articular cartilage, it is unlikely that the chondrocytes contribute significantly to the pool of eicosanoids found in rheumatoid synovial effusions.

From the available evidence it seems likely that the main source of the eicosanoids found in the synovial fluid of the rheumatoid joint is the chronically inflamed synovial lining. In addition to the normal resident population of synovial lining cells (containing a mixture of macrophages and fibroblasts), this tissue contains infiltrating macrophages, fibroblasts and endothelial cells, all of which are capable of synthesizing prostanoids.

CONTROL OF EICOSANOID SYNTHESIS AND THE CELL POPULATIONS INVOLVED

Based upon the findings that explants of rheumatoid synovial lining produce large amounts of prostanoids, compared with normal or non-rheumatoid tissues, the capacity of isolated synovial cells to produce cyclo-oxygenase products has been investigated. In the majority of studies, the rheumatoid synovial lining tissue has been minced and proteolytically disaggregated to produce a mixed cell population. Immediately following isolation, the cultures contain a variable mixture of adherent and non-adherent cells. The adherent cells are large with a stellate/dendritic morphology and lack surface markers associated with the monocyte/macrophage cell population. These stellate/dendritic cells are not to be confused with the antigen-presenting dendritic cells described by Poulter and Janossy[3]. During the first days of culture, these cells produce large quantities of PGE_2[30-32] and 6-keto-$PGF_{1\alpha}$[33]. However, with increasing duration of culture, the adherent cells lose their stellate morphology and the rate of production of PGE_2 falls so that normal and rheumatoid cells produce[32,33] similar but small amounts of PGE_2. This decline in the ability of the rheumatoid adherent stellate cells to synthesize PGE_2 is associated with the disappearance from cultures of cells bearing macrophage markers, such as surface Fc receptors and lysozyme production[30]. This suggests that it is the interaction between the macrophages and the adherent stellate cells that is responsible for the increased PGE_2 synthesis of rheumatoid synovial cell cultures (Figure 7.3).

Cultured human peripheral blood mononuclear cells, which include lymphocytes and monocytes, were found to release a factor which stimulated, up to 200-fold, PGE_2 production by isolated adherent rheumatoid synovial cells. This factor also stimulated collagenase production[31]. The factor responsible for stimulating PGE_2 and collagenase was termed mononuclear cell factor (MCF) and is released by macrophages but not lymphocytes[34]. By a number of criteria, it has been established that MCF is equivalent to interleukin 1 (IL-1)[35,36]. This monokine has been shown to be the central mediator of the acute phase response, causing fever, neutrophilia, production of acute phase proteins, etc.[37]. Other workers have isolated factors such as catabolin from blood monocytes[38] or synovial factor from rheumatoid synovial explants[39], which stimulate PGE_2 and collagenase synthesis by synovial cells. These factors and MCF are identical to IL-1[38-40]. It is clear, therefore, that the monokine IL-1 is

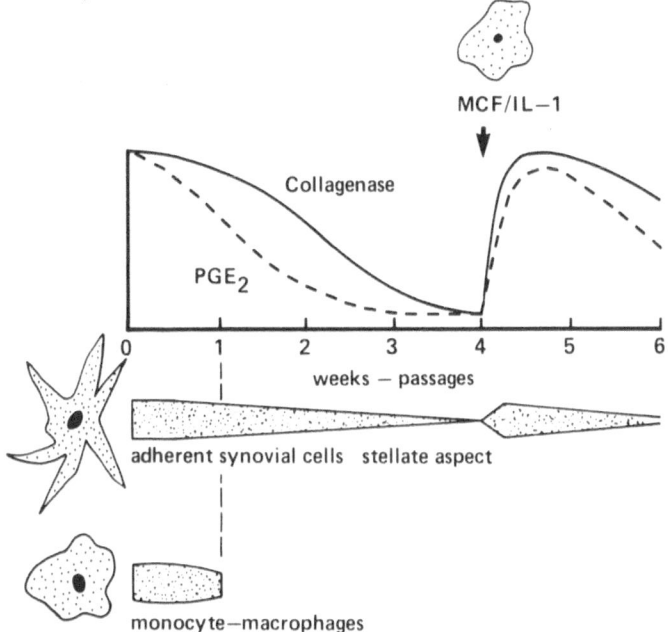

Figure 7.3 Schematic diagram showing the rates of synthesis of PGE$_2$ and collagenase by synovial adherent stellate cells and the influence of time/cell passage on synthesis. With increasing duration of culture, the monocyte-macrophage cells disappear, the adherent cells lose their stellate appearance and the rate of synthesis of PGE$_2$ and collagenase declines. Addition of monocyte-macrophages or MCF/IL-1 to established cells causes them to regain their stellate shape and to synthesize PGE$_2$ and collagenase. (Reproduced from reference 32, with permission)

capable of stimulating the adherent stellate synovial cells to produce PGE$_2$ and collagenase (Table 7.3). The dendritic cells are believed to be synovial fibroblasts and their dendritic/stellate morphology depends upon the indirect action of IL-1. Thus, addition of MCF/IL-1 to adherent rheumatoid synovial cells results in a more stellate morphology. In the presence of this monokine, indomethacin inhibits both PGE$_2$ production and the stellate changes. Addition of PGE$_2$, or the cyclic AMP analogue 8-bromo-cyclic AMP, to cultures, reproduces the stellate changes induced by MCF/IL-1. It appears that the stellate morphology of the rheumatoid synovial fibroblast depends upon PGE$_2$-induced cyclic AMP stimulation[41]. It is not clear what are the functional consequences of this change in cell morphology. There does appear to be some relationship between the morphology of rabbit synovial fibroblasts and the synthesis of metalloproteinases such as collagenase. This relationship is complex and has not been fully explained[42,43].

Interleukin 1 stimulates rheumatoid synovial fibroblasts to synthesize PGE$_2$ and collagenase. The synthesis of these two moieties is not closely connected. Indomethacin will totally inhibit PGE$_2$ production without affecting collagenase synthesis[44]. Synovial fibroblasts, like fibroblasts in all tissues, synthesize types

Table 7.3 Summary of the structural characteristics and activities of IL-1, MCF, synovial factor (SF) and catabolin

	IL-1	MCF	SF	Catabolin (pig)
Mol. wt. (gel filtration)	15 000	15 000	15 000	21000
(cloned)	17 500			
pI	5,6,7	5,7	5,7	5,8.3
Inhibition by phenylglyoxal	+	+	+	+
Pyrogenic activity	+	nd	nd	+
Activity in LAF* assay	+	+	+	+
Stimulation of synovial cell PGE$_2$ synthesis	+	+	+	+
Stimulation of synovial cell collagenase release	+	+	+	+
Cartilage resorbing activity	+	+	+	+

nd — not done
*LAF — lymphocyte activating factor

I and III collagen and fibronectin. Synthesis of these three components of the extracellular matrix is stimulated by MCF/IL-1. Stimulation by this monokine is augmented by indomethacin (14 μmol L^{-1}) and inhibited by addition of PGE$_2$ (IC$_{50}$ 5–10 ng ml^{-1})[45]. This finding is of importance as fibrotic growth of the synovial lining is one of the damaging sequelae of rheumatoid arthritis.

In recent years, purified IL-1 has become available and the molecule has been cloned and two distinct gene products have been isolated[46]. Addition of highly purified IL-1 to human skin fibroblasts[47] results in the stimulation of PGE$_2$ synthesis but only after a lag-phase of 2–4 h. A similar lag-phase is found with MCF-stimulated synovial adherent cells[48]. Anisomycin, an inhibitor of messenger RNA translation, decreased the stimulatory effect of IL-1 indicating that this monokine induces PGE$_2$ production by first activating protein synthesis[47]. Highly purified and recombinant IL-1 has been reported to activate phospholipase A$_2$ in cultured rabbit articular chondrocytes and to stimulate release of enzyme into the culture medium[49]. Large amounts of free phospholipase A$_2$ are found in arthritic synovial fluids[50]. Whether this is a response to IL-1 remains to be determined.

The experiments described in this section support the hypothesis that the production of PGE$_2$ and other prostanoids by the rheumatoid synovial lining is the result of the stimulation of synovial lining fibroblasts by interleukin 1. This stimulation would account for the high levels of prostanoids found in rheumatoid synovial effusions. Further support for this hypothesis comes from the finding that IL-1 is present in rheumatoid synovial fluids[51–53] and is produced by the rheumatoid synovial lining[39,54]. We have only scratched the surface of the complex web of interactions between cells and mediators in the rheumatoid joint which are responsible for the synthesis of eicosanoids. There is a substantial amount of literature, which is often conflicting, on the effects of eicosanoids in the control of immune responses *in vitro*. This is described more fully in Chapter 4. The complexity of this literature stems from the number of distinct eicosanoids generated by cells and the cellular complexity of the immune system. The consensus view is that prostaglandins of the E series provide inhibitory signals for immune reactions. Leukotrienes may also have inhibitory actions but less work has been done with them. The relationship between eicosanoids and IL-1 synthesis and activity is now being investigated. It was first shown by Dinarello and colleagues[55] that the dual inhibitors, ETYA and BW755C, would inhibit the ability of IL-1 to stimulate thymocyte mitogenesis. Inhibitors of cyclo-oxygenase were without effect. ETYA and BW755C were also shown to inhibit IL-1 release from *Staphylococcus albus*-stimulated human monocytes, but only when added prior to the stimulus[56]. The concentrations of inhibitors used were relatively high (IC_{50} for BW755C: $50-100 \mu mol L^{-1}$). Other workers have claimed that: (1) prostanoids inhibit IL-1 synthesis by lipopolysaccharide (LPS)-stimulated monocytes in a dose-dependent manner[57]; and (2) that leukotriene B_4 or D_4 stimulates release of IL-1 from LPS-stimulated monocytes, again in a dose-dependent fashion[58]. The concentrations of PGE_2 and LTB_4 used in these studies were roughly within the range found in rheumatoid synovial fluids. Further work is needed to establish the interactions between eicosanoids and monokines in inflammatory lesions. In a recent study, it was shown that the monokine, tumour necrosis factor (TNF), stimulates rheumatoid synovial adherent cells to secrete PGE_2 and collagenase[59]. The production of monokines, such as the interleukin 1 'family' and TNF, in the rheumatoid synovial lining is in turn dependent upon other protein mediators produced by helper T cells, such as γ-interferon, macrophage activating factor (MAF) and less well-characterized proteins[60]. Cell populations other than stellate cells in the rheumatoid synovial lining responsive to lymphokines include, among others: HLA-DR positive and HLA-DR negative macrophages, the antigen-presenting cells termed dendritic cells, and endothelial cells.

So far, the dicussion has been concerned with the control of eicosanoid synthesis and has described the experimental findings which suggest that prostanoid synthesis in the rheumatoid joint is the consequence of the stimulation of synovial cells by monokines such as IL-1. In the next section, the biological consequences of generating eicosanoids in the rheumatoid joint will be discussed.

INFLUENCE OF EICOSANOIDS ON RHEUMATOID JOINT FUNCTION

Pain, swelling and tissue destruction are the three major elements of the pathology of RA. The NSAIDs such as aspirin and indomethacin are analgesics which make the pain of RA tolerable[61]. This suggests that the prostanoids, and in particular PGE_2 and prostacyclin, which induce hyperalgesia, are responsible for the pain in the rheumatoid joint. Direct evidence supporting this hypothesis has come from the use of a dog model[62] in which bradykinin, injected into the joint cavity, induces a reflex rise in blood pressure which is dose-dependent. This rise in blood pressure was used as a measure of nociceptive activity. The joint cavity became more sensitive to bradykinin as the experiment proceeded, or when small amounts (50 ng min^{-1}) of PGE$_1$ or PGE$_2$ were infused locally. This increase in sensitivity with time was prevented by local infusion of aspirin or indomethacin but these drugs could not block the increased sensitivity produced by exogenous prostaglandins. These experiments support the hypothesis that local synthesis of prostaglandins in the rheumatoid joint sensitizes pain receptors to chemical stimuli.

Prostaglandins synergize with other mediators to cause vascular leakage with concomitant oedema and tissue swelling. Joint swelling is a typical feature in patients with RA. Therefore, it is surprising that there is little clinical evidence that NSAIDs have any influence on joint swelling. This may be a reflection of the joints chosen for measurement. The joints of the fingers, particularly the metacarpophalangeal joints, are the most commonly affected in RA and are certainly the easiest to measure. However, in the established disease, the swelling in these joints is most likely to be due to changes in the bone and synovial lining and not to synovial effusion[61]. In experimental studies, it has been shown that NSAIDs will inhibit the swelling of the knee joints of rabbits with experimental chronic arthritis. However, these agents only inhibit swelling by around 50%[63]. It is not known whether infusion of prostaglandins into the synovial cavity would produce the same magnitude of swelling as seen in chronic arthritis. As joint swelling in chronic arthritis is normally the summation of growth of the synovial lining, changes in bone, and exudation, it is unlikely that the simple injection of PGE$_2$ would mimic chronic swelling.

In addition to producing pain and swelling, prostaglandins have been implicated in the tissue destruction found in the RA joint. A number of *in vitro* studies have demonstrated that prostaglandins, in some cases at heroic concentrations, will inhibit the production of proteoglycan by cartilage explants[64] or isolated chondrocytes[65], or will cause depletion of proteoglycan from cartilage slices[66]. Cartilage is composed of a meshwork of collagen fibres within which are found the enormous, negatively charged, proteoglycans. The proteoglycans bind large amounts of water and so give articular cartilage its stiffness and resilience. Loss of proteoglycan can therefore compromise the normal function of articular cartilage. Prostaglandins have also been implicated in the erosion of subchondral bone, which is a common finding in RA[67].

In spite of these *in vitro* studies, there is no clinical evidence that NSAIDs have any influence on the progression of tissue damage in RA[68]. The only drug to have a limited influence on disease progression is gold[4] which is a weak inhibitor of prostanoid synthesis[27].

CONCLUSIONS

The prostanoids (PGE_2, prostacyclin, TxB_2) and LTB_4 are found in the synovial effusion in the rheumatoid joint. Explants of rheumatoid synovial lining produce these prostanoids and it is suggested that this tissue is the source of the cyclo-oxyenase products found in the synovial fluid. It has not been established whether the rheumatoid synovial lining produces leukotrienes. Rabbit synovial cells (again, mainly fibroblasts) do not produce 5-HETE, 12-HETE or 15-HETE even after stimulation[69] with calcium ionophore A23187. In contrast, explants of inflamed synovial lining from rabbits with chronic arthritis produce[20] small amounts of immunoreactive LTB_4.

It has been established that the prostanoids, particularly PGE_2 and prostacyclin, contribute to the pain and swelling in the rheumatoid joint. These symptoms can be fairly effectively managed by the use of NSAIDs or steroids. Unfortunately, clinicians are currently unable to control the progression of damage to articular cartilage, subchondral bone and other articular structures. During the 1960s and 1970s, the popular hypothesis was that tissue damage was due to the release of degradative enzymes, such as lysosomal hydrolases and collagenase. The prostaglandins were also believed to play a direct role in tissue damage. However, in a very simple experiment, it was shown that, if synovial lining was co-cultured with articular cartilage, there was a marked loss of proteoglycan from living, but not from dead, cartilage[70]. This indicated that the synovial lining released a soluble factor which could stimulate chondrocytes to degrade their own matrix. As has been described, this factor, catabolin, plus mononuclear cell factor (MCF) and synovial factor (SF) have all been shown to be equivalent to IL-1 (Table 7.3). This monokine is now perceived to be one of the key mediators of the pathology of RA. For example, it causes damage to the matrices of cartilage and bone in explant culture, stimulates release of prostanoids and collagenase from various cell populations and stimulates fibroblast cell division and synthesis of extracellular matrix components[71,72]. IL-1 has been shown to be a potent chemoattractant *in vitro* for various inflammatory cell populations[73]. Furthermore, injection of highly purified IL-1 into the knee joints of rabbits causes a massive influx of PMN at 4 h, and by 24 h, there are large numbers of mononuclear cells in the synovial fluid. This cellular infiltrate is associated with damage to the cartilage matrix though it is not established that the two are related. The synovial fluids from IL-1-injected joints did not contain[74] measurable levels of PGE_2 or LTB_4. Thus, it is likely that IL-1 is responsible, at least in part, for the cellular infiltrate in the rheumatoid joint. In contrast, injection of LTB_4 into the knee joint of the dog did not induce an infiltrate in the synovial cavity[75].

With our increasing understanding of the role of IL-1 in RA, there is the suggestion that PGE_2 and other eicosanoids may have important immunomodulatory effects within the chronically inflamed joint. At concentrations in the range found in RA joints, PGE_2 inhibits IL-1 production by macrophages[57] and inhibits the mitogenic effects of IL-1 on T lymphocytes[76]. In contrast, LTB_4 and LTD_4 appear to be able to stimulate IL-1 release[54]. Further, the rheumatoid synovial lining contains a number of macrophage subpopulations

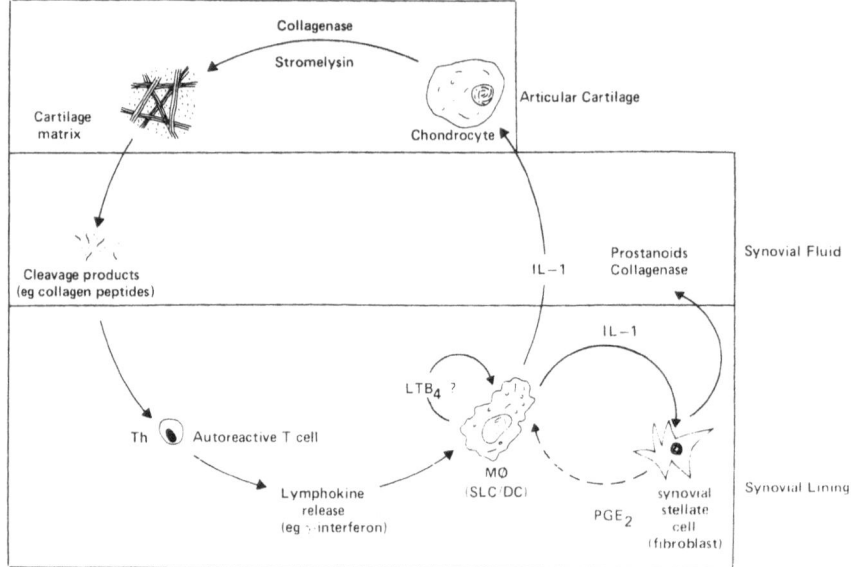

Figure 7.4   Schematic representation of a possible pathological mechanism to account for eicosanoid synthesis, IL-1 production and tissue damage. IL-1 release from synovial macrophages (or synovial lining cells (SLC) or dendritic cells (DC)) would stimulate chondrocytes to release degradative enzymes resulting in cleavage products. Such products have been shown to stimulate collagenase release from rheumatoid synovial lining explants by a mechanism thought to involve T helper cell stimulation[80]. Stimulated autoreactive Th cells will release lymphokines which will stimulate macrophage (SLC/DC) to release IL-1, thus completing the circle. IL-1 will also stimulate synovial adherent cells to produce PGE_2 and collagenase. The PGE_2 may feedback onto macrophage ($M\phi$) to inhibit IL-1 synthesis (----). The role of LTB_4 in this pathological mechanism is not clear. Synovial $M\phi$ are most likely to be able to produce leukotrienes which may in turn stimulate IL-1 synthesis

which can be separated on the basis of their density. Heavy cells are potent antigen-presenting cells and produce little PGE_2. Light cells[77] suppress the process of antigen presentation and produce large quantities of PGE_2. The chronicity of RA is due to the perpetuation of lymphocyte reactivity brought about by the continued process of antigen presentation. As has been argued by others[78,79], the inhibition of prostanoid synthesis within the rheumatoid joint may exacerbate the chronic nature of the disease while suppressing the symptoms. There is, therefore, a pressing need to know more about the interrelationship between eicosanoids and monokines in the pathology of RA. One plausible pathological mechanism to account for the presence of IL-1, PGE_2 and tissue damage in the rheumatoid joint is depicted schematically in Figure 7.4.

REFERENCES

1. Henderson, B. and Pettipher, E.R. (1985). The synovial lining cell: Biology and pathobiology. *Semin. Arthr. Rheum.*, **15**, 1–32
2. Poulter, L.W., Duke, O., Panayi, G.S., Hobbs, S., Raftery, M.J. and Janossy, G. (1985). Activated T lymphocytes of the synovial membrane in rheumatoid arthritis and other arthropathies. *Scand. J. Immunol.*, **22**, 683–690
3. Poulter, L.W. and Janossy, G. (1985). The involvement of dendritic cells in chronic inflammatory disease. *Scand. J. Immunol.*, **21**, 401–407
4. Ianuzzi, L., Dawson, N., Zein, N. and Kushner, I. (1983). Does drug therapy slow radiographic deterioration in rheumatoid arthritis. *N. Engl. J. Med.*, **309**, 1023–1028
5. Watson Buchanan, W., Rooney, P.J. and Rennie, J.A.N. (1983). Aspirin and the salicylates. In Huskisson, E.C. (ed.) *Anti-Rheumatic Drugs*, pp. 55–95. (East Sussex: Praeger Press)
6. Vane, J.R. (1971). Inhibition of prostaglandin synthesis as a mechanism of action for aspirin-like drugs. *Nature (London)*, **231**, 232–235
7. Higgs, G.A., Vane, J.R., Hart, F.D. and Wojtulewski, J.A. (1974). Effects of anti-inflammatory drugs on prostaglandins in rheumatoid arthritis. In Robinson, H.J. and Vane, J.R. (eds.) *Prostaglandin Synthetase Inhibitors*, pp. 165–173. (New York: Raven Press)
8. Robinson, D.R. and Levine, L. (1974). Prostaglandin concentrations in synovial fluid in rheumatic diseases: Action of indomethacin and aspirin. In Robinson, H.J. and Vane, J.R. (eds.) *Prostaglandin Synthetase Inhibitors*, pp. 223–228. (New York: Raven Press)
9. Trang, L.E., Granstrom, E. and Lovgren, O. (1977). Levels of prostalgandins $F_{2\alpha}$ and E_2 and thromboxane B_2 in joint fluid in rheumatoid arthritis. *Scand. J. Rheumatol.*, **6**, 151–154
10. Sturge, R.A., Yates, D.B., Gordon, D., Franco, M., Paul, W., Bray, A. and Morley, J. (1978). Prostaglandin production in arthritis. *Ann. Rheum. Dis.*, **37**, 315–320
11. Egg, D., Gunther, R., Herold, M. and Kerschbaumer, F. (1980). Prostaglandin E_2 und $F_{2\alpha}$ konzentrationen in der Synovia bei rheumatischen und traumatischen Kniegelenker-krankungen. *Z. Rheumatol.*, **39**, 170–175
12. Bombardieri, S., Cattani, P., Ciabattoni, G., Di Munno, O., Pasero, G., Patrono, C., Pinca, E. and Pugliese, F. (1981). The synovial prostaglandin system in chronic inflammatory arthritis: Differential effects of steroidal and nonsteroidal anti-inflammatory drugs. *Br. J. Pharmacol.*, **73**, 893–901
13. Tokunaga, M., Ohuchi, K., Yoshizawa, S., Tsurufuji, S., Rikimaru, A. and Wakamatsu, E. (1981). Change of prostaglandin E level in joint fluids after treatment with flurbiprofen in patients with rheumatoid arthritis and osteoarthritis. *Ann. Rheum. Dis.*, **40**, 462–465
14. Egg, D. (1984). Concentrations of prostaglandin D_2, E_2, $F_{2\alpha}$, 6-keto-$F_{1\alpha}$ and thromboxane B_2 in synovial fluid from patients with inflammatory joint disorders and osteoarthritis. *Z. Rheumatol.*, **43**, 89–96
15. Caruso, I., Moro, E., Patrono, C., Sacchetti, G., Tamassia, V. and Tosolini, G.P. (1980). Plasma and synovial fluid pharmacokinetics and prostaglandin inhibitory effect of indoprofen in patients with rheumatoid arthritis. *Scand. J. Rheumatol.*, **9**, 123–126
16. Klickstein, L.B., Shapleigh, C. and Goetzl, E.J. (1980). Lipoxygenation of arachidonic acid as a source of polymorphonuclear leukocyte chemotactic factors in synovial fluid and tissue in rheumatoid arthritis and spondylarthritis. *J. Clin. Invest.*, **66**, 1166–1170
17. Davidson, E.M., Rae, S.A. and Smith, M.J.H. (1983). Leukotriene B_4 a mediator of inflammation present in synovial fluid in rheumatoid arthritis. *Ann. Rheum. Dis.*, **42**, 677–679
18. Rae, S.A., Davidson, E.M. and Smith, M.J.H. (1982). Leukotriene B_4, an inflammatory mediator in gout. *Lancet*, **1**, 677–679
19. Salmon, J.A., Higgs, G.A., Vane, J.R., Bitensky, L., Chayen, J., Henderson, B. and Cashman, B. (1983). Synthesis of arachidonate cyclo-oxygenase products by rheumatoid and non-rheumatoid synovial lining in nonproliferative organ culture. *Ann. Rheum. Dis.*, **42**, 36–39
20. Henderson, B. and Higgs, G.A. (1987). Synthesis of arachidonate oxidation products by tissues of the synovial joint during the development of chronic erosive arthritis. *Arthr. Rheum.*, **30**, 1149–1157
21. Simmons, P.M., Salmon, J.A. and Moncada, S. (1983). The release of leukotriene B_4 during experimental inflammation. *Biochem. Pharmacol.*, **32**, 1353–1359

22. Crook, D., Collins, A.J., Bacon, P.A. and Chan, R. (1976). Prostaglandin synthetase activity from human rheumatoid synovial microsomes: Effect of 'aspirin-like' drug therapy. *Ann. Rheum. Dis.*, **35**, 327–332
23. Blotman, F., Chaintreuil, J., Poubelle, P., Flandre, O., Crastes de Paulet, A. and Simon, L. (1982). PGE_2, PGF_{2x} and TxB_2 biosynthesis by human rheumatoid synovia. In Samuelsson, B., Ramwell, P.W. and Paoletti, R. (eds.) *Advances in Prostaglandin and Thromboxane Research*. Vol. 8, pp. 1705–1708. (New York: Raven Press)
24. Robinson, D.R., McGuire, M.B. and Levine, L. (1975). Prostaglandins in the rheumatic diseases. *Ann. NY Acad. Sci.*, **256**, 318–329
25. Robinson, D.R., McGuire, M.B., Bastian, D., Kantrowitz, F. and Levine, L. (1978). The effect of anti-inflammatory drugs on prostaglandin production by rheumatoid synovial tissue. *Prostagl. Med.*, **1**, 461–477
26. McGuire, M.K.B., Meats, J.E., Ebsworth, N.M., Harvey, L., Murphy, G., Russell, R.G.G. and Reynolds, J.J. (1982). Properties of rheumatoid and normal synovial tissue *in vitro* and cells derived from them. *Rheumatol. Int.*, **2**, 113–120
27. Higgs, G.A., Harvey, E.A., Ferreira, S.H. and Vane, J.R. (1976). The effect of anti-inflammatory drugs on the production of prostaglandins *in vivo*. In Samuelsson, B. and Paoletti, R. (eds.) *Advances in Prostaglandin and Thromboxane Research*. Vol. 1, pp. 105–110. (New York: Raven Press)
28. Malemud, C.J., Moskowitz, P.W. and Hassid, A. (1981). Prostaglandin biosynthesis by lapine articular chondrocytes in culture *Biochim. Biophys. Acta*, **663**, 480–490
29. Mitrovic, D., McCall, E. and Dray, F. (1982). The *in vitro* production of prostanoids by cultured bovine articular chondrocytes. *Prostaglandins*, **23**, 17–28
30. Dayer, J-M., Krane, S.M., Russell, R.G.G. and Robinson, D.R. (1976). Production of collagenase and prostaglandins by isolated adherent rheumatoid synovial cells. *Proc. Natl. Acad. Sci. USA*, **73**, 945–949
31. Dayer, J-M., Robinson, D.R. and Krane, S.M. (1977). Prostaglandin production by rheumatoid synovial cells: Stimulation by a factor from human mononuclear cells. *J. Exp. Med.*, **145**, 1399–1404
32. Dayer, J-M. (1984). Monokines and connective tissue destruction in rheumatoid arthritis. In Lambert, P.H., Perrin, L. and Izui, S. (eds.) *Recent Advances in SLE*, pp. 195–216. (London: Academic Press)
33. Pietila, P., Moilanen, E., Sepala, E., Nissila, M., Lepisto, P., Laitinen, O. and Vapaatalo, H. (1984). Differences in the production of arachidonic acid metabolites between healthy and rheumatic synovial fibroblasts *in vitro*. *Scand. J. Rheumatol.*, **13**, 243–246
34. Dayer, J-M., Breard, J., Chess, L. and Krane, S.M. (1979). Participation of monocyte-macrophages and lymphocytes in the production of a factor that stimulates collagenase and prostaglandin release by rheumatoid synovial cells. *J. Clin. Invest.*, **64**, 1386–1392
35. Mizel, S.B., Dayer, J-M., Krane, S.M. and Mergenhagen, S.E. (1981). Stimulation of rheumatoid synovial cell collagenase and prostaglandin production by partially purified lymphocyte activating factor (interleukin 1). *Proc. Natl. Acad. Sci. USA*, **78**, 2474–2477
36. Dayer, J-M. (1985). Mononuclear cell factor – Interleukin-1 in rheumatoid arthritis. *Br. J. Rheumatol.*, **24** (Suppl. 1), 15–20
37. Dinarello, C.A. (1984). Interleukin 1. *Rev. Inf. Dis.*, **6**, 51–95
38. Saklatvala, J., Pilsworth, L.M.C., Sarsfield, S.J., Gavrilovic, J. and Heath, J.K. (1984). Pig catabolin is a form of interleukin 1. *Biochem. J.*, **224**, 461–466
39. Elford, P.R., Meats, J.E., Sharrard, R.M. and Russell, R.G.G. (1985). Partial purification of a factor from human synovium that possesses interleukin 1, chondrocyte-stimulating and catabolin-like activities. *FEBS Lett.*, **179**, 247–251
40. Elford, P.R., Richardson, H.J., Sharrard, R.M., Meats, J.E., Skjodt, H., Bunning, R.A.D., Crawford, A. and Russell, R.G.G. (1985). Mononuclear cell factor and synovial factor are closely related to, or identical with, interleukin 1. *Br. J. Rheumatol.*, **24** (Suppl. 1), 55–58
41. Baker, D.G., Dayer, J.M., Roelke, M., Schumacher, H.R. and Krane, S.M. (1983). Rheumatoid synovial cell morphologic changes induced by a mononuclear cell factor in culture. *Arthr. Rheum.*, **26**, 8–14
42. Aggeler, J., Frisch, S.M. and Werb, Z. (1984). Changes in cell shape correlate with collagenase gene expression in rabbit synovial fibroblasts. *J. Cell Biol.*, **98**, 1662–1671
43. Werb, Z., Hembry, R.M., Murphy, G. and Aggeler, J. (1986). Commitment to expression of the metallo-endopeptidases, collagenase and stromelysin: Relationship of inducing events to changes in cytoskeletal architecture. *J. Cell Biol.*, **102**, 697–702

44. Dayer, J.M., Roelke, M.S. and Krane, S.M. (1985). Effects of prostaglandin E_2, indomethacin, trifluoroperazine and drugs affecting the cytoskeleton on collagenase production by cultured adherent rheumatoid synovial cells. *Biochem. Pharmacol.*, **33**, 2893–2899

45. Krane, S.M., Dayer, J-M., Simon, L.S. and Byrne, M.S. (1985). Mononuclear cell-conditioned medium containing mononuclear cell factor (MCF), homologous with interleukin 1, stimulates collagen and fibronectin synthesis by adherent rheumatoid synovial cells: Effect of prostaglandin E_2 and indomethacin. *Collagen Relat. Res.*, **5**, 99–117

46. March, C.J., Mosley, B., Larsen, A., Cerretti, D.P., Braedt, G., Price, V., Gillis, S., Henney, C.S., Kronheim, S.R., Grabstein, K., Conlon, P.J., Hopp, T.P. and Cosman, D. (1985). Cloning, sequence and expression of two distinct interleukin 1 complementary DNA's. *Nature (London)*, **315**, 641–647

47. Bernheim, H.A. and Dinarello, C.A. (1985). Effect of purified human interleukin-1 on the release of prostaglandin E_2 from fibroblasts. *Br. J. Rheumatol.*, **24** (Suppl. 1), 122–127

48. Dayer, J-M., Goldring, S.R., Robinson, D.R. and Krane, S.M. (1979). Effects of human mononuclear cell factor on cultured rheumatoid synovial cells: Interactions of prostaglandin E_2 and cyclic adenosine $3'5'$-monophosphate. *Biochim. Biophys. Acta*, **586**, 87–105

49. Chang, J., Gilman, S.C. and Lewis, A.J. (1986). Interleukin 1 activates phospholipase A_2 in rabbit chondrocytes: A possible signal for IL-1 action. *J. Immunol.*, **136**, 1283–1287

50. Pruzanski, W., Vadas, P., Stefanski, E. and Urowitz, M.B. (1985). Phospholipase A_2 activity in sera and synovial fluids in rheumatoid arthritis and osteoarthritis. Its possible role as a proinflammatory enzyme. *J. Rheumatol.*, **12**, 211–216

51. Wood, D.D., Ihrie, E.J., Dinarello, C.A. and Cohen, P.L. (1983). Isolation of an interleukin-1-like factor from human joint effusions. *Arthr. Rheum.*, **26**, 975–983

52. Nouri, A.M.E., Panayi, G.S. and Goodman, S.M. (1984). Cytokines and the chronic inflammation of rheumatic disease. I. The presence of interleukin-1 in synovial fluid. *Clin. Exp. Immunol.*, **55**, 295–302

53. Nouri, A.M.E., Panayi, G.S., Goodman, S.M. and Waugh, A.P.W. (1985). Cytokines in rheumatoid arthritis: Production of IL-1. *Br. J. Rheumatol.*, **24** (Suppl. 1), 191–196

54. Wood, D.D., Ihrie, E.J. and Hamerman, D. (1985). Release of interleukin-1 from human synovial tissue *in vitro*. *Arthr. Rheum.*, **28**, 858–862

55. Dinarello, C.A., Marnoy, S.O. and Rosenwasser, L.J. (1983). Role of arachidonate metabolism in the immunoregulatory function of human leukocytic pyrogen/lymphocyte-activating factor/interleukin 1. *J. Immunol.*, **130**, 890–895

56. Dinarello, C.A., Bishai, I., Rosenwasser, L.J. and Coceani, F. (1984). The influence of lipoxygenase inhibitors on the *in vitro* production of human leukocytic pyrogen and lymphocyte activating factor (interleukin-1). *Int. J. Immunopharmacol.*, **6**, 43–50

57. Kunkel, S.L., Chensue, S.W. and Phan, S.M. (1986). Prostaglandins as endogenous mediators of interleukin 1 production. *J. Immunol.*, **136**, 186–192

58. Rola-Pleszczynski, M. and Lemaire, I. (1985). Leukotrienes augment interleukin 1 production by human monocytes. *J. Immunol.*, **135**, 3958–3961

59. Dayer, J-M., Beutler, B. and Cerami, A. (1985). Cachectin/tumor necrosis factor stimulates collagenase and prostaglandin E_2 production by human synovial cells and dermal fibroblasts. *J. Exp. Med.*, **162**, 2163–2166

60. Amento, E.P., Kurnick, J.T. and Krane, S.M. (1985). Interleukin 1 production by the human monocyte cell line U937 requires a lymphokine induction signal distinct from interleukin 2 or interferons. *J. Immunol.*, **134**, 350–357

61. Balint, G.P., Marrikakis, M.E., Lee, P., Rooney, P.J. and Buchanan, W.W. (1977). Standardization in clinical measurement. In Dumond, D.C. and Jasani, M.K. (eds.) *The Recognition of Anti-Rheumatic Drugs*, pp. 251–265 (Lancaster: MTP Press)

62. Moncada, S., Ferreira, S.H. and Vane J.R. (1975). Inhibition of prostaglandin biosynthesis as the mechanism of analgesia of aspirin-like drugs in the dog knee joint. *Eur. J. Pharmacol.*, **31**, 250–260

63. Blackham, A. and Radziwonik, H. (1977). The effect of drugs in established rabbit monoarticular arthritis. *Agents Actions*, **7**, 473–480

64. Lippiello, L., Yamamoto, K., Robinson, D. and Mankin, H.J. (1978). Involvement of prostaglandins from rheumatoid synovium in inhibition of articular cartilage metabolism. *Arthr. Rheum.*, **21**, 909–917

65. Mitrovic, D., Lippiello, L., Gruson, F., Aprile, F. and Mankin, H.J. (1981). Effect of various prostanoids on the *in vitro* metabolism of bovine articular chondrocytes. *Prostaglandins*, **22**, 499–511

145

66. Fulkerson, J.P., Ladenbauer-Bellis, I.M. and Chrisman, O.D. (1979). *In vitro* hexosamine depletion of intact articular cartilage by E-prostaglandins. Prevention by chloroquine. *Arthr. Rheum.*, **22**, 1117–1121
67. Robinson, D.R., Tashjian, A.H. and Levine, L. (1975). Prostaglandin-stimulated bone resorption by rheumatoid synovia. *J. Clin. Invest.*, **56**, 1181–1188
68. Rosenbloom, D., Brooks, P., Bellamy N. and Buchanan, W. (1985). *Clinical Trials in the Rheumatic Disease: A Selected Critical Review*. (East Sussex: Praeger Press)
69. Rothenberg, R., Moskowitz, R.W. and Malemud, C.J. (1983). Arachidonic acid metabolism by rabbit synovial cells in culture. Studies of non-cyclooxygenase pathways. *Biochim. Biophys. Acta*, **753**, 257–265
70. Fell, H.B. and Jubb, R.W. (1977). The effect of synovial tissue on the breakdown of articular cartilage in organ culture. *Arthr. Rheum.*, **20**, 1359–1371
71. Nuki, G. and Duff, G. (eds.) (1985). Interleukin 1. *Br. J. Rheumatol.*, **24** (Suppl. 1)
72. Gowen, M., Elford, P.R., Skjodt, H., Richardson, H.J. and Russell R.G.G. (1985). Tissue destruction and its prevention. In Bonta, I.L., Bray, M.A. and Parnham, M.J. (eds.) *Handbook of Inflammation, Vol. 5: The Pharmacology of Inflammation*, pp. 167–178. (North Holland: Elsevier)
73. Luger, T.A., Charon, J.A., Colot, M., Micksche, M. and Oppenheim, J.J. (1983). Chemotactic properties of partially purified human epidermal cell-derived thymocyte-activating factor (ETAF) for polymorphonuclear and mononuclear cells. *J. Immunol.*, **131**, 816–820
74. Henderson, B., Higgs, G.A. and Pettipher, E.R. (1986). Effects of interleukin 1 on leukocyte migration and cartilage destruction *in vivo*. *Br. J. Pharmacol.*, **88** (Proceedings Suppl.), 243P
75. Carlson, R.P., Chang, J. and Lewis, A.T. (1985). Does leukotriene B$_4$ play a role in urate-induced synovitis in dogs. *Br. J. Pharmacol.*, **86** (Proceedings Suppl.), 521P
76. Hayari, Y., Kukulansky, T. and Globerson, A. (1986). Regulation of thymocyte proliferative response by macrophage-derived prostaglandin E$_2$ and interleukin 1. *Eur. J. Immunol.*, **15**, 43–47
77. Klareskog, L., Holmdahl, R., Rubin, K., Victorin, A. and Lindgren, J.A. (1985). Different populations of rheumatoid adherent cells mediate activation versus suppression of T lymphocyte proliferation. *Arthr. Rheum.*, **28**, 863–872
78. Goodwin, J.S., Ceuppens, J.L. and Gualde, N. (1984). Control of the immune response in humans by prostaglandins. In Otterness, I., Capetola, R. and Wong, S. (eds.) *Advances in Inflammation Research*, Vol. 7, pp. 79–92. (New York: Raven Press)
79. Goodwin, J.S. (1985). Immunologic effects of nonsteroidal anti-inflammatory agents. *Med. Clin. N. Am.*, **69**, 793–804
80. Fisher, W.D., Golds, E.E., Van der Rest, M., Cooke, T.D., Lyons, H.E. and Poole, A.R. (1982). Stimulation of collagenase secretion from rheumatoid synovial tissue by human collagen peptides: Evidence of autoimmunity. *J. Bone Jt. Surg.*, **64A**, 546–557

8
Lipoxygenase Inhibitors and Leukotriene Receptor Antagonists

B. J. FITZSIMMONS and J. ROKACH

INTRODUCTION

The object of this chapter is to give the reader an overview of the numerous agents· that directly modulate the effects of the leukotriene section of the arachidonic acid cascade (Figure 8.1). These agents fall into two general categories: enzyme inhibitors and receptor antagonists. Compounds in the former category exercise their effect by reducing or preventing the formation of the biologically active products of this pathway, while those in the latter group do so by competitively occupying the receptor through which a specific leukotriene manifests its action.

The sulphidopeptide leukotrienes (LTC$_4$, LTD$_4$, LTE$_4$)[1,2] are strongly implicated as principal factors in the elicitation of the symptoms of asthma[3] and other pulmonary conditions such as acute respiratory distress. On the other hand, leukotriene B$_4$ (LTB$_4$), a potent chemotactic agent[4], is believed to be involved in diverse inflammatory conditions. However, it must be stressed that, while the body of evidence implying roles for leukotrienes in various disease states is large, their role is just that, implied but not proven. What is known is that leukotrienes are formed by involved tissues under conditions that mimic a disease and that leukotrienes can cause some of the symptoms of a specific disease *in vivo* in both humans and animals. The logical extension to the above results and the proof of the hypothesis, namely the alleviation of clinical symptoms by a specific lipoxygenase inhibitor or receptor antagonist, remains to be shown.

A schematic representation of the arachidonic acid cascade with possible sites for intervention is shown in Figure 8.1. The desirability of a particular intervention is dependent in part on the intended use of the inhibitor. Inhibition of 5-lipoxygenase (site A) or LTA$_4$ synthase (site B) would shut down the entire pathway, while the inhibition of LTA$_4$ hydrolase (site C) or LTC$_4$ synthase (site D) would have a more specific effect, inhibiting the

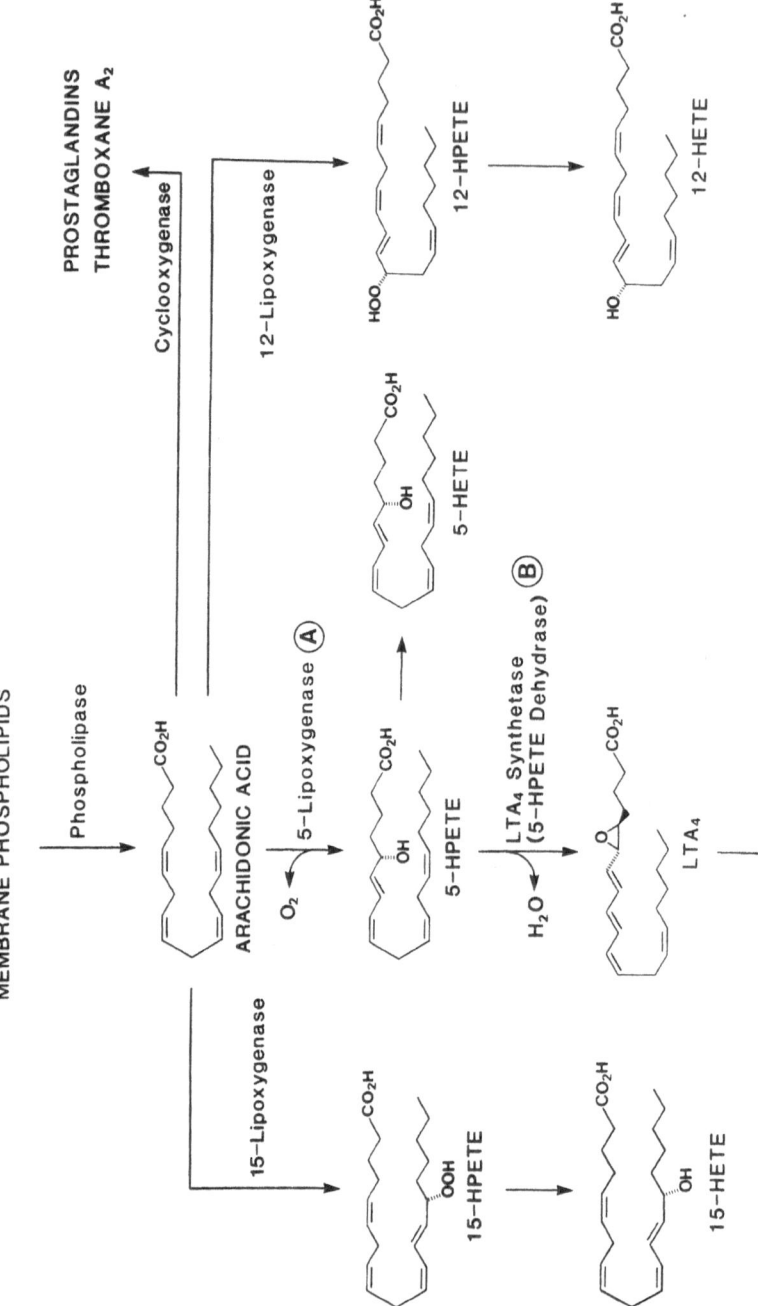

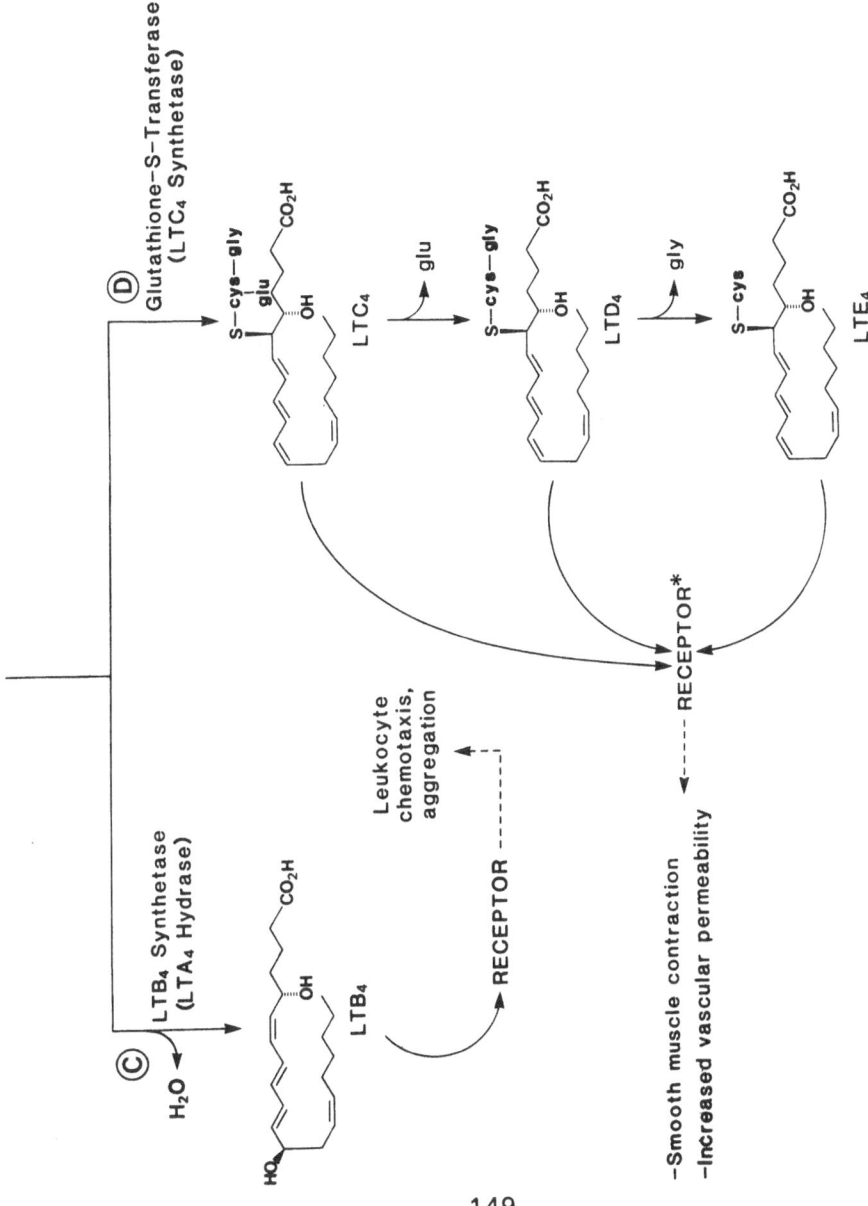

Figure 8.1 The arachidonic acid cascade

formation of LTB_4 or the sulphidopeptide leukotrienes respectively. Conversely, since LTB_4 and sulphidopeptide leukotrienes elicit their effect via receptors[5,6], specific blockade of one of these receptors would negate the effects of that particular leukotriene.

Of the possible target enzymes for inhibition, the lipoxygenases have received most attention. These are the first enzymes specific to the lipoxygenase arm of the arachidonic acid cascade, converting arachidonic acid into the hydroperoxyeicosaenoic acids (HPETEs), and, therefore, inhibition of these enzymes would have the widest possible effect. Research to find inhibitors of the lipoxygenase enzymes is being undertaken in both academia and industry. Inhibitors of the 5-lipoxygenase enzyme have been the most studied from the pharmaceutical standpoint owing to the biological prominence of the products from this pathway. However, inhibitors of 12- and 15-lipoxygenase have also been synthesized in substantial numbers. It is interesting to note, although the 5-lipoxygenase enzyme gives rise to what appears to be the biologically most important leukotrienes, it is the least characterized owing to its instability and requirement of many stabilizing or activation 'co-factors'[7].

Other enzymes which are potential targets for inhibition are LTA_4 synthase (site B), the enzyme which converts LTA_4 into the chemotactic LTB_4 (LTA_4 hydrolase) (site C) or the glutathione-S-transferase which converts LTA_4 into LTC_4 (site D). Inhibition of LTA_4 synthase would have much the same effect as inhibition of 5-lipoxygenase, while the results of inhibition of the other enzymes would be more specific, blocking the formation of the proinflammatory LTB_4 or the spasmogenic sulphidopeptide leukotrienes respectively. While the synthesis of LTA_4 from arachidonic acid by the 5-lipoxygenase/LTA_4 synthase enzyme appears to require activation, the formation of LTB_4 and LTC_4 by their respective enzymes does not. Therefore, regulation of the amount of LTA_4 available will also control the synthesis of LTB_4 and LTC_4. However, if the synthesis of LTB_4 or LTC_4 is blocked selectively, the LTA_4 formed may be redirected to form more of the other leukotrienes. This would be true especially in cell types that possess both LTA_4 hydrolase and LTC_4 synthase. Moreover, recent evidence[8,9] has shown that LTA_4 can be exteriorized by synthesizing cells, and that exogenous LTA_4 can be utilized by non-synthesizing cells to produce LTB_4 or LTC_4. Therefore, inhibition of these latter two enzymes may lead to undesirable effects brought about by the redirection of the LTA_4 to other cells.

The other approach to regulating the effects of the leukotrienes is to develop receptor antagonists. A potential advantage of receptor antagonists is that their action can be much more specific. A receptor antagonist would block the action of a specific leukotriene without affecting the action of the other leukotrienes. As mentioned previously, inhibition of an enzyme may lead to a build up of products prior to the point of blockade and to the redirection of these intermediates. In the simplest sense, a receptor antagonist would be devoid of this feature since it would not affect the levels of any of the leukotrienes, only block the action of a specific one.

Unlike the lipoxygenase inhibitors, the development of receptor antagonists has been almost solely the territory of the pharmaceutical industry. Although this has led to a much smaller volume of published results, this data is more relevant to the design of a drug. In humans, the blockade of putative LTB_4 and LTD_4 receptors may yield beneficial results. Antagonism of the effects of LTB_4 should negate the proinflammatory actions of this molecule, whilst blockade of the LTD_4 receptor would obviate the spasmogenic effects of this sulphidopeptide leukotriene which is thought to be important in bronchospasm. Of these, the latter has received the majority of attention, with only a few sporadic reports of LTB_4 receptor antagonists in the literature. Nevertheless, there is little doubt that many more will be forthcoming due to the therapeutic possibilities for an LTB_4 antagonist.

Despite the presence of specific high-affinity receptors for LTC_4 in lung[10], no concerted effort to develop an antagonist of the action of this sulphidopeptide leukotriene has been reported to date. The reasoning behind the lack of activity in this area is twofold. Firstly, whether LTC_4 uniquely mediates specific biological events is not known at this time. Secondly, the actions of LTC_4 in most preparations can be abolished by an LTD_4 antagonist due to the rapid conversion of LTC_4 to LTD_4 by many tissues. However, if this conversion is inhibited by treatment with serine borate complex, the effects of LTC_4 are unaffected by most LTD_4 receptor antagonists. Therefore, in situations where LTC_4 is not converted to LTD_4, an antagonist of LTC_4 would be of potential value.

Due to the presence of a separate site of action for LTC_4 in some tissues, the importance of this mediator will doubtless be the subject of future research. In time, these studies may lead to a specific LTC_4 receptor antagonist and thus a method to fully evaluate the physiological role of LTC_4.

ENZYME INHIBITORS

Lipoxygenase inhibitors

Upon surveying the myriad of reports in the literature of compounds which are described as lipoxygenase inhibitors, one is confronted with several problems. First, there is an enormous range in the concentrations required to produce 50% enzyme inhibition (IC_{50}) of the reported compounds. Therefore, one is faced with the question of where to draw the upper limit in defining an effective lipoxygenase inhibitor. Secondly, some of the claimed lipoxyenase inhibitors are ill-defined species, such as amniotic fluid. Thirdly, when attempting to compare potencies of reported inhibitors, one finds that this is best done with caution since many different enzyme preparations and assay conditions have been used, occasionally leading to vastly different IC_{50} values for the same compound. This is particularly true for inhibitors of the 5-lipoxygenase enzymes. Lastly, for some compounds reported at conferences and meetings by pharmaceutical firms, the structure is not available. This review will deal with those compounds which have the potential to be, or lead to therapeutically useful agents. Compounds which are unlikely to fulfil this criterion will be omitted. This is not to say that such compounds are not of use, for many such compounds have provided, and will continue to provide, valuable information about the nature and mechanisms of the lipoxygenase enzymes.

151

Both natural products and synthetic compounds have been reported as lipoxygenase inhibitors. The former category encompasses compounds isolated from both animate and inanimate sources, while the latter class is comprised of lipoxygenase substrate and product analogues, synthetically modified natural products and novel structures obtained by total synthesis.

Natural products
There are many reports of natural extracts, and compounds isolated therefrom, possessing potent lipoxygenase inhibitory activity. These compounds range from the simple to the very complex in structure. However, often a common thread binds them together, namely they are one half of a redox pair. In other words, they can behave as antioxidants by being preferentially oxidized themselves or by generating a species which can. Indeed, some of these compounds are also reported as antioxidants in the literature and find use as such in other applications.

Flavonoids
This is the largest and the most thoroughly studied class of natural lipoxygenase inhibitors. Because of the wide distribution of these compounds in nature and thus the availability of many structural analogues, several studies of the features required for lipoxygenase activity have been performed.

S. Yamamoto and co-workers have studied the effects of various flavonoids on 5-lipoxygenase from rat basophilic leukemia (RBL) cells and guinea pig polymorphonuclear leukocytes (PMN)[11,12]. The results of these studies are shown in Table 8.1. Cirsiliol (entry 2) was found to be the most potent $(IC_{50}, 10^{-7}\,mol\,L^{-1})$ of the more than 100 compounds tested, with pedalitin a close second. These studies clearly indicated that a catechol-like structure of the B ring was imperative for activity. In addition, derivatization of the C-5 phenol of cirsiliol also reduced the inhibitory activity.

Being the most potent, the characteristics of the inhibitory action of cirsiliol were studied. According to dialysis, the inhibition was irreversible and non-competitive on the basis of a Lineweaver-Burk plot. The IC_{50} of the synthetic compound, AA-861, (see the section on novel synthetic compounds) under the conditions used in this assay was $8 \times 10^{-7}\,mol\,L^{-1}$. In this study, cirsiliol was also found to inhibit slow reacting substance of anaphylaxis (SRS-A) release at the tissue level $(IC_{50}, 0.4\,\mu\,mol\,L^{-1})$ and to inhibit 12-lipoxygenase from bovine platelets and porcine leukocytes, but the IC_{50} values were about one order of magnitude higher than for the RBL 5-lipoxygenase. On the other hand, cyclo-oxygenase enzyme from the bovine vesicular gland was only slightly inhibited at high concentrations of cirsiliol. A 5-lipoxygenase from guinea pig peritoneal leukocytes was also inhibited by cirsiliol with an IC_{50} of $0.3\,\mu\,mol\,L^{-1}$.

Eupatilin and 4-demethyl eupatilin (Table 8.1, entries 11 and 12) are also reported to be 5-lipoxygenase inhibitors with IC_{50} values of $1.8 \times 10^{-5}\,mol\,L^{-1}$ and $1.4 \times 10^{-5}\,mol\,L^{-1}$ respectively versus a 5-lipoxygenase from cloned mastocytoma P-815 2-E-6 cells. Here again, the relatively low potency of these compounds compared with cirsiliol may be due to the lack of a free catechol subunit.

152

Table 8.1 Inhibition of 5-lipoxygenase by various flavonoids

ENTRY	R1	R2	R3	R4	R5	R6	R7	5-LIPOXYGENASE SOURCE	INHIBITION (CONCENTRATION OF INHIBITOR)
1	-	OCH3	OCH3	-	-	-	-	RBL supernatant	23% (10μM)
2 (cirsiliol)	OH	OCH3	OCH3	-	-	OH	OH	RBL supernatant	92% (1μM)
3 (pedalitin)	OH	OCH3	OCH3	-	-	OH	OH	RBL supernatant	91% (1μM)
4	OH	OCH3	OCH3	OCH3	-	OH	OH	RBL supernatant	83% (1μM)
5	OCH3	OH	OH	-	-	OH	OH	RBL supernatant	67% (1μM)
6	OH	-	OH	-	-	OH	OH	RBL supernatant	50% (1μM)
7 (quercetin)	OH	-	OH	-	OH	OH	OH	RBL supernatant	85% (10μM)
								RBL supernatant	50% (4μM)
								RBL supernatant	50% (2.1μM)
								Rat PMN (intact)	50% (6μM)
8	OH	OCH3	OCH3	-	-	OH	OH	RBL supernatant	64% (10μM)
9	OH	OCH3	OCH3	-	-	OCH3	OCH3	RBL supernatant	22% (10μM)
10	OH	OCH3	OCH3	-	-	OCH3	OCH3	RBL supernatant	8% (10μM)
11 (eupatilin)	OH	OCH3	OH	-	-	OCH3	OCH3	RBL supernatant	50% (98μM)
								P-815 2E6	50% (14μM)
12 (4-demethyl Eupatilin)	OH	OCH3	OH	-	-	OCH3	OH	P-815 2E6	50% (18μM)
13 (Rutin)	OH	-	OH	-	O-Rutinose	OH	OH	P-815 2E6	50% (33μM)
14 (Baicalein)	OH	OH	OH	-	-	-	-	RBL supernatant	50% (1.2μM)
15 (Trihyroxy isoflavin)*	H	OH	OH	-	-	-	OH	Human PMN (intact)	50% (1.6μM)

* lacks double bond and oxo functionality in the oxygen containing ring.

153

Although the potency of the parent compounds is low, the flavonoids may yet yield interesting compounds through subtle modification of their substituents. This is illustrated by the flavones reported by Otsuka to be discussed in a later section. A compound structurally related to the flavonoids is the dihydroxy coumarin, esculetin (**1**). This compound is reported to inhibit RBL and human PMN 5-lipoxygenase and platelet 12-lipoxygenase, with IC_{50} values of 4.5, 0.4 and 10 μ mol L^{-1} respectively[13-15].

1

ESCULETIN

Caffeic acid

The other major class of natural products that have been investigated as lipoxygenase inhibitors are the hydroxylated cinnamic acids. Of these, caffeic acid (**2**) is the most potent of the naturally occurring compounds (see Table 8.4) with an IC_{50} in the micromolar range[16]. The structural simplicity of this molecule lends itself to classical medicinal chemical modifications and thus many synthetic analogues have been investigated as potential lipoxygenase inhibitors. These analogues are reported to be considerably more active and will be discussed in a later section. It is interesting to note that conversion of one of the phenols of caffeic acid to methyl ether to yield ferulic acid substantially reduces the ability to inhibit lipoxygenase. Again, this indicates the possible role of a catechol subunit for lipoxygenase inhibition.

Synthetically prepared inhibitors

In this section, two principal types of lipoxygenase inhibitors will be discussed. These are (a) synthetically modified natural products and (b) novel synthetic compounds.

Much of the effort with synthetic inhibitors has been directed towards the 5-lipoxygenase pathway with a lesser amount of work aimed at the 12-lipoxygenase pathway. This is principally due to the biological prominence of the products of the 5-lipoxygenase pathway. Synthetic inhibitors span a wide range of potential uses, including possible therapeutic agents, pharmacological tools and mechanistic probes of the lipoxygenase enzyme itself. Synthetically modified natural products and novel synthetic compounds are invariably attempts to find a potent therapeutic agent. Naturally, compounds which fail as therapeutic agents often find use as pharmacological tools.

Synthetically modified natural products

As discusssed earlier, two of the most promising natural products in terms of their activity are the flavones and caffeic acid derivatives. The ease of structural modification of these classes of compounds has resulted in their being the subject of numerous synthetic modifications in an effort to further increase their potency.

154

The principal source of data on modified flavones has been patents from Otsuka Pharmaceutical Co. Ltd.[17,18]. The attachment of a lipophilic chain at the hydroxyl at C-6 of the flavone nucleus yielded a series of compounds approximately ten times more potent than cirsiliol. These compounds (3–5) and their reported activities are shown in Table 8.2. The activity of these compounds again illustrates the importance of lipophilicity for lipoxygenase inhibition. It is quite likely that the acetate (4) is active by virtue of being a prodrug of (3) given the importance of the catechol subunit for activity in this series.

It is somewhat surprising that these structures have a methyl ether at C-5 rather than a free hydroxy since the latter case was more potent in the natural flavones.

Research into caffeic acid derivatives has been carried out principally by the Terumo Corporation[19] and the Green Cross Corporation[20,21]. The nature of the modifications carried out by both companies has been the alteration of the carboxylic acid side chain of caffeic (2) or ferulic (6) acid. The Terumo Corporation has reported on derivatives of both caffeic

6

and ferulic acids. They have also claimed some compounds which are modified on the aromatic ring. However, the principal type of change has been to the carboxylate-bearing side chain. This chain has been extended, as in structure (7), and/or different esters and amides of varying complexity have been

Table 8.2 Inhibition of RBL-1 5-lipoxygenase by modified flavones

NUMBER	R	R'	% INHIBITION AT 0.1 μM
3	C_6H_{13}	H	85%
4	C_6H_{13}	Ac	75%
5	$C_{12}H_{25}$	H	95%

prepared. A few representative structures (**7–12**) are given below and the activities against the 5-lipoxygenase of P-815 E6 mouse mastocytoma cells of specific compounds are given in Table 8.3.

The amide groups of the Terumo compounds (**7–12**) are quite complex and contain a large number of nitrogens; this is in direct contrast to the simple compounds reported by Green Cross. These compounds are all derivatives of caffeic acid and fall into four clases; esters, amides, enones and olefins as shown below. Several of these compounds are very potent inhibitors of 5-lipoxyenase with IC_{50} values as low as 10^{-8} mol L^{-1}. A few representative examples of each class are given in Table 8.4.

In summary, synthetic flavone and caffeic acid derivatives have been reported whose potency is sufficient for consideration as therapeutic agents. Whether the promising results of the *in vitro* tests can be eventually translated into a successful drug remains to be seen.

Table 8.3 Inhibitory activity of caffeic and ferulic acid derivatives versus P-815 2E6 5-lipoxygenase

STRUCTURE	IC_{50} (µM)
7	8.0
8	0.2
9	3.0
10	0.003
11	0.3
12	0.04

Table 8.4 Inhibition of guinea pig PMN 5-lipoxygenase by caffeic acid derivatives

PARENT	R	IC_{50} (μM)
2 CAFFEIC ACID		1.00
13 ESTER	$n\text{-}C_4H_9$ $n\text{-}C_2H_5$	0.067 0.165
14 AMIDE	$n\text{-}C_8H_{17}$ $n\text{-}C_{14}H_{29}$	0.042 0.155
15 ENONE	$n\text{-}C_3H_7$ $n\text{-}C_5H_{11}$	0.275 0.035
16 OLEFIN	$n\text{-}C_2H_5$ $n\text{-}C_4H_9$	0.095 0.012

Novel synthetic compounds
This is a structurally diverse group of compounds which have been prepared with the goal of developing a lipoxygenase inhibitor. These compounds are almost exclusively the result of efforts in this field by pharmaceutical companies. Consequently, the genesis of the structural classes being developed is often unclear. Some are based on analyses of previously described natural inhibitors; however the majority were developed from leads obtained from extensive screening of natural and synthetic products. The structures of members of this class of inhibitors often bear little resemblance to each other, but several features are common to all. Most compounds contain an aromatic ring and are structurally less complex and synthetically more straightforward to prepare than the natural products discussed previously. The aromatic ring is usually an electron-rich phenyl moiety and often has at least one heteroatom substituent but examples containing a heterocyclic aromatic ring are not

157

uncommon. Because of the structural diversity of this group of inhibitors, lines of categorization are not obvious; they will be discussed as a whole without subdivision into classes.

One chemical feature common to the inhibitors described previously is their ability to act as antioxidants. Inhibition of lipoxyenase by this type of compound is not surprising since these enzymes catalyze an oxidative process. The challenge here is to make the inhibition specific to a certain lipoxyenase. To this end, classical synthetic antioxidants and their analogues have been evaluated as lipoxygenase inhibitors.

An antioxidant in common use is butylated hydroxytoluene (BHT) (17), as a quick check of the list of ingredients of many food products will show. On its own BHT is a moderately potent inhibitor of 5-lipoxygenase[22] with

17: R=CH₃ BHT
18: R=OCH₃ BHA

an IC_{50} of $2\,\mu\,mol\,L^{-1}$. However, it is not specific and also inhibits 12-lipoxygenase and cyclo-oxygenase enzymes. A related compound butylated hydroxyanisole (BHA) (18) is also reported to be a lipoxygenase inhibitor. Two analogues of BHT which show improved activity of selectivity are R-830 from Riker Laboratories (19)[23] and KME-4 (20)[24,25] from Kanegafuchi. However, these compounds are at least equipotent at inhibition of cyclo-oxygenase. Both of these compounds vary from BHT by the replacement of the methyl group *para* to the phenol with another more lipophilic moiety and are representatives of a large number of related structures. The activities of these compounds are given in Table 8.5.

Both these compounds show *in vivo* effects which classical cyclo-oxygenase inhibitors do not, and which may be due to their inhibition of lipoxygenase. However, this is only one possible explanation and not proof of this hypothesis.

A second class of antioxidant are the polyhydroxylated aromatics, catechol being a representative of this group. We have already seen how this moiety is important for the inhibition of lipoxygenase by flavones and caffeic acid and their derivatives. Catechol (21) by itself is a poor lipoxygenase inhibitor[26] with an IC_{50} of $62\,\mu mol\,L^{-1}$; however, introduction of a lipophilic tail as in compound (22), reported by Yamanouchi Corporation[27], lowers this value dramatically to $54\,nmol\,L^{-1}$. The reader's attention is drawn to the similarities between compound (22) and the olefin compounds of Green Cross discussed earlier (Table 8.4).

Amino phenols and amino thiophenols[28–31] are also reported to be lipoxygenase inhibitors, illustrating that dioxygen substitution is not a basic requirement. Although these compounds are not classically antioxidants, they

158

Table 8.5 Inhibitory activity of the BHT analogues R-830 and KME-4

COMPOUND	ENZYME	IC_{50} (μM)
19 R-830	Bovine Seminal Vesical CO	0.5
	Guinea Pig Lung 5-LO	20*
	RBL-1 5-LO	30
20 KME-4	RBL-1 Sup CO	0.74
	Rabbit Platelet CO	0.44
	RBL-1 Sup 5-LO	1.3
	Guinea Pig PMN Sup. 5-LO	0.85
	Guinea Pig PMN intact 5-LO	11.5
	Rabbit Platelet 12-LO	no inhibition at 100

* substrate linoleic acid

21: R=H
22: R=$(CH_2)_{10}$-CH_2OH

can partake in oxidation–reduction reactions similar to the catechols. Several examples (**23–28**) of this molecular class and their activities are shown below in Table 8.6.

Toluene-3,4-dithiol (**29**) is simply a thiocatechol, and, as such, would be expected to inhibit lipoxygenases. This is indeed the case[32,33] (IC_{50} 5 μmol L^{-1}), however, the inhibition has not been ascribed to its antioxidant properties but to its ability to strongly chelate Fe^{3+}. As with the catechol analogues of arachidonic acid, the mechanism by which the inhibition by toluene dithiol occurs is unclear. Hydroxyamine is another moiety which may inhibit lipoxyenase by virtue of its chelation of iron as observed with substrate and product analogues containing hydroxamic acid moieties. Therefore, this functionality has been incorporated into synthetic compounds in an effort to

159

Table 8.6 Inhibition of 5-lipoxygenase by amino phenols

STRUCTURE	IC_{50} μM
23	15*
24	0.4*
25	3.0+
26	0.14
27	1.0*
28 SERIES	0.5–10

*Also inhibits cyclooxygenase
+Does not inhibit cyclooxygenase

29

prepare lipoxygenase inhibitors. Three series of compounds of this type are shown below: compound (**30**) from Squibb[34], (**31**) from Veb Arzneimittel Dresden[35], (**32**) from Abbott[36] and (**33**) from Sandoz[37]. All are reported to be potent 5-lipoxygenase inhibitors.

A series of compounds related to the catechols are the para-hydroquinones. In contrast to the catechols, the quinone form is generally more stable than

30

31

32

33

the hydroquinone form. Therefore, in many cases, the quinone has been evaluated instead of or in addition to, the hydroquinone. While the quinone itself cannot act as an antioxidant, it can be reduced in the milieu of the assay to the hydroquinone or an intermediate that can act as such. This supposition is supported by the observation that both halves of a quinone–hydroquinone pair have comparable activities in the limited number of cases where such data are available[38]. That quinones are lipoxygenase inhibitors by virtue of the antioxidant properties of a reduced form is at present only a hypothesis which can be confirmed or denied by studies utilizing pure enzyme.

35

COENZYME Q_{10}

The most prominent of the quinones at present is the Takeda compound, AA-861 (34, see Table 8.7)[39,40]. However, several other companies have also reported quinones as lipoxygenase inhibitors. The genesis of these quinones is unclear but the structural similarities between them and coenzyme Q_{10} (35)[41] may provide a clue. The activity of the quinones appears to depend principally on the nature of the long chain and on the electronic density of the quinone. The most studied of the quinones is AA-861 and a summary of its inhibitory properties is given in Table 8.7.

Many other quinones, including analogues of AA-861[38–40,42–45], have been reported as inhibitors of 5-lipoxygenase. These results are summarized in Table 8.8.

Several points with regard to Table 8.8 are worth noting. First is the lack of activity with the AA-861 analogue (45) that cannot participate in a redox pathway. Second is the insensitivity of the potency to changes in the lipophilic

161

Table 8.7 5-lipoxygenase inhibition by AA-861

CELL	INTACT (I) OR SUPERNATANT (S)	IC_{50} µM
Guinea Pig PMN	I	0.8
Rat PMN	I	0.05
RBL-1	S	2.6
Guinea Pig Lung	I	0.1*

*SRS-A Release

chain. Third is the relatively low potency of the quinone parent of AA-861 (**46**), indicating the importance of the lipophilic chain. The other quinone of substantial interest is compond (**50**) and the prodrug (**51**). Both of these compounds show good activity versus 5-lipoxygenase. However, more importantly, compound (**52**) has been reported to be very effective as a topical agent against psoriasis, a disease where lipoxygenase products are thought to play an important role.

Substitution of another heteroatom for one of the oxygens of a quinone/hydroquinone yields a related series of compounds. Examples of this type of compound have been reported by Merck (**54**) and (**55**)[46,47], Sterling (**57**)[48,49] and Upjohn (**57**)[50] and are shown in Table 8.9. The most potent of these are the two series reported by Merck with Sterling's series a close second and the Upjohn compound considerably less active.

As seen earlier with BHT and its derivatives, a quinone/hydroquinone pair is not obligatory for antioxidant activity. Therefore, monoheteroatom-substituted aromatics or multi-substituted aromatics, where derivatization of the hetroatoms blocks quinone (or quinonoid) formation, may also behave as antioxidants. Conversely, such substitution on a lipoxygenase inhibitor does not demand that the inhibition is due to the compound's antioxidant properties, although it must be considered as a possibility. There are many compounds that definitely fall into the above class; however, there are others that are borderline members. Therefore, inclusion or exclusion of some compounds in this section has been strictly arbitrary. The IC_{50} values of these compounds range from 10^{-1} to 10^{-8} mol L^{-1}, with two of the most potent being the benzofuran derivatives of Merck (**58**) and (**59**)[51,52] and the quinoline derivatives of Revlon (**60**)[53]. The latter compound is claimed to be based on 15-HETE, a reported endogenous inhibitor. However, the low activity of compound

162

Table 8.8 5-lipoxygenase inhibition by quinones and hydroquinones

COMPOUND	CELL	IC$_{50}$ (*estimated) (μM)
36 R=CH$_3$', R' =	GP PMN	0.8
37 R-CH$_3$'; R' =	"	0.9*
38 R=CH$_3$; R' =	"	0.8*
39 R=CH$_3$; R' =	"	1.2*
40 R=CH$_3$; R' =	"	75
41 R=OCH$_3$; R' =	"	1.5*
42 R=OCH$_3$; R' =	"	0.5*
43	GP PMN	0.9*

163

44 R=OCH$_3$;
R'= [structure: chain with two triple bonds ending in OH]   "   0.5*

45 [structure: benzene ring with OMe, methyl substituents and chain ending in OH]   "   100

46 R=CH$_3$;
R'=H   "   50*

47 H$_3$C [structure: chain with two triple bonds ending in OH]   "   inactive at 100

48 [structure: quinone with MeO, OMe, CH$_2$ linked dimer]₂   "   0.5*

49 [structure: quinone with long chain with cis double bond]   "   0.3-0.5

50 MeO [structure: naphthoquinone with Cl, two MeO groups]   Rat PMN   0.06
MeO   RBL-1 Super.   0.05-0.1

⁺**51** MeO [structure: naphthalene with OAc, OAc, Cl, two MeO]   Human PMN   20
MeO   Rat PMN   0.02-0.06
                    RBL-1 Super.   0.1-0.5

52 [structure: quinoline quinone with N-phenyl]   NO DATA

53 [structure: quinoxaline quinone with N-(fluorophenyl)]

✝ Prodrug for corresponding quinone.

164

Table 8.9 5-lipoxygenase inhibition by heteroquinones and heterohydroquinones

SERIES	CELL	IC$_{50}$ (μM)
 54 X =Br, Cl, F, OMe Y =H, OMe	RBL-1 supernatant Rat PMN Human PMN	0.03 0.007 0.006
 55	RBL-1 supernatant Rat PMN Human PMN	0.005 0.03 0.5
 56	RBL-1 supernatant	0.09
 57		10

(**60**) in the RBL-1 assay indicates that it may not be acting directly on the enzyme. Some biochemical data for these compounds is given in Table 8.10. Other examples of this class of compounds are shown below[53-64].

Up to this point, all of the inhibitors discussed above have had a six membered aromatic ring as their central feature, and, in most cases, this has

Table 8.10 Inhibition of 5-lipoxygenase IC$_{50}$ (μmol L^{-1})

	58	59	60
RBL-1 supernatant	0.03	0.3	80
Rat PMN	0.05	0.04	0.2-0.5
Human PMN	0.5	0.08	6.0-8.0
Guinea Pig PMN	–	–	0.03

* also a potent cyclooxygenase inhibitor

been a phenyl ring. However, there are a comparable number of inhibitors which are based on five membered heterocycles (61–71). These heterocycles

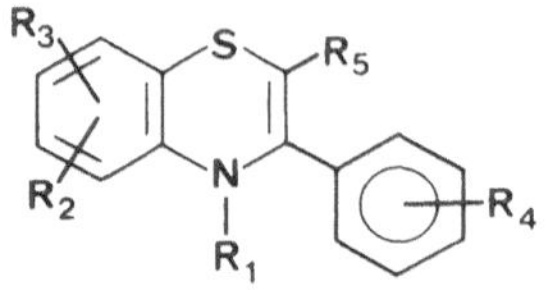

61

BAYER 0.5–1.0µM

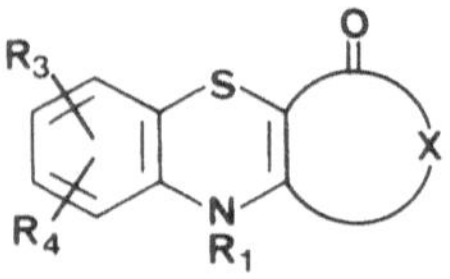

62

BAYER 0.5–1.0µM

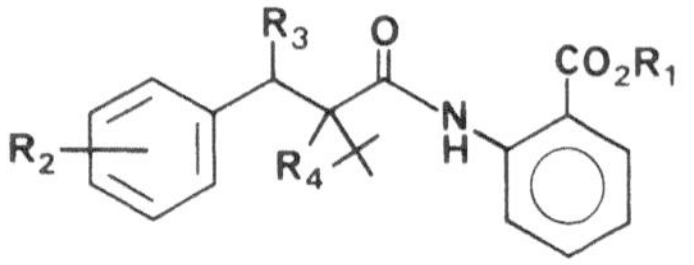

63

KISSEI 10^{-1}–10^{-4}M

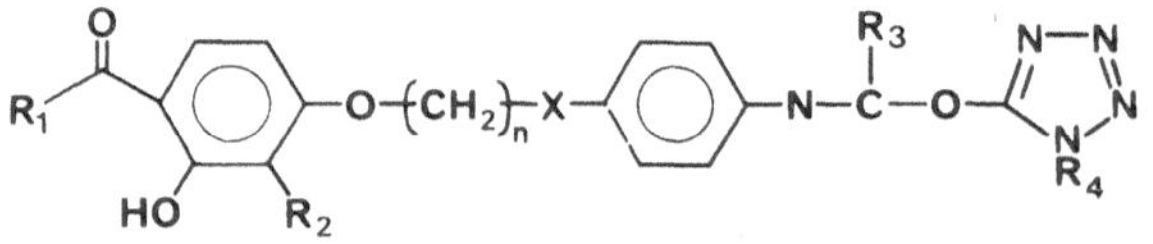

64

LILLY

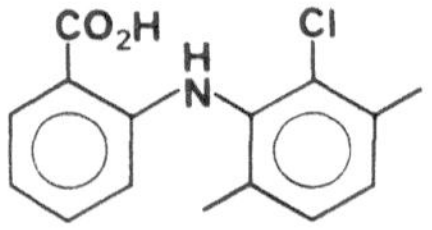

65

MECLOFENAMATE

300uM

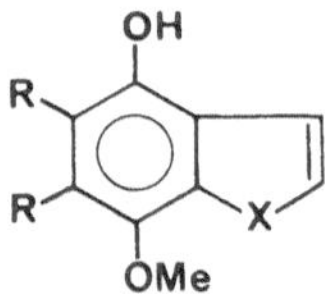

66

X=O, NMe, S

UPJOHN

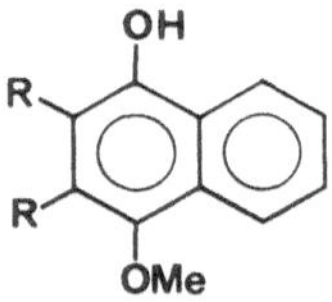

67

UPJOHN

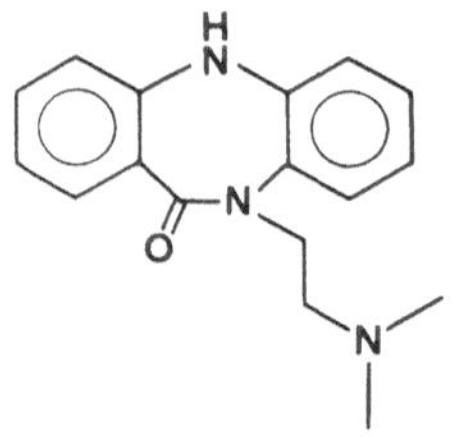

68

TEIKOKU

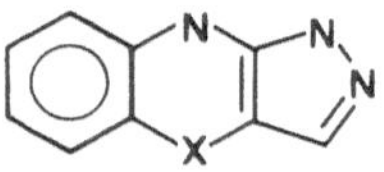

69

X=O, S

BAYER 0.1µM

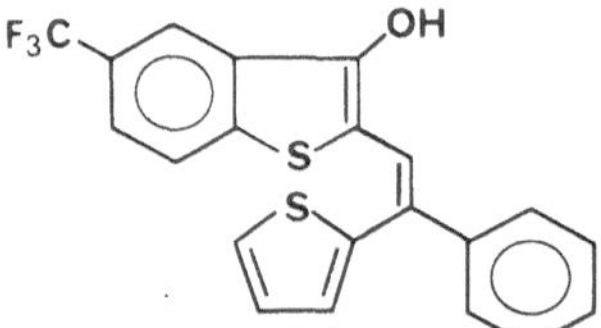

CO 0.5 µM

LO 2.0 µM

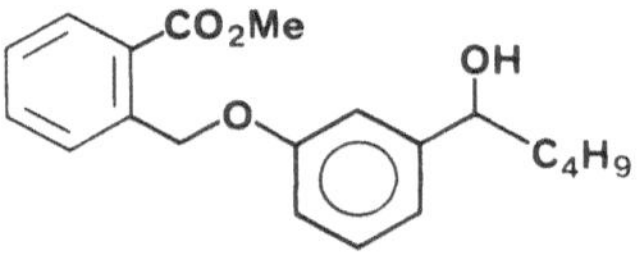

70

MERCK &CO.

71

USV

166

may contain more than one heteroatom, and, while nitrogen is the most common heteroatom, molecules containing oxygen and sulphur are not uncommon. The most widely studied of these compounds are the aminopyrazolines (**72–76**) with the major contribution being from Burroughs-Wellcome.

72-76

The most well known of these compounds is BW 755C (**72**)[65,66] which has found wide use as a pharmacological tool. These compounds also inhibit cyclo-oxygenase with comparable potency. The inhibitory activity of BW 755C and several of its analogues is given in Table 8.11. The genesis of these inhibitors seems to be based on the observation that a commercially used photographic developer, phenidone (**77**)[67,68] inhibited both lipoxygenase and cyclo-oxygenase enzymes.

Similar compounds have been reported by Chinoin Laboratories[69], the major difference being that the nitrogen of the pyrazoline is not attached

Table 8.11 Inhibition of 5-lipoxygenase and cyclo-oxygenase by 3-amino-2-pyrazoline derivatives

	R	IC$_{50}$ (μM)	
		5-LO	CO
72	H (BW 755C)	2.9	3.1
73	Me (BW 540C)	0.4	1.2
74	Pr	0.04	0.3
75	Bu	0.08	0.2
76	Bn	0.1	0.1
77	Phenidone	12	42

directly to an aromatic ring but to an sp³ carbon. These compounds (**78 and 79**) are much less potent than BW 755C, sugesting that direct attachment of the heteroatom to the aromatic ring may be important for inhibitory activity. It is also interesting to note than the Chinoin compounds stimulate rather than inhibit the cyclo-oxygenase enzyme.

78: R=H (KD 679)
79: R=Me (KD 785)

Addition of another double bond into the heterocyclic ring of the pyrazoline gives the corresponding pyrazole (**80**), an aromatic species which has lipoxygenase-inhibiting activity. Fisons have reported compounds in this series analogous to BW 755C which are also inhibitors of lipoxygenase and cyclo-oxygenase[70]. The intrinsic activity of the pyrazole is best illustrated by LC-6 (**81**)[71] which has an IC_{50} of 47 μmol L^{-1} for inhibition of histamine release by human basophils on challenge with antigen E, and of approximately 50 μmol L^{-1} versus soybean 15-lipoxygenase. No data on direct measurement of 5-lipoxygenase inhibitory activity was found; however, LC-6 was equipotent with nordihydroguiaretic acid (NDGA) versus 15-lipoxygenase.

80

81
LC-6

82
IG$_{50}$ ~1μM

83

84

Pyrazole derivatives have also been reported as lipoxygenase inhibitors by Bayer (**82**)[72] and (**83**)[73] and Troponwerke (**84**)[74] and are shown below. Bayer has also reported triazole (**85**)[75] as a 5-lipoxygenase inhibitor with an IC_{50} of 3 μmol L^{-1}. A series of compounds which combine some of the active features of both the pyrazolines and pyrazoles have been prepared at the Institute of Drug Research in Budapest, series (**86**)[76]. While the pyrazole is obviously

168

present, the hydrazide can be considered electronically analogous to a *N*-phenyl pyrazoline.

85

86

X = 3⁻Cl, 4⁻Cl, 4 Me, 3⁻CF

These compounds were found to be up to ten times as potent as BW 755C versus potato 5-lipoxygenase. The analogy between a hydrazone and a pyrazoline may also be the rationale behind the development of BW 755C from the phenidone lead. An analogy can also be seen between *N*-phenyl pyrazoline and the hydrazones CBS 1108 (**87**)[77] and CBS 1114 (**88**)[78] reported by Chauvin Blanche as dual inhibitors with IC_{50} values of 2 and 15 μmol L^{-1} against 5-lipoxygenase, and 2 and 1.5 μmol L^{-1} against cyclo-oxygenase respectively. Upjohn has also reported a series of hydrazones, such as (**89**)[79], as lipoxygenase inhibitors with IC_{50} values from 0.14–140 μmol L^{-1} against 12-lipoxygenase.

87
CBS 1108

88
CBS 1114

89

The pyrrole derivative, piriprost (**90**)[80] is reported by Upjohn to inhibit 5-lipoxygenase with an IC_{50} of 1.8 μmol L^{-1}, while its methyl ester has an IC_{50} of 0.42 μmol L^{-1}. Piriprost is also reported to possibly inhibit LTC$_4$ synthase ($IC_{50} \simeq 1$ μmol L^{-1}). Appending a benzene onto a pyrrole gives an indole. Indoles have been reported as lipoxygenase inhibitors by Merck, Teikoku, Warner-Lambert and Yoshitomi (compounds **91, 92, 93** and **94** respectively)[81–84].

Fenflumazole (**95**)[85], ketoconazole (**96**)[86] and benoxaprofen (**97**)[87–89] have also been reported to inhibit lipoxygenase with IC_{50} values of 6 μmol L^{-1}, 30 μmol L^{-1}, and 5–30 μmol L^{-1} respectively.

Since lipoxygenation is postulated to occur via the formation of a carbon centred radical, compounds that inhibit the formation of this radical, or trap it once formed, would be expected to be lipoxygenase inhibitors. Such

169

90
PIRIPROST

91

92

93

94
IC_{50} 14.5 μM

170

95
FENFLUMAZOLE

96

97
BENOXAPROFEN

compounds often act by formation of a lower energy radical, thus diverting the intended path of the reaction. Disulphides are one such class of molecules and have been found to inhibit lipoxygenases. Bayer's non-symmetrical disulphide (**98**)[90] has an IC_{50} of 3.5 μmol L^{-1} versus thrombocyte 12-lipoxygenase. Several aromatic disulphides based on structure (**99**) were studied as 5-lipoxygenase (RBL-1) inhibitors by Merck[91,92]; the activities of some of these compounds are given in Table 8.12.

98

99

The obvious trend in these data is that electron withdrawing substituents which would destabilize the sulphydryl radical decrease the potency of the compound, while electron donating, radical stabilizing substituents increase the potency. These compounds were found to inhibit 5-lipoxygenase selectively in contrast to cyclo-oxygenase or 15-lipoxygenase. The compounds proved much less active and selective with intact cells, possible due to interference by membrane protein sulphydryl groups.

These are several examples of lipoxygenase inhibitors based on six-membered heterocycles containing one or more nitrogen atom. The best known of these is dipyridamole (**100**)[93] from Abbott Laboratories. Dipyridamole inhibits 5-HETE synthesis by RBL-1 supernatant and in calcium ionophore-stimulated RBL-1 cells with IC_{50} values of 0.6 and 4.3 μmol L^{-1} respectively. Other representatives of this class are shown below[94-97].

Various other structural classes have been reported as lipoxygenase inhibitors. Timegadine (**101**) is an inhibitor of 5-lipoxygenase and cyclo-oxygenase, with IC_{50} values of 7 μmol L^{-1} and 10 μmol L^{-1} respectively[98].

171

Table 8.12 Inhibition of RBL-1 supernatant 5-lipoxygenase by aromatic disulphides

R	IC$_{50}$ (µM)
ortho-CH$_3$	1.3 µM
para-CH$_3$	0.8 µM
ortho-NH$_2$	1.3 µM
H	1.5 µM
ortho-acetamido	22 µM
ortho-aldehydo	27 µM
meta nitro, para carboxyl	250 µM

100

101
TIMEGADINE
IC$_{50}$ (5LO) 0.4–20µM

However, it is apparently more potent when LTB$_4$, rather than 5-HETE, production is monitored (IC$_{50}$, 0.4 µmol L^{-1}). This may indicate inhibition of LTA$_4$ synthase or hydrolase as well.

The last group of compounds to be discussed are those based on a seven-membered carbocyclic ring. The cycloheptatrienes, such as (**102**), are selective 5-lipoxygenase inhibitors[99] with IC$_{50}$ values in the 3 µmol L^{-1} range when tested against the RBL-1 enzyme. The other example of this class is the cycloheptatrienone, 3-methoxytropolone (**103**), which has been reported to selectively inhibit 12-lipoxygenase with IC$_{50}$ values of 1.8 µmol L^{-1} versus bovine platelet 12-lipoxygenase and 280 µmol L^{-1} versus RBL-1 5-lipoxygenase[100].

In summary, a wide range of structurally diverse compounds can act as lipoxyenase inhibitors. These compounds can inhibit the enzyme in many

102

103

different ways, but the most common and most potent ones are those which are potentially good electron donors and thus are possibly acted on by the lipoxygenase enzyme preferentially. Lipoxygenase enzymes may also be inhibited by molecules which chelate iron, implying the presence of iron at the active site. However, it should be reemphasized that due to the poorly understood nature of mammalian 5-lipoxygenase, statements regarding the mode of action of any inhibitor must be regarded as a proposal only and not a definitive answer.

LTA$_4$ synthase or HPETE dehydrase

Due to the uniqueness of the chemical transformation catalysed by this enzyme, it is, on the surface, a very attractive target. However, the current evidence suggests that 5-lipoxygenase activity and LTA$_4$ synthase activity are intimately linked, thus making the prospect of finding a specific LTA$_4$ synthetase inhibitor less than bright. There are, however, scattered reports of compounds which do not inhibit the formation of 5-HPETE (or 5-HETE) but do inhibit the formation of LTB$_4$ and/or LTC$_4$, or give differential inhibition of the formation of 5-HETE and the latter products. Inhibition of the synthesis of both would indicate blockage of the formation of LTA$_4$, while inhibition of one without the other would suggest an effect further down the pathway. The only compound reported which does not inhibit the formation of 5-HETE but effectively reduces the formation of LTB$_4$ and LTC$_4$ is diethylcarbamazine (**104**) (IC$_{50}$ 7 μmol L^{-1})[101,102]. However, this compound also inhibits glutathione-S-transferase (LTC$_4$ synthase)[103], albeit at high concentrations. 5-Amino-salicylic acid (**105**) inhibits the synthesis of LTB$_4$ but not 5-HETE, possibly indicating inhibition of LTA$_4$ synthase[104]. However, its effect on LTC$_4$ production has not been reported.

104

105

173

LTA$_4$ hydrolase (LTB$_4$ synthase)

This enzyme has potential as a site for intervention and has been well characterized[105]. However, very little work towards finding an inhibitor has been reported. In fact, the only compounds which are definite LTB$_4$ synthase inhibitors are the LTA$_4$ analogues, LTA$_3$ (**106**) and related compounds[106] shown in Table 8.13 reported by Merck Frosst. The inhibition by LTA$_3$ was shown to be due to the LTA$_3$ having a good affinity for the active site but being a very poor substrate[107]. The result of this combination is that the enzyme becomes alkylated by the reactive allylic epoxide moiety, thus giving irreversible inhibition. It is interesting to note that the methano-analogue of LTA$_4$ is not a good inhibitor of the hydrolase, implying a requirement for the epoxide moiety for active site affinity.

Glutathione-S-transferase (LTC$_4$ synthase)

This enzyme is interesting as a target for inhibition since blocking it would only affect the levels of the sulphidopeptide leukotrienes. However, this class of enzyme is ubiquitous and very important to detoxification of compounds. Therefore, selective inhibition of LTC$_4$ synthesis originally appeared very difficult. However, recent evidence has brightened the prospect for selective moderation of this enzyme, since it now appears that LTC$_4$ synthase is a

Table 8.13 Inhibition of LTA$_4$ hydrolase by LTA$_4$ analogues

COMPOUND	% INHIBITION VS vs 25 µM LTA$_4$
106 LTA$_3$	100 (IC$_{50}$ ≈ 0.3 µM)
107	100 (IC$_{50}$ ≈ 0.5 µM)
108	70
109	36
110	0

specific glutathione-S-transferase. Piriprost (**90**)[108] and diethylcarbamazine (**104**)[103] both inhibit the synthesis of LTC_4. However the degree of inhibition is dependent not only on the cellular source of the enzyme preparation but also on the particular isoenzymes in the preparation. As it is not known which enzyme is most important for the synthesis of LTC_4 the IC_{50} values obtained are difficult if not impossible to compare.

Summary

In recent years, numerous potent inhibitors of lipoxygenases have been reported. Due to the newness of this area of research, the therapeutic potential of inhibitors is yet to be determined, although some preliminary data in animal models and man looks very encouraging. The main thrust of this work has been the development of inhibitors of 5-lipoxygenase predicated by the perceived biological prominence of the products of this pathway.

The development of this class of therapeutic agent has not been without difficulties. Many of these have resulted from the problems associated with working with the extremely unstable 5-lipoxygenase enzyme. However, the field has progressed rapidly despite these difficulties and progress continues to be made. Since the exact properties of many of the best lipoxygenase inhibitors are not immediately disclosed due to their proprietary nature, the true picture of the state of the area is difficult to determine. However, it is most likely that the next five years will be a watershed for this field of endeavour.

Inhibition of the other enzymes in the 5-lipoxygenase pathway has not been studied extensively. In fact, many of the compounds reported to inhibit these enzymes were prepared for other purposes. The inhibition of the steps subsequent to lipoxygenase has therefore been, in general, a fortuitous finding. The lack of activity in this area is by no means an indication of lack of potential but a reflection of the concentrated effort on inhibition of 5-lipoxygenase. In all likelihood, inhibitors of these enzymes will be represented in the second wave of enzyme inhibitors directed against the lipoxygenase pathway.

In conclusion, the tip of the iceberg has barely been scratched in this area of endeavour. Thus, the future will undoubtedly hold new discoveries and ideas that will be of great interest and intellectually stimulating.

RECEPTOR ANTAGONISTS

The history of leukotriene receptor antagonists predates the determination of their structure by several years. The interest in this field was predicated on the spasmogenic properties of a mysterious substance known as the Slow Reacting Substance of Anaphylaxis or SRS-A. Although SRS-A was first discovered more than 40 years ago, structural elucidation was only accomplished approximately seven years ago. Because of the extreme potency of SRS-A, it is present in minute quantities and its structure was, of necessity, determined by comparison of the natural substance(s) with well characterized

synthetic material. The active components of the SRS-A are the sulphidopeptide leukotrienes LTC_4, LTD_4 and LTE_4. The name leukotriene is derived from
the strong triene U.V. chromophore possessed by these compounds, and from
their initial cellular source in leukocytes.

Sulphidopeptide leukotriene antagonists

The principal pharmacological effects of SRS-A include contraction of smooth
muscle and increased vascular permeability, thus implying a possible role in
allergic asthma. Of the leukotrienes, LTD_4 is the most potent spasmogen and
is believed to be of primary importance in humans. In this section, the term
'leukotriene antagonist' will be used to describe SRS-A antagonists.

Despite the lack of characterization of SRS-A, several antagonists of its
action were developed in the mid to late seventies by using biologically
generated SRS-A. Since this material was a mixture of LTC_4, LTD_4 and LTE_4
in varying ratios, plus possibly other factors, comparison of the potency of
these compounds with that of compounds studied using pure synthetic
leukotrienes should be made cautiously. Where possible, the data presented
for a compound will be that generated using pure material. The activities of
a leukotriene antagonist are much more conducive to comparison than those
of the lipoxygenase inhibitors. This is, in part, due to a single assay system,
the guinea-pig ileum, being used predominantly. Also, data on antagonists
may be translated into PA_2 values which are less variable than IC_{50} values
and will be quoted when available.

Of the early antagonists, one compound stands out; FPL-55712[109-112] (**111**)
from Fisons which was developed as an offshoot of their Intal program. While
FPL-55712 was quite potent *in vitro*, this activity could not be translated *in
vivo* due to the very short half-life of the compound. Fisons have subsequently
reported other related compounds with improved *in vivo* properties, such as
FPL-59257 (**112**)[113]. The structure of FPL-55712 is well worth noting since
portions of it have been incorporated into many of the leukotriene antagonists
reported to date. This is especially true of the propyl hydroxyacetophenone
'left half'. Since FPL-55712 was the first potent SRS-A antagonist, it quickly
obtained the status of the standard for determination of the involvement of
SRS-A in *in vitro* experiments and this status has continued to the present
day. Due to the wide usage of FPL-55712 as a standard, results obtained by
different workers are much easier to compare. To this end, where possible,
the potency of compounds will be listed with the value obtained for FPL-
55712 (Table 8.14). Two related series were reported by Glaxo[114] and
Beecham[115] in the late 1970s, compounds (**113**) and (**114**) respectively. The
Beecham compound was claimed to be approximately ten times more potent
than FPL-55712 versus SRS-A-induced contraction of the guinea pig ileum.

The elucidation of the structure of the active components of SRS-A in
1979–80 greatly stimulated research in this area. Knowledge of the structure
of the agonist led to the preparation of analogues that would bind to the
receptor but not trigger it; that is, be antagonists. Comparing the antagonist,
FPL-55712, with the structure of LTD_4, workers at Merck Frosst deduced

that the chromone portion of the antagonist was possibly binding to the receptor where the peptide portion of LTD_4 binds. Therefore, they prepared the LTD_4 analogue (**115**) in which the peptide was replaced with the chromone portion of FPL-55712. This compound proved to be a potent antagonist of LTD_4 in the guinea-pig ileum assay with a PA_2 of 7.3 (FPL-55712 $PA_2 \simeq$ 7.0), thus lending credence to the rationale behind its preparation. In an effort to simplify the structure of this analogue, the linear backbone was partially replaced by a phenyl ring, as in compound (**116**). These compounds also proved to be potent LTD_4 antagonists with IC_{50} values of approximately $0.3\,\mu\text{mol}\,L^{-1}$ (FPL-55712 $0.2\,\mu\text{mol}\,L^{-1}$). Many other reports of antagonists based on the leukotriene structure have also appeared[116-120].

Although the leukotriene analogues provided clues to the requirements of the receptors and were, on the whole, intellectually satisfying exercises, the probability of the development of drug candidates from these leads is small. Therefore, the development of a pharmaceutical leukotriene antagonist fell to more traditional medicinal chemistry methods. It is here that the importance of the structure of FPL-55712 becomes apparent. For, despite extensive effort on the part of many pharmaceutical companies, a large percentage of potent sulphidopeptide leukotriene antagonists incorporate the hydroxyaceto-phenone portion of FPL-55712. Several examples of these compounds are shown in Table 8.14. Of these compounds, LY 171883 (**122**)[121] and LY 163443 (**123**) from Eli Lilly and L-649,923 (**125**) and L-648,051 (**126**)[122] from Merck Frosst have been the most thoroughly studied.

Table 8.14 Hydroxy-acetophenone containing peptido leukotriene antagonists

			R=		ACTIVITY – GUINEA PIG ILEUM % INHIBITION OF CONTRACTION @ CONCENTRATION
			COMPANY/CODE	pA_2	(ILEUM)
111			FISONS (FPL-55712)	7.1	50% @ 0.01
112			FISONS (FPL-59257)	7.8	–

113   CO$_2$H

Glaxo   –   –

114   OH NO$_2$

Beecham   –   50% @ 0.006

117   NH$_2$ / CN

American Home
Products   –   –

118

Beecham   –   50% @ 0.4

119   Me / Cl

CIBA–GEIGY (CGP 35 949)   8.2*

120   CO$_2$H

Hoffmann–LaRoche   –   –

121   CO$_2$H

Hoffmann–LaRoche   –   50% @ 0.2

122

Eli Lilly (LY-171883)   7.2   100% @ 3

Table 8.14 — *continued*

LIPOXYGENASE INHIBITORS

123	Eli Lilly (LY-163443)	8.1	–
124	Eli Lilly	–	92% @ 100
125	Merck Frosst	8.1	–
126	Merck Frosst	7.7	–
127	Merck Frosst	–	100% @ 2
128	Merck Frosst	–	100% @ 2
129	Merck Frosst	–	100% @ 2
130	Wyeth (WY-44329)	–	–
131	Yamanouchi (YM-16638)		50% @ 1

Table 8.14 — *continued*

179

113

114

115

116

The predominance of FPL substructure in the reported LTD_4 (or SRS-A) antagonists is by no means a reflection of the necessity for this type of structure for potent antagonism. More correctly, it is the result of the combination of several factors. First, FPL-55712 is a potent compound, indicating a good fit on the receptor. Thus, improvement of potency and structural divergence is more difficult. Secondly, the proven potency of the FPL 'left half' provided an easy entry for first generation LTD_4 antagonists. Lastly, because this area of research has been the province of the pharmaceutical industry, there has been a certain time lag before the structure of these compounds and their activities were reported.

A partial divergence from the FPL type structures is seen in the series of compounds (**132**)[123,124] reported by the Ono Pharmaceutical Company as potent LTD_4 antagonists. The most potent of these compounds are approximately one thousand times more potent than FPL-55712 (eg: RS-411: PA_2 10.4 vs. 7.69). While these compounds do not incorporate the hydroxyacetophenane portion of FPL-55712, they do have an equivalent to

180

132
RS-411

the chromone portion. The potency of these compounds and the chromone LTD$_4$ analogue (**115**) prepared by Merck Frosst illustrate that this substructure, as well as the more studied hydroxyacetophenone, has substantial potential activity associated with it.

Two totally structurally unrelated compounds, the thio acetals (**133**) and (**134**)[125] and Amoxanox (**135**)[126], are reported to be equipotent to FPL-55712, indicating that none of the latter structure is a basic requirement for potency. Recently, Smith, Kline and French have reported the thio ether (**136**)[127], developed from the thioacetal lead, as being 100 times more potent than FPL-55712.

133: R = Bu
134: R = Ph

135
AMOXANOX

136

LTB$_4$ antagonists

The other leukotriene whose actions it would be of interest to antagonize is leukotriene B$_4$ (LTB$_4$). This dihydroxy fatty acid has very different properties from the sulphidopeptide leukotrienes and thus antagonists of its action would be targeted at other physiological conditions. LTB$_4$ is a potent chemotactic agent and has been implicated in psoriasis and inflammatory conditions. While these are areas of great interest for drug therapy, the reports of LTB_4 receptor antagonists are few and far between. This is partially due to the newness of the field; however, it is also the result of the research priorities being weighted in favour of 5-lipoxygenase inhibitors and sulphidopeptide leukotriene antagonists.

The four compounds (**120,137–9**) are reported to be LTB_4 receptor antagonists[120,129,130,131]; however, comparison of their potency is not possible due to the scarcity of data. Compound (**120**) is also reported to antagonize the actions of the sulphidopeptide leukotrienes.

While there is little to report or discuss in this area of research at present, it is very likely that this subject will be the focus of considerable attention, and, consequently, it will see great progress in the future.

137

138

139

Summary

While receptor antagonists have yet to demonstrate their therapeutic usefulness in disease, it is probably only a matter of time. In fact, initial clinical studies using Merck Frosst's LTD_4 antagonist, L-648,051 (**126**), against antigen challenge in man have yielded encouraging results. The future in this area of endeavour is open for the taking and will doubtless see great strides being made. As time progresses, more and more potent sulphidopeptide leukotriene antagonists which bear no resemblance to FPL-55712 will appear as second generation antagonists are disclosed. The progress in the development of drugs will go hand in hand with that at the molecular biology level, with better knowledge of the processes involved as the result. This will doubtless include more detailed knowledge of the receptors' structures and requirements.

Therefore, it is not unfair to say that the potential of this area of research has just begun to be realized and will be the source of considerable interest and effort in the next few years.

CONCLUSION

Research in the areas of leukotriene synthesis inhibitors and receptor antagonists is in its infancy. However, since the structural elucidation of the leukotrienes, the interest and effort in research into these compounds has increased dramatically in both academia and industry. The therapeutic potential of compounds which block the synthesis of the leukotrienes or their receptors remains to be conclusively demonstrated and requires further study. Considerable research remains to be done on the characterization and properties of the enzymes involved in the biosynthesis of the leukotrienes, such as the differences between enzymes from different sources and the question of regulation at the cellular level. Even now, the level of understanding is increasing daily as new techniques and approaches are investigated.

Finally, the desire for leukotriene biosynthesis inhibitors and antagonists is predicated on the hypothesis, based on a large volume of indirect evidence with animal models, that these compounds play a major role in various disease states. While several compounds have been shown to be potent *in vivo* as lipoxygenase inhibitors or receptor antagonists, future developments will be influenced by the demonstration of efficacy against disease in clinical trials.

REFERENCES

1. Corey, E.J., Clark, D.A., Goto, G., Marfat, A., Mioskowski, C., Samuelsson, B. and Hammarström, S. (1980). Stereospecific total synthesis of a 'slow reacting substance' of anaphylaxis, leukotriene C-1. *J. Am. Chem. Soc.*, **102**, 1436–9 and p3663
2. Morris, H.R., Taylor, G.W., Rokach, J., Girard, Y., Piper, P.J., Tippins, J.R. and Samhoun, M.N. (1980). Slow reacting substance of anaphylaxis, SRS-A: assignment of the stereochemistry. *Prostaglandins*, **20**, 601–607
3. Samuelsson, B. (1983). Leukotrienes: a new class of mediators of immediate hypersensitivity reactions and inflammation. In Samuelsson, B., Ramwell, P.W. and Paoletti, R. (eds.) *Advances in Prostaglandin, Thromboxane and Leukotriene Research*, Vol. 11, pp. 1–13
4. Ford-Hutchinson, A.W. (1983). The role of leukotriene B$_4$ as a mediator of leukocyte function. *Agents Action*, **12** (Suppl.), 154–165
5. Mong, S., Wu, H.L., Scott, M.O., Lewis, M.A., Clark, M.A., Weichman, B.M., Kinzig, C.M., Gleason, J.G. and Crooke, S.T. (1985). Molecular heterogeneity of leukotriene receptors: correlation of smooth muscle contraction and radioligand binding in guinea pig lung. *J. Pharmacol. Exp. Ther.*, **234**, 316–325
6. Goldman, D.W. and Goetzl, E.J. (1984). Heterogeneity of human polymorphonuclear leukocyte receptors for leukotriene B$_4$. Identification of a subset of high affinity receptors that transduce the chemotactic response. *J. Exp. Med.*, **159**, 1027–1041
7. Rouzer, C.A. and Samuelsson, B. (1985). On the nature of the 5-lipoxygenase reaction in human leukocytes: Enzyme purification and requirement for multiple stimulatory factors. *Proc. Natl. Acad. Sci. USA*, **82**, 6040–6044
8. Dahinden, C.A., Clancy, R.M., Gross, M., Chiller, J.M. and Hugli, T.E. (1985). Leukotriene C$_4$ production by murine mast cells: Evidence for a role for extracellular leukotriene A$_4$. *Proc. Natl. Acad. Sci. USA*, **82**, 6632–6636

9. McGee, J. and Fitzpatrick, F. (1985). Enzymic hydration of leukotriene A_4. Purification and characterization of a novel epoxide hydrolase from human erythrocytes. *J. Biol. Chem.*, **260**, 12832–12837

10. Pong, S.S., Dehaven, R.N., Kuehl, F.A. Jr. and Egan, R.W. (1983). Leukotriene C_4 binding to rat lung membranes. *J. Biol. Chem.*, **258**, 9616–9619

11. Yoshimoto, T., Furukawa, M., Yamamoto, S., Horie, T. and Watanabe-Kohno, S. (1983). Flavonoids: potent inhibitors of arachidonate 5-lipoxygenase. *Biochem. Biophys. Res. Commun.*, **116**, 612–618

12. Yamamoto, S., Yoshimoto, T., Furukawa, M., Horie, T. and Watanabe-Kohno, S. (1984). Arachidonate 5-lipoxygenase and its new inhibitors. *J. Allergy Clin. Immunol.*, **74**, 349–352

13. Panossian, A.G. (1984). Inhibition of arachidonic acid 5-lipoxygenase of human polymorphonuclear leukocytes by esculetin. *Biomed. Biochim. Acta*, **43**, 1351–1355

14. Neichi, T., Koshihara, Y. and Murota, S. (1983). Inhibitory effect of esculetin on 5-lipoxygenase and leukotriene biosynthesis. *Biochim. Biophys. Acta*, **753**, 130–132

15. Sekiya, K., Okuda, H. and Arichi, S. (1982). Selective inhibition of platelet lipoxygenase by esculetin. *Biochim. Biophys. Acta*, **713**, 68–72

16. Koshihara, Y., Neichi, T., Murota, S., Lao, A., Fujimoto, Y. and Tatsuno, T. (1984). Caffeic acid is a selective inhibitor for leukotriene biosynthesis. *Biochim. Biophys. Acta*, **792**, 92–97

17. Otsuka Pharmaceutical Co. Ltd. (1984). Flavone derivatives. *Jpn. Pat. S 60-100,570, (1985) Chem. Abstr.*, **103**, 178100r

18. Otsuka Pharmaceutical Co. Ltd. (1985). Flavone derivative preparation as inhibitors of arachidonic acid 5-lipoxygenase for the treatment of asthma. *Jpn. Pat. S 60-25,923, (1985) Chem. Abstr.*, **103**, 59301

19. Wakabayashi, T., Takai, M., Ichikawa, S., Arai, J. and Murota, S. (1986). Amide derivatives and 5-lipoxygenase inhibitors containing them as active ingredients. *Jpn. Pat. S61,22057 (1986). EP 157420A2 Chem. Abstr.*, **104**, 168177C

20. Watanabe, M., Sugiura, M., Fukaya, C., Kondo T. and Yokoyama, K. (1984). Selective inhibition of 5-lipoxygenase by caffeic acid derivatives. *Abstract. p. 178.* Presented at the *Kyoto Conference on Prostaglandins*, November 26–28, Kyoto, Japan

21. Yokoyama, K., Fukaya, C., Sugiura, M., Naito, Y. and Suyama, T. (1985). Lipoxygenase inhibitor. *Eur. Pat. Appl. EP 85106390 (1985)*

22. Reddana, P., Rao, M.K. and Reddy, C.C. (1985). Inhibition of 5-lipoxygenase by vitamin E. *FEBS Lett.*, **193**, 39–43

23. Moore, G.G.I. and Swingle, K.F. (1982). 2,6-Di-tert-butyl-4-(2'-thenoyl)phenol(R-830): a novel nonsteroidal anti-inflammatory agent with antioxidant properties. *Agents Actions*, **12**, 674–683

24. Hidaka, T., Hosoe, K., Ariki, Y., Takeo, K., Yamashita, T., Katsumi, I., Kondo, H., Yamashita, K. and Watanabe, K. (1984). Pharmacological properties of a new anti-inflammatory compound, α-(3,5-di-tert-butyl-4-hydroxybenzylidene)-γ-butyrolactone (KME-4), and its inhibitory effects on prostaglandin synthetase and 5-lipoxygenase. *Jpn. J. Pharmacol.*, **36**, 77–85

25. Hidaka, T., Takeo, K., Hosoe, K., Katsumi, I., Yamashita, T. and Watanabe, K. (1985). Inhibition of polymorphonuclear leukocyte 5-lipoxygenase and platelet cyclooxygenase by α-(3,5-di-tert-butyl-4-hydroxybenzylidene)-γ-butyrolactone (KME-4), a new anti-inflammatory drug. *Jpn. J. Pharmacol.*, **38**, 267–272

26. Hope, W.C., Welton, A.F., Nagy, C.F. and Coffey, J.W. (1981). Quercetin inhibits SRS-A biosynthesis and lipoxygenase activity *in vitro. Fed. Proc.*, **40** (Abstr.), 4488

27. Murase, K., Arima, H., Mase, T. and Tomioka, K. (1985). Catechol derivatives. *Eur. Pat. 0125919. Chem. Abstr.*, **102**, 113041g

28. Miyamoto, T. and Obata, T. (1983). New inhibitors of 5-lipoxygenase. *Int. Congr. Ser. Excerpta Med.*, **623**, 78–80

29. Arai, Y., Wakatsuka, H., Mohri, T., Obata, T. and Miyamoto, T. (1985). Aminophenol derivative: a potent inhibitor for 5-lipoxygenase. In Hayaishi, O. and Yamamoto, S. (eds.) *Advances in Prostaglandin, Thromboxane and Leukotriene Research*. Vol. 15, p. 313. (New York: Raven Press)

30. Miyamoto, T., Mohri, T., Shimoi, K., Wakatsuka, H., Itoh, H., Hayashi, M. and Hashimoto, S. (1983). 2-Aminophenol derivatives. *Eur. Pat. EP 81321 A (1983), Chem. Abstr.*, **99**, 104990H

31. Miyamoto, T., Watsuka, H., Hashimoto, S., Itoh, H., Mohri, T., Hayashi, M. (1983). Aminoresorcinol derivatives. *Eur. Pat. EP 79141 (1983), Chem. Abstr.,* **99**, 121998j

32. Aharony, D., Smith, J.B. and Silver, M.J. (1981). Inhibition of platelet lipoxygenase by toluene-3,4-dithiol and other ferric iron chelators. *Prostagl. Med.,* **6**, 237−242

33. Peterson, D.A. and Gerrard, J.M. (1983). Inhibition of platelet lipoxygenase by toluene-3,4-dithiol and other ferric iron chelators. *Prostagl. Leuk. Med.,* **10**, 107−108

34. Karanewsky, D.S. and Haslanger, M.F. (1986). Arylydroxamates. *Eur. Pat. EP 161939A2 (1986), Chem. Abstr.,* **104**, 148549x

35. Veb Arzneimittelwerk Dresden (1985). ω-(2-Naphythoxy) alkylhydroxamic acids. *Jpn. Pat. JP 59/205345 (1984), Chem. Abstr.,* **102**, 166495g

36. Summers, J.B., Holms, J.H., Ayer, R.D., Carter, G.W. and Summers, J.B., Mazdiyasni, H., Ratazezyk, J.D., Dyer, R.D. and Carter, G.W. (1986). Hydroxamic acid inhibitors of 5-lipoxygenase I: structure activity relationships in simple hydroxamic acids. Abstracts MEDI19,20. Presented at *The American Chemical Soc. Natl. Meeting.* September 7−12, Anaheim, California

37. Strasser, M. (1985). N-(naphthylalkyl)hydroxylamines. *Eur. Pat. Appl. EP 149,588 (1984), Chem. Abstr.,* **103**, 215016r

38. Yoshimoto, T. Yokoyama, C. Ochi, K., Yamamoto, S., Maki, Y., Ashida, Y., Terao, S. and Shiraishi, M. (1982). 2,3,5-Trimethyl-6-(12-hydroxy-5,10-dodecadiynyl)-1,4-benzoquinone (AA861), a selective inhibitor of the 5-lipoxygenase reaction and the biosynthesis of slow-reacting substance of anaphylaxis. *Biochim. Biophys. Acta,* **713**, 470−473

39. Ashida, Y., Saijo, T., Kuriki, H., Makino, H., Terao, S. and Maki, Y. (1983). Pharmacological profile of AA-861, a 5-lipoxygenase inhibitor. *Prostaglandins,* **26**, 955−972

40. Ishihara, Y., Kitamura, S. and Takaku, F. (1983). Effect of lipoxygenase inhibitors, AA-861 and T-22083, on chemical mediators released from sensitized guinea pig lung tissue. *Prostaglandins,* **26**, 623−629

41. Ishihara, Y., Uchida, Y., Kitamura, S. and Takaku, F. (1985). Effect of coenzyme Q_{10}, a quinone derivative, on guinea pig lung and tracheal tissue. *Arzneim-Forsch.,* **35**, 929−933

42. Fleisch, J.H., Haisch, K.D., Spaethe, S.M., Rinkema, L.E., Cullinan, G.J., Schmidt, M.J. and Marshall, W.S. (1984). Pharmacologic analysis of two novel inhibitors of leukotriene (slow reacting substance) release. *J. Pharmacol. Exp. Ther.,* **229**, 681−689

43. Murthy, D.V.K., Kruseman-Aretz, M., Rouhafza-Fard, S., Bedord, C.J., Young, J.M., Jones, G. and Venuti, M. (1985). Selective inhibition of arachidonic acid (AA) 5-lipoxygenase by a novel anti-psoriatic agent. *Fed. Proc.,* **44**, 886 (Abstr. 2774)

44. Iwaki, H., Fukuyama, Y. and Matsui, K. (1986). 1,4-Benzoquinone derivatives and benzene derivatives. *Eur. Pat. Appl. EP 151,995 (1985), Chem. Abstr.,* **104**, 33861q

45. Otsuka Pharmaceutical Co. Ltd. Predominantly Z-substituted allylic alcohols and their uses. *Jpn. Pat. JP 56-075442A*

46. Guindon, Y., Girard, Y., Maycock, A., Ford-Hutchinson, A.W., Atkinson, J.G., Bélanger, P.C., Dallob, A., DeSousa, D., Dougherty, H., Egan, R., Ham, E., Fortin, R., Hamel, P., Hamel, R., Lau, C.K., Leblanc, Y., McFarlane, C.S., Piechuta, H., Thérien, M., Yoakim, C. and Rokach, J. (1987). L-651,392, a novel, potent and selective 5-lipoxygenase inhibitor. In Samuelsson, B., Paoletti, R. and Ramwell, P.W. (eds.) *Advances in Prostaglandin, Thromboxane and Leukotriene Research.* Vol. 17A, pp. 554−557. (New York: Raven Press)

47. Guindon, Y., Fortin, R., Lau, C.K., Rokach, J. and Yoakim, C. (1984). Phenothiazene derivatives and analogs. *Eur. Pat. Appl. EP 115,394 (1984), Chem. Abstr.,* **101**, 230555t

48. Bailey, D.M. (1985). Substituted aminobenzamides and their use as agents which inhibit lipoxygenase activity. *U.S. Pat. US 4,510,139 (1985), Chem. Abstr.,* **103**, 71072f

49. Bailey, D.M. (1985). Substituted aminobenzoates and their use. *U.S. Pat. US 4,515,980 (1985), Chem. Abstr.,* **103**, 123174n

50. Lin, C.H. (1985). Pyridinylmethylamino-arylic acids. *Eur. Pat. Appl. EP 114,734 (1984), Chem. Abstr.,* **102**, 62086r

51. Bonney, R.J., Hand, K., Opas, E.E., Olson, B., Dallob, A., Argenbright, L. and Humes, J.L. (1986). L-651,896 A novel dual inhibitor of prostaglandin and leukotriene synthesis that possesses potent topical antiinflammtory and analgesic activity. *J. Invest. Dermatol.,* **86**, 465

52. Atkinson, J.G., Guindon, Y. and Lau, C.K. (1985). Lipoxygenase inhibitors. *Eur. Pat. Appl. EP 146243A1 (1985), Chem. Abstr.,* **103**, 21515f

53. Khandwala, A., Coutts, S., Amin, D. and Sutherland, C. (1984). Rev. 5901 – A specific inhibitor of 5-lipoxygenase: comparison of *in vitro* activity profile with non-steroidal antiinflammatory drugs. Abstr., 183 (Theme 26). *III Internal Congress of Inflammation.* September 3–7, Paris

54. Niemers, E., Gruetzmann, F., Mardin, M., Brusse, W.D. and Meyer, H. (1984). 4H-1, 4-benzothiazine lipoxygenase inhibitors. *Ger. Offen. DE 3,229,121 (1984), Chem. Abstr.,* **100,** 209852g

55. Niemers, E., Gruetzmann, R., Mardin, M., Brusse, W.D. and Meyer, H. (1984). Annellated 4H-1, 4-benzothiazine lipoxygenase inhibitors. *Ger. Offen. DE 3,229,122 (1984). Chem. Abstr.,* **100,** 185787m

56. Momose, D. (1986). Halocarboxanilides as antiallergics. *Japan Kokai Tokkyo Koho JP 60,146,856 (1985), Chem. Abstr.,* **104,** 33891k

57. Momose, D., Naito, A. and Kitazawa, M. (1985). Halocarboxanilide derivatives as antiallergics. *Jpn. Kokai Tokkyo Koho JP 60,146,857. Chem. Abstr.,* **104,** 33892m

58. Steggles, D.J. and Verge, J.P. (1986). 1H-tetrazole-5-carboxamides and their pharmaceutical use. *Eur. Pat. Appl. EP 147,973 (1985), Chem. Abstr.,* **104,** 340085n

59. Baumann, J., Bruchhausen, F.V. and Wurm, G. (1980). Flavonoids and related compounds as inhibitors of arachidonic acid peroxidation. *Prostaglandins,* **20,** 627–639

60. Yamashita, A. (1985). Substituted naphthalenes, indoles, benzofurans, and benzothiophenes as lipoxygenase inhibitors. *Eur. Pat. Appl. EP 146,348 (1985), Chem. Abstr.,* **103,** 196418e

61. Teikoku Hormone Mfg. Co. Ltd. (1984). Dibenzazepine-2-acetic acids. *Jpn. Kokai Tokkyo Koho JP 58,146,568 (1983), Chem. Abstr.,* **100,** 85603e

62. Mardin, M., Sunderman, R., Hoffmeister, F., Busse, W.D., Horstmann, H. and Raddatz, S. (1983). Pyrazolooxazines, -thiazines, -quinolines, and their use as drugs. *Chem. Abstr.,* **99,** 175781b

63. Bailey, B., Dallob, A., Dougherty, H., Bonney, R., Humes, J., Tishler, A., Davies, P., Goldenberg, M. and Moore, V . (1986). A dual cyclooxygenase/5-lipoxyenase inhibitor. Presented at the *6th International Conference on Prostaglandins and Related Compounds.* (Abstr. 406). June 3–6, Florence, Italy

64. Rapoport, S., Haertel, B. and Hausporf, G. (1984). Methionine sulfoxide formation: the cause of self-inactivation of reticulocyte lipoxygenase. *Eur. J. Biochem.,* **139,** 573–576

65. Musser, J.H. and Chakraborty, U.R. (1984). Antiinflammatory and antiallergic benzyl phenyl ethers. *Eur. Pat. Appl. EP 110405 (1984), Chem. Abstr.,* **101,** 170878p

66. Copp, F.C., Islip, P.J. and Tateson, J.E. (1984). 3-N-Substituted-amino-1-(3-(trifluoromethyl)phenyl)-2- pyrazolines have enhanced activity against arachidonate 5-lipoxygenase and cyclooxyenase. *Biochem. Pharmacol.,* **33,** 339–340

67. Blackwell, G.J. and Flower, R.J. (1978). 1-Phenyl-3-pyrazolidone: an inhibitor of arachidonate oxidation in lung and platelets. *Br. J. Pharmacol.,* **63,** 360P

68. Blackwell, G.J. and Flower, R.J. (1978). 1-Phenyl-3-pyrazolidone: an inhibitor of cyclooxygenase and lipoxygenase pathways in lung and platelets. *Prostaglandins,* **16,** 417–425

69. Robak, J. and Dunniec, Z. (1982). The influence of some 3-amino-2-pyrazoline derivatives on cyclooxygenase and lipoxidase activities. *Biochem. Pharmacol.,* **31,** 1955–1959

70. Appleton, R.A., Burford, S.C., Hardern, D.N. and Wilkinson D. (1986). Antiinflammatory 3-aminopyrazoles. *Australian Patent AU 8542275A, Eur. Pat. Appl. EP 178035A1 (1986). Chem. Abstr.,* **105,** 42796f

71. Magro, A.M. and Hurtado, I. (1983). The orally active antiallergic compound, LC-6 (trans-2,3b,4,5,7,8b,9,10-octahydronaphtho(1,2-C:5,6-C)dipyrazole) inhibits the arachidonate lipoxygenase enzyme. *J. Immunopharmacol.,* **5,** 191–202

72. Strasser, T., Fischer, S. and Weber, P.C. (1985). Inhibition of leukotriene B$_4$ formation in human neutrophils after oral nafazatrom (BAY g 6575). *Biochem. Pharmacol.,* **34,** 1891–1894

73. Bayer, A.G. (1985). Therapeutic pyrazolone derivatives as lipoxygenase inhibitors. *Jpn. Kokai Tokkyo Koho JP 59,175,469 (1984), Chem. Abstr.,* **102,** 56154v

74. Fruchtmann, R., Horstmann, H., Opitz, W., Pelster, B., Raddatz, S. and Mardin, M. (1984). Pyrazolo (4,3-b) (1,4)oxazines and their use as lipoxygenase inhibitors. *Ger. Offen. DE 3246148A1 (1984), Chem. Abstr.,* **101,** 171270w

75. Busse, W.D., Krauthausen, E. and Mardin, M. (1983). Sulfenamides for use in pharmaceuticals. *Chem. Abstr.*, **98**, 143446j

76. Tihanyi, E., Fehér, O., Gàl, M., Janàky, J., Tolnay, P. and Sebestyén, L. (1986). Pyrazolecarboxylic-acid hydrazides as antiinflammatory agents new selective lipoxygenase inhibitors. *Eur. J. Med. Chem. – Chim. Ther.*, **19**, 433–439

77. Bertez, C., Miquel, M., Coquelet, C., Sincholle, D. and Bonne, C. (1984). Dual inhibition of cyclooxygenase and lipoxygenase by 2 acetyl thiophene 2 thizolyl hydrazone CBS-1108 and effect on leukocyte migration in-vivo. *Biochem. Pharmacol.*, **33**, 1757–1762

78. Bertez, C., Conduzorgues, J.P., Sincholle, D. and Bonne, C. (1984). CBS1114(N-phenyl-benzamidrazone chloride), a dual inhibitor of cyclooxygenase and lipoxygenase. Abstract 115. (Theme 26). Presented at *III International Congress of Inflammation*, September 3–7, Paris

79. Wallach, D.P. and Brown, V.R. (1981). A novel preparation of human platelet lipoxygenase. Characteristics and inhibition by a variety of phenyl hydrazones and comparisons with other lipoxygenases. *Biochim. Biophys. Acta*, **663**, 361–372

80. Sun, F.F. and McGuire, J.C. (1983). Inhibition of human neutrophil arachidonate 5-lipoxygenase by 6,9-deepoxy-6,9-phenylimino-$\Delta^{6,8}$ prostaglandin I$_1$ (U-60257). *Prostaglandins*, **26**, 211–221

81. Guindon, Y., Gillard, J.W., Yoakim, C., Jones, T.R. and Fortin, R. (1986). Indole-2-alkanoic acids and their use as prostaglandin antagonists. *Eur. Pat. Appl. EP 166591A2 (1986), Chem. Abstr.*, **105**, 78827f

82. Teikoku Hormone Mfg. Co. Ltd. (1984). 1-Substituted-2-phenylindoles. *Jpn. Kokai Tokkyo Koho JP58,162,573 (1983), Chem. Abstr.*, **100**, 68179u

83. Tahara, I., Ikebe, T., Maruyama, Y., Yaoka, O. and Miura, Y. (1986). 3-Indolecarboxamide compounds. *Eur. Pat. Appl. EP 150,505 (1985), Chem. Abstr.*, **104**, 5787n

84. Boctor, A.M., Eickholt, M.M., Hovinga, M.E. and Pugsley, T.A. (1984). Modulation of arachidonic metabolism by the anti-allergy compound CI-922 (4H-furo(3,2-B)indole-2-carboxamide, 3,7-dimethoxy-4-phenyl-N-1H-tetrazole-5-yl). *Pharmacologist*, 26, 155 (Abstr. 137)

85. Corell, T., Hasselmann, G., Splawinski, J. and Wojtaszek, B. (1983). Fenflumizole: interactions with the arachidonic acid cascade. *Acta Pharmacol. Toxicol.*, **53**, 297–303

86. Beetens, J.R., Loots, W., Somers, Y., Coene, M.C. and DeClerck, F. (1986). Ketoconazole inhibits the biosynthesis of leukotrienes in vitro and in vivo. *Biochem. Pharmacol.*, **35**, 883–891

87. Boot, J.R., Sweatman, W.J.F., Cox, B.A., Stone, K. and Dawson, W. (1982). The antiallergic activity of benoxaprofen (2-(4-chlorophenyl)-α-methyl-5-benzoxazole acetic acid), a lipoxygenase inhibitor. *Int. Arch. Allergy Appl. Immunol.*, **67**, 340–343

88. Harvey, J., Parish, H., Ho, P.P.K., Boot, J.R. and Dawson, W. (1983). The preferential inhibition of 5-lipoxygenase formation by benoxaprofen. *J. Pharm. Pharmacol.*, **35**, 44–45

89. Walker, J.R. and Dawson, W. (1979). Inhibition of rabbit PMN lipoxygenase activity by benoxaprofen. *J. Pharmacol.*, **31**, 778–779

90. Busse, W.D., Krauthausen, E. and Mardin, M. (1983). Use of disulfides as lipoxygenase inhibitors and pharmaceuticals containing them. *Ger. Offen. DE 3,118,128A1 (1982), Chem. Abstr.*, **98**, 95663d

91. Egan, R.W. and Gale, P.H. (1985). Inhibition of mammalian 5-lipoxygenase by aromatic disulfides. *J. Biol. Chem.*, **260**, 11554–11559

92. Egan, R.W., Tischler, A.N., Baptista, E.M., Ham, E.A., Soderman, D.D. and Gale, P.H. (1983). Specific inhibition and oxidative regulation of 5-lipoxygenase. In Samuelsson, R., Ramwell, P.W. and Paoletti, R. (eds.) *Advances in Prostaglandin, Thromboxane and Leukotriene Research.* Vol. 11, pp. 151–157. (New York: Raven Press)

93. Carter, G.W., Dyer, R. and Young, P. (1985). Dipyridamole: a potent and specific 5-lipoxygenase inhibitor. *Fed. Proc.*, **44**, 904 (Abstr. 2880)

94. Lammattina, J.L. (1985). 2-Amino-5-hydroxy-4-methylpyrimidine derivatives. *Eur. Pat. Appl. EP 138,464A2 (1985). Chem. Abstr.*, **103**, 142000u

95. Kitamura, S., Hashizume, K., Iida, T., Miyashita, E. Shirahata, K. and Kase, H. (1986). Studies on lipoxygenase inhibitors. II. KF8940 (2N-heptyl-4-hydroxyquiniline-N-oxide), a potent and selective inhibitor of 5-lipoxygenase, produced by *Pseudomonas methanica*. *J. Antibiot.*, **39**, 1160–1166

187

96. Schulte, K., Puetter, S. and Loew, D. (1986). Antiinflammatory pharmaceutical. *Ger. Offen. DE 3,409,415 (1985), Chem. Abstr.*, **104**, 33897s

97. Clémence, F. LeMartret, O., Delevallée, F. and Benzoni, J. (1984). New 4-hydroxy-3-quinolinecarboxamides, potent inhibitors of both lipoxygenase and cyclooxygenase with anti-arthritic activities. Presented at the *VIIIth International Symposium on Medicinal Chemistry*, August 27–31, Uppsala, Sweden

98. Ahnfelt-Ronne, I. and Arrigoni-Martelli, E. (1980). A new anti-inflammatory compound timegadine *N*-cyclohexyl-*N'*-4-2-methylquinolyl- *N'*-2-thiazolylguanidine which inhibits both prostaglandin and 12-hydroxyeicosatetraenoic acid (12-HETE) formation. *Biochem. Pharmacol.*, **29**, 3265–3270

99. Durette, P.L. and Gallapher, T.F. (1985). Lipoxygenase inhibitors. *United States Patent: US 4526999 A, 1985*

100. Kitamura, S., Iida, T., Shirahata, K. and Kase, H. (1986). Studies on lipoxygenase inhibitors. I. MY3-469 (3-methoxytropolone) a potent and selective inhibitor of 12-lipoxygenase, produced by Streptoverticillium hadonense KY11449. *J. Antibiot.*, **39**, 589–593

101. Mathews, W.R. and Murphy, R.C. (1982). Inhibition of leukotriene biosynthesis in mastocytoma cells by diethylcarbamazine. *Biochem. Pharmacol.*, **31**, 2129–2132

102. Piper, P.J. and Temple, D.M. (1981). The effect of lipoxygenase inhibitors and diethylcarbamazine on the immunological release of slow reacting substance of anaphylaxis (SRS-A) from guinea pig chopped lung. *J. Pharm. Pharmacol.*, **33**, 384–386

103. Bach, M.K. and Brashler, J.R. (1986). Inhibition of the leukotriene synthetase and rat basophil leukemia cells by diethylcarbamazine, and synergism between diethylcarbamazine and piriprost, a 5-lipoxygenase inhibitor. *Biochem. Pharmacol.*, **35**, 425–433

104. Stenson, W.F. and Lobos, E. (1982). Sulfasalazine inhibits the synthesis of chemotactic lipids by neutrophils. *J. Clin. Invest.*, **69**, 494–497

105. Evans, J.F., Dupuis, P. and Ford-Hutchinson, A.W. (1985). Purification and characterization of leukotriene A₄ hydrolase from rat neutrophils. *Biochim. Biophys. Acta*, **840**, 45–50

106. Evans, J., Nathaniel, D., Charleson, S., Léveillé, C., Zamboni, R., Leblanc, Y., Frenette, R., Fitzsimmons, B.J., Leger, S., Hamel, P. and Ford-Hutchinson, A.W. (1986). Neutrophil LTA₄ hydrolases and leukotriene B₄ receptors: effects of leukotriene epoxides and their enzymatic products. *Prostagl. Leuk. Med.*, **23**, 167–171

107. Evans, J.F., Nathaniel, D.J., Zamboni, R.J. and Ford-Hutchinson, A.W. (1985). Leukotriene A₃. A poor substrate but a potent inhibitor of rat and human neutrophil leukotriene A₄ hydrolase. *J. Biol. Chem.*, **260**, 10966–10970

108. Bach, M.K., Brashler, J.R., Peck, R.E. and Morton, D.R. (1984). Leukotriene C synthetase, a special glutathione S-transferase: properties of the enzyme and inhibitor studies with special reference to the mode of action of U-60,257, a selective inhibitor of leukotriene synthesis. *J. Allergy Clin. Immunol.*, **74**, 353–357

109. O'Donnell, M. and Welton, A.F. (1984). Pharmacologic properties of FPL 55712 administered by aerosol. *Agents Actions*, **14**, 43–48

110. Chand, N. (1979). FPL-55712 an antagonist of slow reacting substance of anaphylaxis (SRS-A): a review. *Agents Actions*, **9**, 133–140

111. Jones, T., Denis, D., Hall, R. and Ethier, D. (1983). Pharmacological effects of leukotrienes C₄, D₄, E₄, F₄ on guinea pig trachealis: interaction with FPL-55712. *Prostaglandins*, **26**, 833–843

112. Appleton, R.A., Bantick, J.R., Chamberlain, T.R., Hardern, D.N., Lee, T.B. and Pratt, A.D. (1977). Antagonists of slow reacting substance of anaphylaxis. Synthesis of a series of chromone-2-carboxylic acids. *J. Med. Chem.*, **20**, 371–379

113. Holroyde, M.C. and Ghelani, A.M. (1983). Kinetics of action of two leukotriene antagonists on guinea pig ileum. *Eur. J. Pharmacol.*, **90**, 251–255

114. Oxford, A.W. and Ellis, F. (1982). Phenoxyalkoxyphenyl derivatives. *U.K. Pat. Appl. GB 2058785A (2981). Chem. Abstr.*, **96**, 51977p

115. Buckle, D.R., Outred, D.J., Ross, J.W., Smith, H., Smith, R.J. and Spicer, B.A. (1979). Aryloxyalkyloxy- and aralkyloxy-4-hydroxy-3-nitrocoumarins which inhibit histamine release in the rat and also antagonize the effects of a slow reacting substance of anaphylaxis. *J. Med. Chem.*, **22**, 158–168

116. Snyder, D.W., Bernstein, P.R. and Krell, R.D. (1985). Pharmacology of chemically stable analogs of peptide leukotrienes (LT). *Fed. Proc.*, **44**, 901 (Abstr. 2863)

LIPOXYGENASE INHIBITORS

117. Weichman, B.M., Wasserman, M.A., Holden, D.A., Osborn, R.R., Woodward, D.F., Ku, T.W. and Gleason, J.G. (1983). Antagonism of the pulmonary effects of the peptidoleukotrienes by a leukotriene D_4 analog. *J. Pharmacol. Exp. Ther.*, **227**, 700–705

118. Gleason, J.G., Ku, T.W., Kinzig, C.M., McCarthy, M.E., Perchonock, C.D., Kuzinskas, I., Berkowitz, B. and Weichman, B.M. (1984). In the *Second SCI-RSC Medicinal Chemistry Symposium*, 257–267 (Special Publication 50: London: Royal Society of Chemistry)

119. Perchonock, C.D. Uzinskas, I., Ku, T.W., McCarthy, M.E., Bondinell, W.E., Volpe, B.W., Gleason, J.G., Weichman, B.M., Muccitelli, R.M., DeVan, J.F., Tucker, S.S., Vickery, L.M. and Wasserman, M.A. (1985). Synthesis and LTD$_4$-antagonist activity of desamino-2-nor-leukotriene analogs. *Prostaglandins, 29*, 75–81

120. Saksena, A.K., Green, M.J., Mangiaracina, P., Wong, J.K., Kreutner, W. and Gulbenkian, A.R. (1985). Synthesis of 7,8-acetylenic analogs of hexahydroleukotriene-E$_4$ with agonist and antagonist activities: convenient stereoselective routes to E- and Z-enzymes. Synthesis of 4,4'-(4E,6Z,9Z-pentadecatrien-2-ynylidenedithio) dibutanoic acid with leukotriene-like activity: novel acetylenic acetals and dithioacetals as antagonists of leukotriene C$_4$. *Tetrahedron Lett.*, **26**, 6423–6426 and 6427–6430

121. Fleisch, J.H. Rinkema, L.E., Haisch, K.D., Swanson-Bean, D., Goodson, T., Ho, P.P.K. and Marshall, W.S. (1985). LY171883, 1-[2-hydroxy-3-propyl-4-(1H-tetrazo-5-yl) butoxy] phenyl] ethanol, an orally active leukotriene D4 antagonist. *J. Pharmacol. Exp. Ther.*, **233**, 148–157

122. Young, R.N., Jones, T.R., Atkinson, J.G., Bélanger, P., Champion, E., Denis, D., DeHaven, R.N., Ford-Hutchinson, A.W., Fortin, R., Frenette, R., Gauthier, J.Y., Gillard, J., Guindon, Y., Kakushima, M., Masson, P., Maycock, A., McFarlane, C.S., Piechuta, H., Pong, S.S., Rokach, J., Williams, H., Yoakim, C. and Zamboni, R. (1987). Novel arylthio- and arylsulfonylpropyloxyacetophenones: design and synthesis of L-648,051 and L-649,923, potent antagonists of leukotriene D$_4$. In Samuelsson, B., Paoletti, R. and Ramwell, P.W. (eds.) *Advances in Prostaglandin, Thromboxane and Leukotriene Research.* Vol. 17A. pp. 544–548. (New York: Raven Press)

123. Obata, T., Katsube, N. Miyamoto, T., Toda, M., Okegawa, T., Nakai, H., Kosuge, S., Konno, M., Arai, Y. and Kawasaki, A. (1985). New antagonists of leukotrienes: ONO-RS-411 and ONO-RS-347. In Hayaishi, O. and Yamamoto, S. (eds.) *Advances in Prostaglandin, Thromboxane and Leukotriene Research.* Vol. 15, pp. 229–231. (New York: Raven Press)

124. Toda, M., Nakai H., Kosuge, S., Konno, M., Arai, Y., Miyamoto, T., Obata, T., Katsube, N. and Kawasaki, A. (1985). A potent antagonist of the slow reacting substance of anaphylaxis. In Hayaishi, O. and Yamamoto, S. (eds.) *Advances in Prostaglandins, Thromboxane and Leukotriene Research.* Vol. 15, pp. 307–308. (New York: Raven Press)

125. Perchonock, C.D., McCarthy, M.E., Erhard, K.F., Gleason, J.G., Wasserman, M.A., Muccitelli, R.M., DeVan, J.F., Tucker, S.S., Vickery, L.M., Kirchner, T., Weichman, B.M., Mong, S., Crooke, S.T. and Newton, J.F. (1985). Synthesis and pharmacological characterization of 5-(2-dodecylphenyl)-4,6-dithianonanedioic acid and 5-(2-(8-phenyloct-yl)phenyl)-4,6-dithianonanedioic acid: prototypes of a novel class of leukotriene antagonists. *J. Med. Chem.*, **28**, 1145–1147

126. Saijo, T. Kuiriki, H. Ashida, Y., Makino, H. and Maki, Y. (1985). Inhibition of amoxanox (AA-673) of the immunoloically, leukotriene D4- or platelet-activating factor-stimulated bronchoconstriction in guinea pigs and rats. *Int. Arch. Allergy Appl. Immunol.*, **77**, 315–321

127. Mong, S., Hall, R.F., Gleason, J.C. and Crooke, S.T. (1986). SKF 104353, an antagonist binding to human and guinea pig lung leukotriene D$_4$ (LTD$_4$) receptors and inhibition of cyclooxygenase dependent effect. Presented at the *6th International Conference on Prostaglandins and Related Compounds*, June 3–6, Florence, Italy (Abstr. 356)

128. Von Sprecher, A., Ernst, I., Main, I., Beck, A., Breitenstein, W., Marki, J., Poray, M.A., Wenk, P., Niederhauser, U., Kuhan, M. and Sallman, A. (1986). Novel leukotriene antagonists: structure activity of analogs of LTD$_4$. Replacement of the 1-carboxylic group by a methyl group ('Methyl Principle') results in leukotriene antagonists and phospholipase inhibitors. Presented at the *6th International Conference on Prostaglandins and Related Compounds*, June 3–6, Florence, Italy

129. Ono Pharmaceutical Co. Ltd. (1984). Leukotriene B$_4$-related compounds. *Jpn. Kokai Tokkyo Koho JP5995249 (1984), Chem. Abstr.*, **101**, 230229q

189

130. Showell, H.J., Otterness, I.G., Marfat, A. and Corey, E.J. (1982). Inhibition of leukotriene B$_4$-induced neutrophil degranulation by leukotriene B$_4$-dimethylamide. *Biochem. Biophys. Res. Commun.*, **106**, 741–747

131. Namiki, M., Igarashi, Y., Sakamoto, K., Nakamura, T. and Koga, Y. (1986). Pharmacological profiles of a potential LTB$_4$-antagonist. SM-9064. *Biochem. Biophys. Res. Commun.*, **138**, 540–546

9
Experimental Models of Pulmonary and Joint Inflammation and Their Relevance to Man

A. N. PAYNE, G. DE NUCCI and E. R. PETTIPHER

INTRODUCTION

For ethical and practical considerations, the study of human disease processes has relied heavily on the use of experimental models in laboratory animals. Inflammation is no exception. By their very nature, the actual relevance of such models to the clinical situation, and consequently their likely predictive value, is open to question. With this point in mind, in this chapter, we will consider the relevance of a variety of experimental models of inflammation in which the contribution of eicosanoids has been investigated. We have chosen, as examples, animal models of asthma, other pulmonary diseases and rheumatoid arthritis.

ASTHMA

Both the pathogenesis of asthma and current concepts as to the putative role of eicosanoids in this disease have already been described in some detail in Chapter 5. Briefly, asthma is typified by intermittent spasmodic episodes of airway obstruction that resolve either spontaneously or following treatment with agents such as inhaled sympathomimetics. Sometimes, the initial 'tonic' reduction in airway calibre may be followed by a more persistent 'phasic' reduction largely unrelated to smooth muscle spasm. A parallel has been drawn between this 'late asthmatic reaction' and the 'late cutaneous reaction' provoked by intradermal injection of antigen[1]. The late reaction in skin is characterized by infiltration of numerous cell types, including neutrophils, eosinophils, basophils and lymphocytes[2]. Similarly, in the late asthmatic response, there is evidence of generalized oedema, cellular infiltration (of both the bronchial mucosa and submucosa) together with the presence of a viscous exudate in the airway lumen[3,4]. The presence of this inflammatory lesion may be synonymous with the clinical expression of airway hyperreactivity[5]. Whilst there is some evidence that the primary event in the acute asthmatic reaction is mast cell degranulation[6], the underlying mechanism of the late asthmatic response is less certain. However, the likelihood that eicosanoids[7], particularly leukotrienes[8], are important mediators of both phases is reflected, for example, in the present interest in lipoxygenase inhibitors as potential therapeutic agents in asthma (see preceding chapter). It follows that a primary determinant for implied relevance of an animal model of asthma is, according to contemporary thinking, a demonstrable role of eicosanoids and an element of airway hyperreactivity, particularly in models of the late response. Further, to establish a clinical parallel, models have been sought in which either sodium cromoglycate (SCG) or steroids are effective inhibitors.

Animal models of asthma

Experimental models of both early and late 'quasi-asthmatic' pulmonary dysfunction have been established in a wide variety of laboratory animals. Most of these models depend on a classical type I immediate hypersensitivity reaction, even though, in some species, for example rats and monkeys, the lungs may not be the major target organ of anaphylaxis[9]. In some instances, a naturally occurring immunity can be exploited such as that to *Ascaris suum* in dogs, monkeys and sheep (see below). Alternatively, various methods of artificial sensitization (either active or passive) can be employed. Commonly used antigens include ovalbumin, either alone or conjugated to haptens, and extracts obtained from either nematodes or plants. Protein conjugates of diisocyanates have also been used in an attempt to generate experimental models of the occupational asthma displayed by manufacturing workers in the polyurethane foam industries[10,11]. Sometimes, additional procedures, such as the use of Freund's adjuvant, are adopted to promote the production of reaginic IgE rather than IgG antibody in an attempt to simulate more closely the human situation[12,13]. The predominant antibody type may be an important predeterminant of the characteristics of the anaphylactic reaction and its inhibition by drugs[14]. Pharmacological studies of pulmonary anaphylaxis *in vitro* have been reviewed recently[9].

The most frequently used route of animal immunization is by intraperitoneal (ip) injection, which bears little relationship to the human situation. Immunization with inhaled aerosols of antigen has been tried, mainly in rodents, with varying degrees of success. As with ip sensitization, there are numerous procedural differences (e.g. duration and/or frequency of exposure) between the methods of individual investigators.

Similarly, the route of antigen challenge, like that of immunization, is also an important consideration in equating the relevance of a particular animal model of asthma to man. For technical reasons, it is generally easier to derive quantitative data about airway mechanics in anaesthetized rather than conscious animals. Conversely, in this state, it is technically more difficult to administer antigen by the plausibly more relevant inhaled route rather than by the intravenous (iv) route, particularly in small animals.

Although most experimental models of asthma are anaphylactic in nature, the use of non-immunological techniques has also been explored. In the acute situation, these techniques include the use of non-specific stimuli such as ionophore A23187, either *in vitro*[15] or *in vivo*[16], to stimulate eicosanoid production, and simply administering the precursor, arachidonic acid[17,18]. In models of chronic lung inflammation, agents such as ozone and hyperbaric oxygen have been employed[19]. Ozone exposure also causes bronchomotor hyperresponsiveness in man[20] and has been used as an experimental stimulus with which to investigate the possible link between airway inflammation and airway hyperreactivity.

Eicosanoid synthesis and the actions of inhibitors in selected models of the early and late asthmatic response

Early response
Guinea-pig: Probably the best counterpart to the pathology of human asthma so far described is that in sensitized guinea-pigs following aerosol challenge, either with ovalbumin or other foreign proteins[21]. Within 10 minutes of first exposure to a sub-lethal dose of aerosolized antigen, there is evidence of the peribronchial vessels being infiltrated by eosinophils. After repeated challenge, cough, viscous oropharyngeal secretions and occlusion of the bronchial lumen with mucus plugs are apparent. However, in contrast to man, the predominant homocytotropic antibody in this species is usually IgG, rather than IgE[22]. In addition, the usual method of experimental challenge is by the intravenous route. Histamine is clearly the primary anaphylactic mediator of the well-characterized allergic bronchoconstriction and accompanying hyperinflation[23]. It may not be so in human asthma as evidenced by the lack of therapeutic utility of currently available antihistamines. However, the putative secondary involvement in guinea-pig anaphylaxis of eicosanoids, particularly leukotrienes[24], has encouraged the continued use of sensitized guinea-pigs as an experimental simulation of allergic bronchoconstriction. This is despite the lack of activity of SCG and steroids in this model except under specialized immunization or challenge conditions[25,26] not used by the majority of investigators.

Recently, various pharmacological manipulations of guinea-pig bronchial anaphylaxis have been described with the intention of 'directing' the immunologically stimulated synthesis of eicosanoids through the lipoxygenase pathway and thus accentuating the contribution of leukotrienes[27-29]. Following pretreatment with the histamine H_1 antagonist mepyramine, the 5-hydroxy-tryptamine (5-HT) antagonist methysergide, and the muscarinic cholinergic antagonist atropine, together with cyclo-oxygenase blockade by indomethacin, there is a slow in onset, but thereafter rapid and sustained, rise in ventilatory pressure after challenge with either intravenous or aerosolized antigen. This can be inhibited by the SRS-A antagonist, FPL 55712, and has been shown to be directly related to the appearance of biologically active SRS-A in the plasma[29]. In this way, 'directed' or presumably 'leukotriene-dependent' anaphylaxis has been used to evaluate the anti-asthmatic potential of numerous lipoxygenase inhibitors *in vivo*. The peak increases both in ventilatory pressure and plasma SRS-A are reduced in a dose-dependent manner by phenidone[29]. Similar results, although not necessarily coupled with measurement of plasma SRS-A levels, have been reported[28] with the dual cyclo-oxygenase/lipoxygenase inhibitor BW755C and U-60,257 (piriprost) a reportedly selective inhibitor of 5-lipoxygenase product release[30].

We have recently described a simple aerosol method of provoking 'histamine-independent' bronchial anaphylaxis in anaesthetized guinea-pigs and in the analogous *in vitro* situation[31]. This dual capability (Figure 9.1) should facilitate the detailed pharmacological investigation of the profile of mediator release (and inhibition) following antigen challenge by an obviously more relevant route.

Rat: Systemic anaphylaxis in rats is characterized by vascular engorgement of the heart and small intestine[32]. Although some degree of respiratory distress may be evident, this is not always the case. At first sight, therefore, rat anaphylaxis seems entirely inappropriate as a model for human asthma

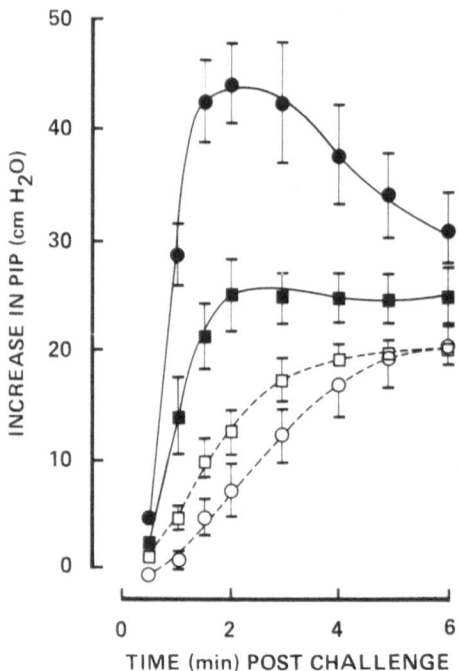

Figure 9.1 Increase in pulmonary inflation pressure (PIP) following antigen challenge *in vivo* and *in vitro* with aerosolized ovalbumin (10 mg ml^{-1}, 5 s) in actively sensitized control animals (●, *in vivo: n = 5*; ■, *in vitro, n = 8*) and in those pretreated with mepyramine (*in vivo*, 2 mg kg^{-1} iv; *in vitro*, 4 μg ml^{-1}, continuous infusion) 10 min before challenge (○, *in vivo: n = 5*, □, *in vitro, n = 8*). Each point represents the mean (±SEM) from *n* as indicated

even though the antibodies responsible are of the IgE class[33]. However, Church and co-workers[34] were able to demonstrate that intravenous antigen (*Nippostrongylus brasiliensis* extract) challenge in actively sensitized rats did provoke severe bronchoconstriction. This was measured as a decrease in tracheal air flow. The reduction in flow was markedly inhibited (by up to nearly 70%) following pretreatment with methysergide, indicating that 5-HT was the predominant anaphylactic mediator involved. This amine, however, does not appear to be a significant primary mediator in human asthma. Of potentially more relevance, therefore, was the finding in the same study that anaphylactic bronchoconstriction in rats can be inhibited by both a corticosteroid (dexamethasone) and SCG, although, curiously, in the latter instance, the dose-response curve was bell-shaped. The inhibitory effect of steroids and SCG in rat bronchial anaphylaxis has been confirmed in more recent studies[35].

In contrast, Church *et al.*[34] found no protective effect of meclofenamate $(1 \, mg \, kg^{-1})$ suggesting that cyclo-oxygenase-derived eicosanoids were not involved in rat anaphylaxis. Experiments with isolated perfused lungs *in vitro* broadly support this view[36]. Nevertheless, it has been argued from results *in vivo* that an as yet unidentified product of the cyclo-oxygenase/thromboxane synthase pathway may be important[37]. In addition, indomethacin has been shown to attenuate the bronchoconstriction provoked by intravenous challenge of rats previously sensitized by aerosolized antigen[38]. However, in this particular model, the predominant antibody type appears to be IgG rather than IgE. Under these circumstances the possible role of platelet-derived substances, e.g. thromboxanes, is controversial[39]. On the basis of *in vitro* evidence, the importance of leukotrienes in rat bronchial anaphylaxis is potentially complicated by interstrain differences and whether passive or active sensitization is employed[40]. Following pretreatment with methysergide, both BW755C[41] and baicalein[42] have been found to inhibit anaphylactic bronchospasm following intravenous and aerosol antigen challenge respectively. However, whilst FPL55712 clearly protects rats against the fatal anaphylactic effect of intravenous challenge, this action appears to reflect an antagonism of the cardiovascular rather than bronchial sequelae. In addition, the inhibitory effect of BW755C noted above depends on the magnitude of the provocation stimulus[41].

Rabbit: Neonatal immunization of rabbits with horseradish peroxidase antigen (HRP) induces the synthesis of specific HRP antibodies of the IgE class[43]. Subsequent intravenous challenge with HRP provokes bronchoconstriction and a marked increase in pulmonary vascular resistance. This is accompanied by a temporally-related systemic hypotension. Haematological changes include acute thrombocytopaenia, due to platelet aggregation, and intravascular pulmonary sequestration, together with neutropenia and basopenia. Some of the physiological and haematological effects of intravenous antigen challenge are reproduced by systemic administration of platelet-activating factor (PAF-acether)[44] which has been shown to be released during anaphylaxis in this species[45]. However, it is clear that neither PAF-acether, platelets, or histamine are responsible for either the tachypnoea or fall in dynamic lung compliance following antigen challenge. Histamine does seem, however, to be primarily responsible for the antigen-induced increase in airway resistance which is blocked by pretreatment with a histamine H_1-antagonist[46]. Following intravenous antigen challenge, a rise in plasma thromboxane B_2 (TxB_2) levels is evident with a maximal increase occurring 120 to 180 s after challenge[47]. This rise in TxB_2 levels, some of which may be due to stimulation of circulatory platelets by PAF-acether, is completely blocked by pretreatment with aspirin (100 mg kg^{-1})[47], but the haematological effects are not blocked, the lethality of the challenge being increased by aspirin pretreatment. It has been suggested, therefore, that in this experimental model, cyclo-oxygenase metabolites may exert a protective role. Intravenously infused PGI_2 ($1-2$ μg kg^{-1}) does not modify the effect of antigen challenge on lung function despite substantial inhibition of platelet aggregation and secretion[44].

Dog: The dog is said to be the only mammal to share man's ability to develop respiratory pollenosis[48]. This finding, together with its apparent IgE-mediated nature, has stimulated the evaluation of canine bronchial anaphylaxis as a model of human asthma. Paradoxically, most studies of allergic bronchoconstriction in dogs have, up to now, employed *Ascaris* antigen as the provocation stimulus, rather than an antigen of plant origin. This is because of the relatively common natural incidence of *Ascaris* sensitivity in the canine population. However, it should be recognized that a polypeptide causing non-immunological histamine release in rat peritoneal mast cells has recently been isolated from crude extracts of *Ascaris* worm[49]. Whilst there is concern that a similar effect may occur *in vivo*, this has been dismissed as unlikely by others[50]. Active sensitization procedures have been described using antigens such as ovalbumin[51], bovine serum albumin[52], ragweed pollen[53] and toluene diisocyanate[54]. These appear to be more successful in newborn inbred strains than in adult animals[52,55]. Both intravenous and aerosol challenge in either naturally sensitive or actively sensitized dogs provokes acute bronchoconstriction that bears some resemblance to human asthma[51–54,56,57].

As yet, the actual mediators involved in canine bronchial anaphylaxis, particularly *in vivo*, have not been fully characterized. Studies using passively sensitized fragmented canine lung *in vitro* point to histamine being the predominant non-eicosanoid mediator[58]. An 'SRS-A'-like material has also been identified[58] which contracts guinea-pig ileum *in vitro*, an effect blocked by FPL 55712. The *in vitro* production of canine SRS-A, but not the release of histamine, is reportedly enhanced by indomethacin[58]. In studies using *Ascaris* antigen, SCG has not been found either to prevent the release of anaphylactic mediators *in vitro* or to modify the pulmonary effects of antigen challenge *in vivo*[57]. Interpretation of this result is complicated because of the possibility that non-specific release of mediators could have occurred in these studies. Whether or not SCG inhibits canine bronchial anaphylaxis provoked by other antigens remains to be established. Bronchial lavage has shown an influx of neutrophils 6 h after aerosol challenge[59]. This is associated with increased responsiveness to inhaled acetylcholine and may be indicative of a late phase response. There is conflicting evidence as to whether sensitized animals exhibit inherent airway hyperreactivity[53,60]. This may depend on the actual strain used.

Sheep: A naturally-occurring hypersensitivity to *Ascaris* antigen has been described in cohorts of adult ewes[61]. Aerosol challenge of animals having a demonstrable cutaneous reaction to this antigen results in acute bronchoconstriction and hyperinflation. This is characterized by an increase in airways resistance and thoracic gas volume coupled with a decrease in dynamic lung compliance and PaO_2 levels[62]. The principal mediator of this allergic response is believed to be histamine as evidenced by the protective effect of pretreatment with the H_1-antagonist, chlorpheniramine[63]. SCG also has a protective effect but not FPL 55712[63]. Interestingly, both the acute allergic bronchoconstriction and the decrease in PaO_2 are sensitive to inhibition by the steroid, methylprednisolone, but only if it is administered at least 3 h before challenge[64]. A temporary enhancement of airways reactivity to histamine, lasting up to 24 h after antigen challenge, has been described[65]. However, *Ascaris*-sensitive sheep seem overtly more responsive to histamine initially[66]. Recently, the description of a late phase bronchoconstrictor response in allergic sheep following antigen challenge[62] has stimulated its consideration as a possible model for the late asthmatic response (see next section).

Cat: For a considerable time, cats were thought to be immunologically incompetent because of their apparent lack of response to immunization with foreign proteins. However, more recent studies have shown cats to possess a wide range of immunological reactions, including acute anaphylactic shock[67]. The ensuing bronchoconstriction can be ameliorated by either intravenous aminophylline or isoprenaline[67]. In our own studies, mepyramine, either alone or in conjunction with both atropine and methysergide, did not modify anaphylactic bronchoconstriction *in vivo* and no rise in plasma LTB_4 (taken as an index of lipoxygenase products) was detected[68]. In contrast, bronchoconstriction was accompanied by a temporally related and progressive rise in plasma TxB_2 levels. Both the rise in plasma TxB_2 and bronchoconstriction were blocked by indomethacin. These results indicate that eicosanoid involvement in feline anaphylactic bronchospasm, certainly following intravenous challenge, is cyclo-oxygenase orientated. However, the release of feline SRS-A (and histamine) has been observed following antigen challenge of chopped sensitized cat lung *in vitro*[69]. Consequently, there may be a different profile of mediator release following aerosol challenge which has yet to be exploited, if it can be, in this species.

Monkey: Ascaris antigen-induced bronchoconstriction in monkeys has been used for the preclinical investigation of numerous potential anti-asthma drugs. A natural IgE-mediated sensitivity to this antigen exists in certain rhesus and cynomolgus monkeys which are closely related species of the genus *Macaca*[70,71]. The bronchoconstrictor response to *Ascaris* antigen in sensitive monkeys has some similarity to the response of humans challenged with ragweed pollen[48]. However, there are some notable physiological differences, which, to some extent, probably reflect different measurement techniques. For example, in monkeys, there is a predominance of rapid shallow breathing with little air trapping[48] which contrasts with the, often considerable, air-trapping and increased residual lung volumes in human asthma[72]. Also, whilst the immediate response has been widely studied in monkeys, the appearance of a late phase response following allergic challenge has yet to be convincingly demonstrated.

Allergic bronchoconstriction in monkeys appears to be only partially inhibited by SCG, when given either intravenously or as an aerosol prior to antigen challenge[73]. Neither histamine nor cholinergic mechanisms appear to play a major role in the airway response although they may have a modulatory function[74,75]. Similarly, cyclo-oxygenase-derived eicosanoids do not appear to be predominant bronchoactive mediators as shown by the very variable and overall relative lack of effect of pretreatment with indomethacin[76]. In contrast, there is good evidence of spasmogenic involvement of lipoxygenase products. Anaphylactic bronchospasm in allergic monkeys is reportedly blocked by 5,8,11,14-eicosatetraynoic acid (ETYA)[77], BW755C and U-60,257[79]. Also, the SRS-A antagonist, FPL 55712, when given by aerosol, significantly increases the threshold dose of antigen required to provoke changes in dynamic compliance[77]. Furthermore, some, but not all, of the anaphylactic change in lung function in monkeys can be reproduced by aerosol provocation with synthetic leukotrienes[80]. The release of immunoreactive leukotrienes from passively sensitized fragmented rhesus monkey lung following challenge with antihuman IgE has been described[81]. This effect is inhibited by the mixed cyclo-oxygenase/lipoxygenase inhibitor, nordihydroguaretic acid, as well as ETYA. In the same study, indomethacin potentiated the release of immunoreactive leukotrienes by an average of 27.6%.

There is some evidence of intrinsic airway hyperreactivity to various spasmogens (carbachol, $PGF_{2\alpha}$, histamine) in monkeys giving a positive allergic response to *Ascaris* antigen[71,82]. Whether eicosanoid synthesis inhibitors, in particular lipoxygenase inhibitors, or antagonists will inhibit this phenomenon remains to be investigated and has obvious relevance to the human situation. A potential problem of such a study is the apparent spontaneous underlying change in sensitivity to antigen, and thus possibly hyperreactivity, and the resulting variation in pulmonary responses that seems to be a frequent finding in naturally allergic monkeys.

Late response
Guinea-pig: Conventional challenge procedures in sensitized guinea-pigs provoke a marked, and often fatal, immediate response with no prolonged or late reaction. A new approach has recently been described in this species using particulate rather than soluble antigen[83]. Intratracheal instillation of ovalbumin covalently coupled to sepharose beads (100 μm in diameter) provokes a severe immediate response in sensitized animals which resolves in about 90 min. This immediate response is followed, approximately 6 h later, by a secondary increase in respiratory resistance, peaking about 20 h after the initial challenge and remitting some 50 h later. Histological studies show evidence of a focal inflammation around the sepharose beads at 20 h, with high local concentrations of polymorphonuclear leukocytes and eosinophils. At the same time, a significant rise in leukocyte numbers is evident in bronchoalveolar lavage fluid. There is, however, no evidence of obvious oedema or epithelial denudation. It has been suggested that the dual response

of guinea-pigs to antigen presented in this way may be a product of frustrated phagocytosis within the airway lumen. The synthetic corticosteroid, budesonide, inhibits the secondary response by up to 75% when given either at the same time or even a couple of hours after intratracheal challenge[64], consistent with the inhibition of an inflammatory component. The effect of selective cyclo-oxygenase and lipoxygenase inhibitors in this model will be interesting.

Persistent intrabronchial antigenic stimulation in the guinea-pig has also been used as model of the chronic inflammation seen in other airway disease entities, such as chronic bronchitis and cystic fibrosis[84].

Rabbit: An IgE-dependent model of the late asthmatic response in the rabbit was originally described by Shampain and co-workers[85]. They found that aerosol challenge of animals, neonatally sensitized to an extract from the mould *Alternaria tenuis*, provoked an obvious biphasic pulmonary response. *Alternaria* and other saprophytic moulds have a documented history of causing both immediate and late human cutaneous and bronchial allergic reactions. In the rabbit, late allergic bronchospasm is characterized by a secondary and prolonged (6 h and beyond) fall in dynamic compliance together with an equally persistent secondary rise in lung resistance. This is in contrast to the initial acute response which lasts only for about 30 min in total. Intravenous infusion of isoprenaline does not reverse the secondary phase which appears to be modulated by antigen-specific IgG[86]. There is histological evidence of progressive pulmonary inflammation beginning at 6 h post-challenge. This takes the form of submucosal vessel dilatation and subsequent cellular infiltration and thickening of both bronchiolar and arterial walls during later stages. In a subsequent modification of the original experimental model, late phase pulmonary responses have also been described in rabbits passively sensitized to ragweed extract[87]. An element of airway hyperreactivity to histamine is evident following the late allergic response[87]. Furthermore, there is a time-related association between this increased airway reactivity and an increased presence of both polymorphonuclear and mononuclear cells in bronchoalveolar lavage fluid. Whether the cellular infiltration itself is responsible for this phenomenon has yet to be proven.

Sheep: As well as acute bronchoconstriction, a temporally separated late pulmonary response has also been observed in *Ascaris*-sensitive sheep following aerosol challenge[62,88]. This delayed response (Figure 9.2) is characterized by a secondary rise in specific lung resistance and a fall in both dynamic compliance and arterial PaO_2 occurring between 6 and 7 h after the initial challenge and is associated with an inflammatory lesion in the airways[89]. Neither β_2-adrenoceptor stimulants nor antihistamines, either alone or with atropine, inhibit the late pulmonary response in sheep although both give some degree of protection from the immediate bronchoconstriction[88]. However, SCG blocks both the immediate and the late response suggesting a common role for mast cell-derived mediators in both cases[88]. FPL55712, which does not block but may shorten the immediate response, inhibits the late phase if given 60 to 90 min before its predicted onset[88]. In the same model, inhaled FPL 55712 has also been found to partially reverse an ongoing

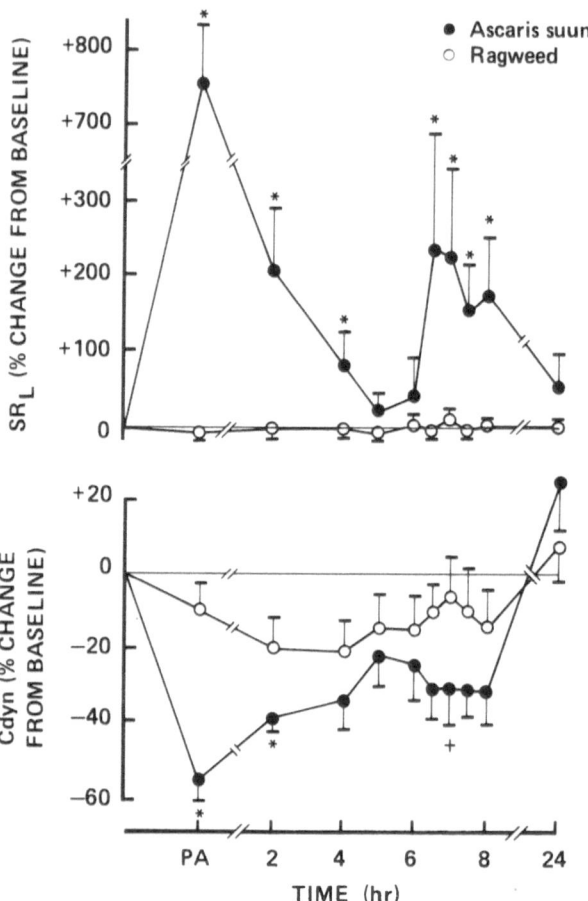

Figure 9.2 Time course of the dual changes in specific lung resistance (SR_L) and dynamic lung compliance (C_{dyn}) after inhalation challenge of *Ascaris*-sensitive sheep with *Ascaris suum* extract. Ragweed antigen was used as a procedural control. Each point represents the mean ($\pm$ SEM) from results in 8 animals (* = $p < 0.05$; + = $p < 0.1$) with respect to changes observed with ragweed antigen. From ref. 62 with permission of the authors and publishers

late phase reaction[88]. The orally active LTD_4/E_4 antagonist, LY171883, given 2 h before challenge, reduces the severity of the acute response to inhaled antigen and completely blocks the late response[90]. In sheep, therefore, peptido-leukotrienes appear to have a predominant role in the late phase and a lesser role in the initial phase of pulmonary anaphylaxis. Indeed, increased airway responsiveness to LTD_4 has been suggested as one factor which distinguishes those sheep showing an early and late response from those only giving an acute reaction[91]. The late phase reaction is inhibited by either intravenous prednisolone[62] or inhaled budesonide[89], both of which are used therapeutically in man. However, the involvement of a generalized inflammatory lesion in the late phase in sheep is far from clear. Histological studies (bronchoalveolar lavage and lung biopsies) do not show a difference between inflammatory cell numbers in untreated animals and those receiving either SCG or steroid[92]. Thus the late pulmonary response in this species may in fact be dependent on the initial release of mediators rather than the subsequent development of airway inflammation. Although enhanced sensitivity to inhaled carbachol is evident after the late phase reaction, this is not inhibited by acute pretreatment with budesonide[64]. The effect of chronic pretreatment with this steroid on airway hyperreactivity in this model has yet to be determined.

Non-immunological pulmonary release of eicosanoids

In addition to antigen challenge, the release of eicosanoids from isolated lungs *in vitro* can be triggered by several stimuli including bradykinin[93], rabbit aorta contracting substance-release factor[94], calcium ionophore A23187[95], SRS and SRS-A[95,96], leukotrienes[97], PAF-acether[98] and mechanical trauma[99]. Exogenous arachidonic acid (AA) infused into guinea-pig isolated lungs also promotes the release of rabbit aorta contracting substance[100], shown subsequently[101] to be a mixture of prostaglandin endoperoxides and TxA_2. Both PGD_2 and TxB_2 are generated by human dispersed lung cells after activation with ionophore A23187 or anti-IgE[102]. There are, however, important quantitative and qualitative differences in the biological activation of AA between species[103,104]. In addition, we have recently shown that the profile of release of eicosanoids from guinea-pig isolated lungs is stimulus dependent[15]. We also found bradykinin to be the only stimulus that releases more 6-oxo-$PGF_{1\alpha}$ than TxB_2, and only calcium ionophore shared the ability of antigen challenge to release leukotriene-like material[15].

Exogenous AA *in vivo* has been found to cause varying degrees of bronchoconstriction depending on its route and speed of administration[17,104–106]. In most instances, however, this is inhibited by cyclo-oxygenase blockade suggesting that exogenous AA is metabolized preferentially through this pathway, although an indirect action of *de novo* synthesized lipoxygenase products through the same pathway[107] cannot be wholly discounted.

In monkeys, aerosolized doses of A23187 and AA, given separately, results in no airway response[16]. In contrast, when given simultaneously by aerosol, there is an increase in respiratory frequency and airways resistance and a decrease in lung compliance, peak expiratory flow rate and tidal volume, qualitatively similar to an antigen-induced response. However, whilst the mixed inhibitor ETYA inhibits this response, so does indomethacin. In contrast, the SRS-A antagonist FPL 55712 does not. This suggests once again that cyclo-oxygenase rather than lipoxygenase metabolites are the predominant mediators under these circumstances[16].

Experimental models of other pulmonary diseases

Increasing experimental and clinical evidence suggests that both immune and inflammatory processes are involved in other airway disease entities apart from asthma[108,109]. These include adult respiratory distress syndrome (ARDS), sarcoidosis, chronic bronchitis, cystic fibrosis and extrinsic allergic alveolitis. Attempts to simulate these diseases in experimental animals have met with varied success. Two examples are described below.

ARDS

ARDS, also referred to as shock lung syndrome, is a severe form of acute lung injury consisting of a triad of gross intrapulmonary shunting with relative or absolute hypoxemia, a decreased pulmonary compliance, and chest X-ray findings consistent with diffuse bilateral pulmonary oedema[110,111].

Numerous specific incidents or illnesses may be complicated by or associated with ARDS, such as bacteraemia and endotoxaemia, aspiration of gastrointestinal contents, severe trauma (thoracic or extrathoracic), fat embolization, smoke or toxic gas inhalation (including O_2), surface burns, long-chain hydrocarbon ingestion, anaphylactic reaction to drugs and blood, neurogenic pulmonary oedema, toxic drugs and poison (e.g. paraquat), Goodpasture's syndrome, pneumonias induced by viral, mycoplasma or bacterial agents, Legionnaire's disease, and radiation of the thorax. The most common causes of ARDS, however, are generally associated with sepsis and trauma[112–114].

This syndrome has been estimated to occur in 150 000 patients each year in the United States, often in previously healthy individuals, and is associated with a mortality rate exceeding 50%[115]. In Britain, there may be 10 000–15 000 cases each year[116] with a fatality rate typically of 60%, and even 90% where sepsis is predominant[117].

The most striking histopathological features of ARDS is the presence of interstitial oedema associated with leukocyte migration. The animal models employed to study ARDS can be divided into two major groups. These consist of those models based on stimuli that resemble those found in clinical settings and those models based on stimuli which cause a pathological feature similar to the ones found clinically.

Models of ARDS based on stimuli found in clinical setting

Sepsis: Sepsis, together with trauma, are the major causes of ARDS. Injection of gram-negative bacteria or endotoxin in sheep[118,119] and dogs[120] induces transient pulmonary hypertension which is followed by interstitial pulmonary oedema, probably due to increased vascular permeability. Eicosanoids administered to animals can induce most of the pathophysiological findings in ARDS, such as pulmonary hypertension (PGA_2, B_2, D_2, E_2, $F_{2\alpha}$, H_2, TxB_2)[121], changes in lung mechanics (LTB_4 and D_4)[121–123], hypoxaemia (PGE_1)[124], increased permeability (LTC_4 and D_4)[125,126] and enhanced neutrophil adherence (LTB_4)[127]. Cyclo-oxygenase inhibitors have been reported to block the experimental syndrome in certain animal models[128,129] but these results are still controversial, since pretreatment with salicylic acid or indomethacin have no effect on the leukocyte sequestration in the pulmonary capillaries or other histological abnormalities seen in endotoxin shock in monkeys[130]. There is no clinical evidence for prevention or treatment of ARDS with cyclo-oxygenase inhibition, although a rigorous clinical trial has yet to be carried out.

Measurements of several eicosanoids in lung lymph over the course of the endotoxin response in sheep indicate an interesting temporal sequence of eicosanoid release from the lung[121]. Concentrations of TxB_2 peak early, coincident with the maximum pulmonary hypertension and changes in lung mechanics. Shortly thereafter, 6-oxo-$PGF_{1\alpha}$ levels reach a maximum value as pulmonary artery pressure begins to decline and the changes in lung mechanics begin to wane. Later, together with the changes in lymph protein clearance which indicate increased microvascular permeability, concentrations of the lipoxygenase products, 5-HETE and 12-HETE, increase[121,131].

The data on the effect of corticosteroids in prevention and development of ARDS models are also controversial[130,132]. The apparent protective role of corticosteroid treatment in ARDS[133,134] suggests that eicosanoids could be involved but it is not yet proven that the mechanism of corticosteroid action in ARDS is through phospholipase A_2 inhibition[135].

Oxygen toxicity: Many of the morphological changes caused by normobaric hyperoxia, such as interstitial oedema and endothelial cell damage, are similar to those occurring in ARDS[136,137]. Oxygen toxicity has been studied in several species[138,139]. We have recently shown[140] that dexamethasone had an inhibitory effect on bradykinin-induced eicosanoid release from isolated lungs of guinea-pigs exposed to O_2 yet had no effect on the release induced from lungs of control guinea-pigs[141]. This led us to propose the concept that whereas cells in normal lungs are protected from certain stimuli because of the integrity of the endothelium, these cells are now exposed in ARDS due to endothelial cell damage[140]. The clinical implications of this concept in the therapy of ARDS have been detailed elsewhere[142].

Pancreatitis: Some of the common and most lethal complications of acute pancreatitis involve ARDS. Experimental pancreatitis induced by injection of trypsin (10 000–20 000 U) into the pancreactic duct has been studied in dogs[143] and rats[144]. The histopathological studies in lungs of dogs following injection of trypsin showed that the lung biopsies of the pancreatitic dogs differed from those of the control dogs by only two criteria, atelectasis and vascular congestion, with the pancreatitic dogs demonstrating more severe pathologic changes. However, there was no observation of hyaline membranes or pulmonary oedema in either the control or the pancreatitic animals' lungs[143].

Models of ARDS unrelated to stimuli in clinical settings
In the rat, α-naphthylthiourea (ANTU) has been shown to induce pulmonary oedema with destruction and rounding up of endothelial cells[145,146]. In isolated lungs from rats treated with ANTU, synthesis of eicosanoids induced by endogenous or exogenous stimulation of arachidonic acid metabolism was increased[147]. Although these results support a role for eicosanoids in ANTU-induced oedema, from the time course of the observed effect, the increase in eicosanoids observed was probably a response to the initial damage rather than a cause of the oedema. Other models of the acute lung injury of ARDS have been described in a variety of species using agents ranging from oleic acid to paraquat[148,149].

Extrinsic Allergic Alveolitis (EAA)

EAA, or hypersensitivity pneumonitis, is characterized by an immunologically driven diffuse chronic inflammation of the peripheral airways[150]. Usually the aetiology is known (e.g. bird fancier's disease, farmer's lung). Infiltration of both intra-alveolar and interstitial spaces by macrophages and lymphocytes is accompanied in the worst prognosis by non-caseating granulomas and fibrotic lung damage. The acute inflammatory lesion of EAA is thought to be caused by immune complex disease (ICD). The chronic phase appears more indicative of cell-mediated immunity (CMI). Experimental models of both phases of EAA have been described in numerous animal species, including mice, rat, guinea-pigs, rabbits, dogs and monkeys[151]. Previously immunized guinea-pigs develop pulmonary ICD after just one subsequent exposure to an aerosol of the initial sensitizing antigen[152]. The development of ICD is followed by gradual pulmonary inflammation and CMI after repeated daily challenge for 2 weeks. Similarly, in rabbits, aerosol exposure for 2 to 3 weeks to the initial sensitizing antigen (soluble pigeon dropping extract) causes the development of chronic granulomatous pulmonary inflammation[153]. This is associated with demonstrable CMI in bronchoalveolar cells. Interestingly, further exposure of these animals to the antigen causes a refractory state which sometimes occurs in human EAA[153]. So far, emphasis in experimental models of EAA has been placed on reproducing the pathology of the disease rather than identifying possible treatments of disease.

RHEUMATOID ARTHRITIS

Rheumatoid arthritis (RA) is a chronic inflammatory disease of unknown aetiology. It affects mainly the peripheral synovial joints which become painful and swollen. In addition, there is progresive damage to joint tissues.

The synovial tissue is infiltrated with macrophages, lymphocytes (T and B cells) and plasma cells[154]. The histology of the rheumatoid synovial lining has been likened to a delayed-type hypersensitivity reaction in the skin, in that T lymphocytes are found associated with HLA-DR expressing macrophage/dendritic cells. These HLA-DR-expressing macrophage/dendritic cells isolated from the synovial lining can mediate T cell activation[155]. In contrast, the predominant cell infiltrating the synovial fluid is the polymorphonuclear leucocyte (PMN) with a lower number of mononuclear cells[154]. This is reminiscent of a PMN-dependent Arthus-like reaction and immune complexes do occur in the synovial fluids of patients with RA[156]. However, it is unlikely that immune complexes play a major role in the pathogenesis of RA because (1) the incidence of RA is common in patients with agammaglobulinaemia (where the levels of IgG are low and therefore where immune complex formation is less likely to occur[157]) and (2) plasmapheresis (which removes immune complexes) does not reduce the severity of the disease[158].

Animal models of RA

Little is known about the biochemical processes occuring in the human rheumatoid joint. Much of our information about what might be occurring in the arthritic joint has to be extrapolated from animal models of inflammation.

Adjuvant arthritis in the rat

One of the models most commonly used for testing anti-inflammatory drugs is adjuvant arthritis in the rat[159]. Briefly, a polyarthritis develops in several joints 2–3 weeks after injection of Freund's complete adjuvant. Interestingly, it has not been possible to induce arthritis in this manner in any other species so far tested. The lesion is characterized by swelling, periostitis and bone remodelling. Any cartilage degradation that does occur appears to be secondary to the bone resorption and there is no evidence of a direct attack on cartilage as an initiating event[160]. Non-steroidal anti-inflammatory drugs (NSAID), such as aspirin or indomethacin, which inhibit the formation of prostaglandins[161], alleviate the symptoms and halt the progression of the disease in this model, suggesting a role for prostaglandins in the disease process. However, this must be seen as a limitation of adjuvant arthritis as a model of RA since NSAID only inhibit the symptoms of the disease in man and do not arrest its development. The suggestion of a role for prostaglandins in adjuvant arthritis is complicated by the finding that systemic administration of high doses of prostaglandin E_2 (PGE_2)[162] and PGE_1[163] suppressed paw swelling in rats with adjuvant arthritis. However, the actions of pharmacological doses of PGE_2 given systemically will undoubtedly be different from the much lower concentrations produced locally in the joint.

Collagen-induced arthritis in the rat and mouse

Immunization with type II collagen induces an arthritis in rats[164] and mice[165]. Histologically, there is inflammatory synovitis with cartilage and bone erosion[164]. Collagen-induced arthritis has been claimed to be an appropriate model of human RA because patients with RA exhibit both humoral[166] and cellular[167] immunity to collagen. However, the fact that this model is sensitive to aspirin-like drugs[159] is again a limitation. Indomethacin was shown to inhibit the paw swelling and the bony ankylosis[168] suggesting a role for prostaglandins not only in the oedema but also in the connective tissue changes. This may be related to the finding that PGE_2 stimulates bone resorption in culture[169]. An involvement of prostaglandins in collagen-induced arthritis in the mouse is supported by the finding that mice which had been fed fish oil (rich in eicosapentaenoic acid) showed a reduction in the incidence and severity of the disease[170]. This was accompanied by a reduction in PGE_2 and PGI_2 production from peritoneal macrophages of these animals. In contrast, Prickett and colleagues[171] found that rats which had been fed fish oil had an increased susceptibility to collagen-induced arthritis. In addition, there was no significiant difference in the severity of the joint inflammation even though the synthesis of PGE_2 by the synovium was reduced by 75–80% compared with controls. These authors attributed these findings to the removal of the immunosuppressant activity of PGE_2.

The relevance of experiments implicating cyclo-oxygenase products in the degradative processes in adjuvant and collagen-induced arthritis to the pathology of RA is questionable. This is because cyclo-oxygenase inhibitors, such as indomethacin, while suppressing the symptoms of inflammation, do not halt the erosive process.

205

Antigen-induced arthritis in the rabbit

A more relevant model of RA is the Dumonde-Glynn model of antigen-induced arthritis (AIA) in the rabbit. The disease is induced by sensitizing rabbits to antigen, usually ovalbumin, in Freund's complete adjuvant and then injecting a sterile solution of antigen into one knee joint. The contralateral knee joint is injected with saline and serves as a 'within animal' control. This monoarticular disease is similar to RA in that it is chronic (lasting the life of the rabbit) and there is progressive cartilage and bone erosion. The histology of the lesion is indistinguishable from that of the rheumatoid joint[172]. Unlike many other animal models of arthritis, the Dumonde–Glynn model responds to drug therapy in a manner similar to the rheumatoid patient. The NSAIDs, such as indomethacin, reduce joint swelling without affecting joint histopathology[173]. Prednisolone, when given prophylactically or to animals with established disease, reduces joint swelling and has some effect on joint histopathology[173]. This parallels the clinical situation. The disease-modifying drug, D-penicillamine, is also active in this model and, like the clinical situation, has a slow onset of action[173].

The chronicity, the histological features of the disease and the response to drug therapy suggest that this is the most relevant model of RA to investigate the role of eicosanoids in the development of the symptoms and the histopathology. Blackham and co-workers[174] were the first to investigate the role of eicosanoids in this model. They showed that the PGE-like activity (measured by bioassay) in arthritic joints peaked at 19 h after the onset of the disease, at a level equivalent to 10 ng PGE_2 per joint, but was lower in the chronic stages. More recently, Henderson and Higgs[175] have detected a level of approximately 10 ng ml^{-1} PGE_2 (measured by radioimmunoassay) 1 day after joint challenge and also found the levels much reduced in chronic stages of the disease. It had been found previously that treatment with indomethacin reduced the prostaglandin E-like activity which correlated with a reduction in joint swelling[174]. However, the number of infiltrating leukocytes and histopathology of the joint tissues were unaffected by indomethacin treatment. Therefore, the presence of PGE_2 in the synovial fluid of arthritic joints, coupled with the finding that indomethacin reduced joint swelling but not the erosions, suggests that prostaglandins may be involved in the development of the symptoms of the disease but not the disease process *per se*.

Immunoreactive LTB_4 has recently been detected in the synovial fluid of rabbits with acute antigen-induced arthritis[175]. Leukotriene B_4 has been shown to be chemotactic for PMN *in vivo*[176] and may, in part, be responsible for the presence of PMN in the synovial fluid. However, LTB_4 was only detected at day 1 in this model and not in the chronic stages. The concentration of PGE_2 in joint washes remained high enough to contribute to joint swelling in the chronic stages of the lesion (see Figure 9.3). However, the absence of LTB_4 after day 1 indicates that this eicosanoid is unlikely to influence the sustained recruitment of inflammatory leukocytes.

A lipid mediator which is not derived from arachidonic acid, platelet activating factor (PAF-acether), has been detected in the antigen-induced arthritis model[177]. The levels of PAF-acether in joint washings show a similar pattern to those of LTB_4; PAF-acether was present at biologically active levels

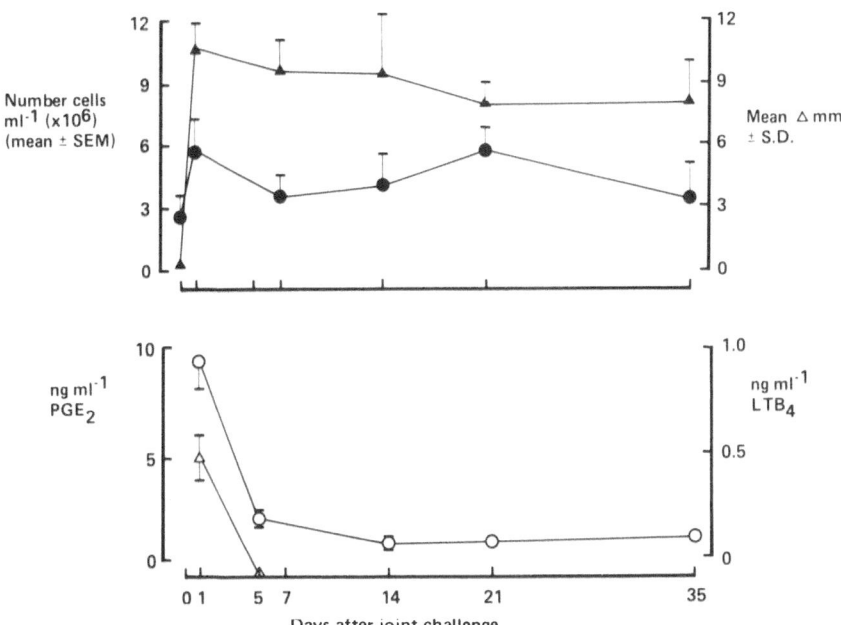

Figure 9.3 The upper panel shows leukocyte infiltration (▲) and joint swelling (●) as antigen-induced arthritis develops in the rabbit. The lower panel shows the corresponding concentrations of PGE$_2$ (○) and LTB$_4$ (△) in the joint fluid as the lesion progresses. The first time point shown is 4 h

at day 1 but was not detectable in the chronic stages of the lesion. The biologically inactive precursor and metabolite of PAF-acether, lyso-PAF, was elevated in arthritic joints in the early stages of the disease but had returned to similar levels to those of control joints by day 14.

The presence of LTB$_4$ and PAF-acether and elevation of PGE$_2$ in arthritic joints at day 1 in this model is consistent with the occurrence of a PMN-dependent Arthus-like reaction in the joint space at this time. Indeed, prostaglandins and PAF-acether have been implicated in Arthus-like reactions because indomethacin[178] and PAF antagonists[179] reduce oedema associated with the reverse passive Arthus reaction. Although it is widely held that an Arthus reaction occurs in the early stage of the lesion in the Dumonde–Glynn model[173], it has been suggested, from experiments utilizing different immunization procedures, that a delayed hypersensitivity reaction is necessary to mediate the chronicity of the disease[180]. The most important pathological events, namely cartilage and bone erosion, occur in the chronic phase of the lesion; the absence of LTB$_4$ and PAF-acether at this stage suggests that these mediators are not involved in the damage to joint tissues. However, the continued presence of PGE$_2$ in the chronic stages could contribute to joint swelling, and the reduction of chronic joint swelling by indomethacin supports this view.

207

CONCLUDING REMARKS

Pharmacological studies *in vitro* have a limited usefulness. For example, they can only suggest what a novel chemical entity might do *in vivo*. Thus there is a need for animal models both for *in vivo* testing and also for the development of hypotheses regarding the treatment of human disease. Experimental models do have a potential advantage over the clinical situation in that the aetiology is known and sometimes well defined. In addition, there is a predetermined time course of disease progression under some degree of control by the investigator. Furthermore, and of particular importance in the context of inflammation, is the ability to correlate physiological events with pathological changes. However, these advantages count for nothing if the model itself is entirely irrelevant to the human situation. Unfortunately, such is the potential for mediator redundancy in inflammation that it is difficult to assess the relative merits of one experimental model versus another when considering this aspect. What may be an important mediator in man and perhaps certain animal species may have no role whatsoever in other species. Thus the relevance to man of models of inflammation where conditions arc geared to accentuate the contribution of one mediator to the exception of others is particularly uncertain in the absence of supportive clinical data. However, the approach of studying the effects of single-component mediators rather than mimicking the disease in its entirety does at least allow specific questions to be addressed such as the likely role of certain eicosanoids[181] and other lipid mediators, e.g. PAF-acether[182,183] in airway hyperreactivity. The advent of more versatile and sensitive assay techniques that allow the models themselves to be better characterized in terms of the mediators involved will help in this respect.

REFERENCES

1. Kaliner, M. (1984). Editorial: Hypotheses on the contribution of the late-phase allergic responses to the understanding and treatment of allergic diseases. *J. Allergy Clin. Immunol.*, **73**, 311–315
2. Dolovich, J., Hargreave, F.E., Chalmers, R., Shier, K.J., Gauldie, J. and Bienenstock, J. (1973). Late cutaneous allergic responses in isolated IgE dependent reactions. *J. Allergy Clin. Immunol.*, **52**, 38–46
3. Dunnill, M.S. (1960). The pathology of asthma with special reference to changes in the bronchial mucosa. *J. Clin. Pathol.*, **13**, 27–33
4. Monchy, J.G.R., Kauffman, H.F., Venge, P., Koeter, G.H., Jansen, H.M., Sluiter, H.J. and De Vries, K. (1985). Bronchoalveolar lavage eosinophilia during allergen-induced late asthmatic reactions. *Am. Rev. Respir. Dis.*, **131**, 373–376
5. Boushey, H.A., Holtzman, M.J., Sheller, J.R. and Nadel, J.A. (1980). Bronchial hyperreactivity. *Am. Rev. Respir. Dis.*, **121**, 389–413
6. Holgate, S.T. and Kay, A.B. (1985). Mast cells, mediators and asthma. *Clin. Allergy*, **15**, 221–234
7. Robinson, C. and Holgate, S.T. (1985). Mast-cell dependent inflammatory mediators and their putative role in bronchial asthma. *Clin. Sci.*, **68**, 103–112
8. Lewis, R.A. (1985). A presumptive role for leukotrienes in obstructive airway disease. *Chest*, **88**, 98S–102S
9. Ogunbiyi, P.O. and Eyre, P. (1985). Pharmacological studies of pulmonary anaphylaxis in vitro: A review. *Agents Actions*, **17**, 158–174

10. Chen, S.E. and Bernstein, I.L. (1982). The guinea-pig model of diisocyanate sensitization. I: Immunologic studies. *J. Allergy. Clin. Immunol.*, **70**, 383–392
11. Bernstein, L., Splansky, G.L., Chen, S.E. and Vinegar, A. (1982). The guinea-pig model of diisocyanate sensitization. II. Physiological studies. *J. Allergy Clin. Immunol.*, **70**, 393–398
12. Ishizaka, T. (1984). IgE-mediated triggering signals for mediator release from human mast cells and basophils. In Kay, A.B., Austen, K.F. and Lichtenstein, L.M. (eds.) *Asthma: Physiology, Immunopharmacology and Treatment.* Third Int. Symposium, pp. 39–54. (London: Academic Press)
13. Kulczycki, A. (1981). Role of immunoglobulin E and immunoglobulin E receptors in bronchial asthma. *J. Allergy, Clin. Immunol.*, **68**, 5–14
14. Undem, B.J., Buckner, C.K., Harley, P. and Graziano, F.M. (1985). Smooth muscle contraction and release of histamine slow-reacting substance of anaphylaxis in pulmonary tissues isolated from guinea-pigs passively sensitized with IgG, or IgE antibodies. *Am. Rev. Respir. Dis.*, **131**, 260–266
15. Bakhle, Y.S., Moncada, S., de Nucci, G. and Salmon, J.A. (1985). Differential release of eicosanoids by bradykinin, arachidonic acid and calcium ionophore A23187 in guinea-pig isolated perfused lung. *Br. J. Pharmacol.*, **86**, 55–62
16. Patterson, R., Harris, K.E. and Greenberger, P.A. (1979). Ionophore and arachidonic acid stimulation of airway responses in Rhesus monkeys. *J. Clin. Invest.*, **64**, 49–55
17. Spanhake, E.W., Hyman, A.L. and Kadowitz, P.J. (1980). Dependence of the airway and pulmonary effects of arachidonic acid upon route and rate of administration. *J. Pharmacol. Exp. Ther.*, **212**, 584–590
18. Burka, J.F. (1985). Pharmacological modulation of responses of guinea-pig airways contracted with arachidonic acid. *Br. J. Pharmacol.*, **85**, 421–426
19. Holtzmann, M.J. (1985). Inflammation of the airway epithelium and the development of airway hyperresponsiveness. *Prog. Respir. Res.*, **19**, 165–172
20. Golden, J.A., Nadel, J.A. and Boushey, H.A. (1978). Bronchial hyperirritability in healthy subjects after exposure to ozone. *Am. Rev. Respir. Dis.*, **118**, 287–294
21. Kallos, P. and Kallos, L. (1984). Experimental asthma in guinea-pigs revisited. *Int. Arch. Allergy Appl. Immunol.*, **73**, 77–85
22. Benacerraf, B. (1968). Properties of immunoglobulins which mediate the release of vasoactive amines in experimental animals. In Schild, H.O. (ed.) *Third International Pharmacological Meeting 1966. Vol. II, Immunopharmacology*, pp. 3–13. (London: Pergamon Press)
23. Collier, H.O.J. and James, G.W.L. (1967). Humoral factors affecting pulmonary inflation during acute anaphylaxis in the guinea-pig in vivo. *Br. J. Pharmacol. Chemother.*, **30**, 283–301
24. Morris, H.R., Taylor, G.W., Piper, P.J. and Tippins, J.R. (1980). Structure of slow-reacting substance of anaphylaxis from guinea-pig lung. *Nature (London)*, **285**, 104–108
25. Andersson, P. (1980). Antigen-induced bronchial anaphylaxis in actively sensitized guinea-pigs: anti-anaphylactic effects of sodium cromoglycate and aminophylline. *Br. J. Pharmacol.*, **69**, 467–472
26. Andersson, P. and Brattsand, R. (1982). Protective effects of the glucocorticoid Budenoside on lung anaphylaxis in actively sensitized guinea-pigs: inhibition of IgE but not IgG mediated responses. *Br. J. Pharmacol.*, **76**, 139–147
27. Blumenthal, A., Dervinis, A. and Lewis, A. (1981). In vivo assessment of SRS-A activity and production in the guinea-pig. *Fed. Proc.*, **40**, 1024
28. Ritchie, D.M., Sierchio, J.N., Capetola, R.J. and Rosenthale, M.E. (1981). SRS-A mediated bronchospasm by pharmacologic modification of lung anaphylaxis in vivo. *Agents Actions*, **11**, 396–401
29. Andersson, W.H., O'Donnell, M., Simko, B.A. and Welton, A.F. (1983). An *in vivo* model for measuring antigen-induced SRS-A mediated bronchoconstriction and plasma SRS-A levels in the guinea-pig. *Br. J. Pharmacol.*, **78**, 67–74
30. Bach, M.K., Griffin, R.L. and Richards, I.M. (1985). Inhibition of the presumably leukotriene dependent component of antigen-induced bronchoconstriction of the guinea-pig by piriprost (U-60,257). *Int. Arch. Allergy Appl. Immunol.*, **77**, 264–266
31. Payne, A.N. and de Nucci, G. (1987). Anaphylaxis in guinea-pigs induced by ovalbumin aerosol: *in vivo* and *in vitro* methods. *J. Pharmacol. Meth.*, **19**, 83–90

32. Sanyal, R.K. and West, G.B. (1958). Anaphylactic shock in the albino rat. *J. Physiol. (London)*, **142**, 571–584
33. Jones, V.E. and Edwards, A.J. (1971). Preparation of an antiserum specific for rat reagin. *Immunology*, **21**, 383–385
34. Church, M.K., Collier, H.O.J. and James, G.W.L. (1972). The inhibition by dexamethasone and disodium cromoglycate of anaphylactic bronchoconstriction in the rat. *Br. J. Pharmacol.*, **46**, 56–65
35. Ufkes, J.G.R. and Ottenhof, M. (1984). Characterisation of various antiallergic agents using a new method for inducing systemic anaphylaxis in the rat. *J. Pharm. Meth.*, **11**, 219–226
36. Ottenhof, M., Ufkes, G.R. and van Rooij, H.J.H. (1985). The effect of prednisolone and ketotifen on the antigen-induced bronchoconstriction and mediator release in rat isolated lungs. *Br. J. Pharmacol.*, **86**, 627–636
37. Dahlback, M., Bergstrand, H. and Sorenby, L. (1984). Bronchial anaphylaxis in actively sensitized Sprague-Dawley rats: studies on the mediators involved. *Acta Pharmacol. Toxicol.*, **55**, 57–64
38. Ahlstedt, S., Smedegard, G., Nygren, H. and Bjorkstein, B. (1983). Immune responses in rats sensitized with aerosolised antigen. *Int. Arch. Allergy Appl. Immunol.*, **72**, 71–78
39. Damas, J., Remacle-Volon, G., Radermecker, M. and Lecomte, J. (1983). The participation of platelets in anaphylactic shock in the rat. *Arch. Int. Physiol. Biochim.*, **91**, 465–469
40. Brunet, G., Charleson, S. and Ford Hutchinson, A.W. (1985). Antigen-induced leukotriene release from rat lung in vitro. *Prostaglandins*, **29**, 921–932
41. Dahlback, M. and Sorenby, L. (1982). Antigen-induced bronchial anaphylaxis in SD rats: Possible mediators involved. *Br. J. Pharmacol.*, **77**, 395P
42. Everitt, B.J., Oliver, W.R., Spiegel, W.D. and Lever, W.O. (1984). Anti-anaphylactic effects of Baicalein in guina-pig and rat lung. *IUPHAR 9th International Congress of Pharmacology*, Abstract 253P
43. Halonen, M., Fisher, H.K., Blair, C., Butler, C. and Pinckard, R.N. (1976). IgE-induced respiratory and circulatory changes during systemic anaphylaxis in the rabbit. *Am. Rev. Respir. Dis.*, **114**, 961–970
44. Halonen, M., Lohman, C., Dunn, A.M., McManus, L.M. and Palmer, J.D.C. (1985). Participation of platelets in the physiologic alterations of the AGEPC response and of IgE anaphylaxis in the rabbit. *Am. Rev. Respir. Dis.*, **131**, 11–17
45. Pinckard, R.N., Farr, R.S. and Hanahan, D.J. (1979). Physiochemical and functional identity of rabbit platelet activating factor (PAF) released in vivo during IgE anaphylaxis with PAF released in vitro from IgE sensitized basophils. *J. Immunol.*, **123**, 1847–1857
46. Halonen, M., Lohman, J.C. and Palmer, J.D. (1984). The role of histamine in the physiologic alteration of IgE anaphylaxis in the rabbit. *Immunopharmacology*, **7**, 77–87
47. McManus, L.M., Shaw, J.O. and Pinckard, R.N. (1980). Thromboxane B₂ (TxB₂) release during IgE anaphylaxis in the rabbit. *J. Immunol.*, **125**, 1950–1954
48. Patterson, R. (1969). Laboratory models of reaginic allergy. *Prog. Allergy*, 12, 332–407
49. Uvnas, B. and Wold, J. (1967). Isolation of a mast cell degranulating polypeptide from Ascaris suis. *Acta Physiol. Scand.*, **70**, 269–276
50. Mjorndal, T.O., Chesrown, S.E., Frey, M.S., Reed, B.R., Lazarus, S.C. and Gold, W.M. (1983). Effect of beta-adrenergic stimulation on experimental canine anaphylaxis in vivo. *J. Allergy Clin. Immunol.*, **71**, 62–70
51. Kepron, W., James, J.M., Kirk, B., Sehon, A.H. and Tse, K.S. (1977). A canine model for reaginic hypersensitivity and allergic bronchoconstriction. *J. Allergy Clin. Immunol.*, **59**, 64–69
52. McConnell, L.H., Arkins, J.A. and Fink, J.N. (1973). Induced homocytotrophic antibody to bovine serum albumin in neonatal dogs. *J. Allergy Clin. Immunol.*, **52**, 47–54
53. Mapp, C., Hartiala, J., Frick, O.L., Shields, R.L. and Gold, W.M. (1985). Airway responsiveness to inhaled antigen, histamine and methacholine in inbred, ragweed-sensitized dogs. *Am. Rev. Respir. Dis.*, **132**, 292–298
54. Patterson, R., Zeiss, C.R. and Harris, K.E. (1983). Immunologic and respiratory responses to airway challenges of dogs with toluene diisocyanate. *J. Allergy Clin. Immunol.*, **71**, 604–611
55. Bice, D.E. and Muggenburg, B.A. (1985). Effect of age on antibody responses after lung immunisation. *Am. Rev. Respir. Dis.*, **132**, 661–665

56. Snapper, J.R., Braasch, P.S., Loring, S.H., Ingram, R.H. and Drazen, J.M. (1980). Comparison of the responsiveness to histamine and to Ascaris suum challenge in dogs. *Am. Rev. Respir. Dis.*, **122**, 775–780

57. Krell, R.D., Chakrin, L.W. and Wardell, J.R. (1976). *In vivo* canine and Rhesus monkey models of allergic asthma. In Rosenthal, M. and Mansmann, H. (eds.) *Immunopharmacology*, pp. 125–148. (New York: Spectrum)

58. Krell, R.D. and Chakrin, L.W. (1978). Pharmacologic regulation of antigen-induced mediator release from canine lung. *Int. Arch. Allergy Appl. Immunol.*, **56**, 39–47

59. Chung, K.F., Becker, A.B., Lazarus, S.C., Frick, O.L., Nadel, J.A. and Gold, W.M. (1985). Antigen-induced airway hyperresponsiveness and pulmonary inflammation in allergic dogs. *J. Appl. Physiol.*, **58**, 1347–53

60. Hirshman, C.A., Malley, A. and Cownes, H. (1980). Basenji-Greyhound dog model of asthma: reactivity to Ascaris worm, citric acid and methacholine. *J. Appl. Physiol.*, **49**, 953–957

61. Wanner, A., Metzy, R.J., Reinhard, M.E. and Eyre, P. (1979). Antigen-induced bronchospasm in conscious sheep. *J. Appl. Physiol.*, **47**, 917–922

62. Abraham, W.M., Delehunt, J.C., Yerger, L. and Marchette, B. (1983). Characterisation of a late phase pulmonary response after antigen challenge in allergic sheep. *Am. Rev. Respir. Dis.*, **128**, 839–844

63. Abraham, W.M., Oliver, W. Jr., King, M.M., Yerger, L. and Wanner, A. (1981). Effect of pharmacological agents on antigen-induced decreases in specific lung conductance in sheep. *Am. Rev. Respir. Dis.*, **124**, 554–558

64. Hogg, J.C., Venge, P., Morley, J., Abraham, W.M. and Brattsand, R. (1985). Glucocorticoids, Inflammation and Bronchial Hyperreactivity. In Herzog, H. and Perruchod, A.P. (eds.) *Asthma and Bronchial Hyperreactivity, Progress in Respiratory Research*, Vol. 19, pp. 461–475 (Karger: Basel)

65. Delehunt, J.C., Yercer, L. and Abraham, W.M. (1981). The time course of antigen-induced airway hyperreactivity to histamine in allergic sheep: role of H_2 receptors. *Physiologist*, **24**, 29

66. Ahmed, T., Krainson, J.P. and Yerger, B.S. (1983). Functional depression of H_2 histamine receptors in sheep with experimental allergic asthma. *J. Allergy Clin. Immunol.*, **72**, 310–320

67. Barch, G.K. and Talbot, M.W. (1976). Allergic bronchoconstriction and its drug-induced reversal in anaesthetised ovalbumin-sensitised cats. *Res. Commun. Chem. Pathol. Pharm.*, **13**, 623–633

68. Adcock, J.J., Payne, A.N. and Salmon, J.A. (1983). The role of cyclo-oxygenase metabolites of arachidonic acid in feline anaphylactic bronchospasm. *Br. J. Pharmacol.*, **80**, 440P

69. Lulich, K.M., Mitchell, H.W. and Sparrow, M.P. (1976). The cat lung strip as an in vitro preparation of peripheral airways; a comparison of β-adrenoceptors aganists, autacoids and anaphylactic challenge on the lung strip and trachea. *Br. J. Pharmacol.*, **58**, 71–79

70. O'Neil, R.M. and Goodman, F.R. (1981). Respiratory responses to Ascaris antigen in rhesus and cynomolgus monkeys. *J. Allergy Clin. Immunol.*, **67**, 229–236

71. Patterson, R., Harris, K.E., Suszko, I.M. and Roberts, M. (1976). Reagin-mediated asthma in rhesus monkeys and relation to the bronchial cell histamine release and airway reactivity to carbocholine. *J. Clin. Invest.*, **57**, 586–593

72. Bouhuys, A., Hunt, U.R., Kim, B.M. and Zapletal, A. (1969). Maximum expiratory flow rates in induced bronchoconstriction in man. *J. Clin. Invest.*, **48**, 1159–1168

73. Patterson, R., Talbot, C.H. and Brandfonbrener, M. (1971). The use of IgE mediated responses as a pharmacologic test system. The effect of disodium cromoglycate in respiratory and cutaneous reactions and on the electrocardiograms of rhesus monkeys. *Int. Arch. Allergy Appl. Immunol.*, **41**, 592–603

74. Patterson, R. and Harris, K.E. (1976). The effect of cholinergic and anticholinergic agents on the primate model of allergic asthma. *J. Lab. Clin. Med.*, **87**, 65–72

75. Patterson, R. and Booth, B.H. (1971). Animal models of immediate type respiratory allergy. *NY State J. Med.*, **71**, 755–759

76. Patterson, R. and Harris, K.E. (1981). An inhibitor of the lipoxygenase and cyclooxygenase pathways of arachidonic acid. 5,8,11,14-eicosatetraenoic acid, inhibits immunoglobulin E mediated antigen induced monkey asthma and skin reactions. *Trans. Assoc. Am. Physicians*, **93**, 317–325

77. Mielens, Z.E. and Gormann, W.G. (1984). Effects of FPL55712, ETYA and aminophylline upon ascaris-induced bronchoconstriction in Cynomolgus monkeys. *Int. Arch. Allergy Appl. Immunol.*, **75**, 368–374

78. Patterson, R., Pruzansky, J.J. and Harris, K.E. (1981). An agent that releases basophil and mast cell histamine but blocks cyclooxygenase and lipoxygenase metabolism of arachidonic acid inhibits immunoglobulin E-mediated asthma in rhesus monkeys. *J. Allergy Clin. Immunol.*, **67**, 444–449

79. Johnson, H.G., McNee, M.L., Bach, M.K. and Smith, H.W. (1983). The activity of a new novel inhibitor of leukotriene synthesis in Rhesus monkey Ascaris reactors. *Int. Arch. Allergy Appl. Immunol.*, **70**, 169–173

80. Patterson, R., Harris, K.E., Smith, L.J., Greenberger, P.A., Shaughnessy, M.A., Bernstein, P.R. and Krell, R.D. (1983). Airway response to leukotriene D_4 in rhesus monkeys. *Int. Arch. Allergy Appl. Immunol.*, **71**, 156–160

81. Weichman, B.M., Muccitelli, R.M., Tucker, S.S. and DeVan, J.F.C. (1985). Effect of calcium antagonists on the biosynthesis and contractile effects of peptidoleukotrienes in rhesus monkey lung. *J. Pharmacol. Exp. Ther.*, **233**, 345–351

82. Krell, R.D. (1976). Airway hyper-reactivity to pharmacologic agents in rhesus monkey cutaneously hypersensitive to ascaris antigen. *Life Sci.*, **19**, 1977–1982

83. Wieslander, E., Andersson, P., Linden, M., Axelsson, B., Kallstrom, L., Brattsand, R. and Paulsson, I. (1985). Importance of particulate antigen for the induction of dual bronchial reaction in guinea-pigs. *Agents Actions*, **16**, 37–38

84. Wallace, J.M., Catanzaro, A., Batcher, S. and Abraham, J.L. (1983). A guinea-pig model to study effects of persistent intrabronchial antigenic stimulation and inflammation. *Am. Rev. Respir. Dis.*, **128**, 1077–1083

85. Shampain, M.P., Behrens, B.L., Larsen, G.L. and Henson, P.M. (1982). An animal model of late pulmonary responses to alternaria challenge. *Am. Rev. Respir. Dis.*, **126**, 493–498

86. Behrens, B.L., Clark, R.A.F., Marsh, W. and Larsen, G.L. (1984). Modulation of the late asthmatic response by antigen-specific immunoglobulin G in an animal model. *Am. Rev. Respir. Dis.*, **130**, 1134–1139

87. Marsh, W.R., Irvin, C.G., Murphy, K.R., Behrens, B.L. and Larsen, G.L. (1985). Increases in airway reactivity to histamine and inflammatory cells in bronchoalveolar lavage after the late asthmatic response in an animal model. *Am. Rev. Respir. Dis.*, **131**, 875–879

88. Delehunt, J.C., Perruchoud, A.D., Yerger, L., Marchette, B., Stevenson, J.S. and Abraham, W.M. (1984). The role of slow-reacting substance of anaphylaxis in the late bronchial response after antigen challenge in allergic sheep. *Am. Rev. Respir. Dis.*, **130**, 748–754

89. Abraham, W.M., Perruchoud, A.P., Sielczak, M.W., Yerger, L.D. and Stevenson, J.S. (1985). Airway inflammation during antigen-induced late bronchial obstruction. In Herzog, H. and Perruchoud, A.P. (eds.) *Asthma and Bronchial Hyperreactivity, Progress Respiratory Research*, Vol. 19, pp. 48–55 (Karger: Basel)

90. Abraham, W.M., Wanner, A., Stevenson, J.S. and Chapman, G.A. (1986). The effect of an orally active leukotriene D_4/E_4 antagonist LY 171883 on antigen-induced airway responses in allergic sheep. *Prostaglandins*, **31**, 457–467

91. Abraham, W.M., Lanes, S., Wanner, A., Stevenson, J.S., Codias, E. and Yerger, L.D. (1986). Differences in airway responsiveness to leukotriene D_4 in allergic sheep with and without late bronchial responses. *Prostaglandins*, **31**, 445–455

92. Abraham, W.M., Sielczak, M.W., Perruchoud, A.P., Yerger, L.D. and Stevenson, J.S. (1984). The role of airway inflammation in late phase allergic bronchial obstruction. *Am. Rev. Respir. Dis.*, **129**, A4

93. Piper, P.J. and Vane, J.R. (1969). Release of additional factors of anaphylaxis and its antagonism by anti-inflammatory drugs. *Nature (London)*, **223**, 29–35

94. Nijkamp, F.P., Flower, R.J., Moncada, S. and Vane, J.R. (1976). Partial purification of rabbit aorta contracting substance-releasing factor and inhibition of its activity by anti-inflammatory steroids. *Nature (London)*, **263**, 479–482

95. Al-Ubaidi, F. and Bakhle, Y.S. (1980). Differences in biological activation of arachidonic acid in perfused lungs from guinea-pig, rat and man. *Eur. J. Pharmacol.*, **62**, 89–96

96. Seale, J.P. and Piper, P.J. (1978). Stimulation of arachidonic acid metabolism by human slow-reacting substances. *Eur. J. Pharmacol.*, **52**, 125–128

97. Piper, P.J. and Samhoun, M.N. (1982). Stimulation of arachidonic acid metabolism and generation of thromboxane A_2 in guinea-pig lung in vitro. *Br. J. Pharmacol.*, **77**, 267–275

98. Lefort, J., Rotilio, D. and Vargaftig, B.B. (1984). The platelet-independent release of thromboxane A_2 by PAF-acether from guinea-pig lungs involves mechanisms distinct from those for leukotriene. *Br. J. Pharmacol.*, **82**, 565–575

99. Palmer, M.A., Piper, P. and Vane, J.R. (1973). Release of rabbit aorta contracting substance (RCS) and prostaglandins induced by chemical or mechanical stimulation of guinea-pig lungs. *Br. J. Pharmacol.*, **49**, 226–242

100. Vargaftig, B.B. and Dao, N. (1971). Release of vasoactive substances from guinea-pig lungs by slow-reacting substance C and arachidonic acid. *Pharmacology*, **6**, 99–108

101. Hamberg, M., Svensson, J., Hedqvist, P., Strandberg, K. and Samuelsson, B. (1976). Involvement of endoperoxides and thromboxanes in anaphylactic reactions. In Samuelsson, B and Paoletti, R. (eds.) *Advances in Prostaglandin Research*, Vol. 1, pp. 495–501. (New York: Raven Press)

102. Harvey, J., Holgate, S.T., Peters, B.J., Robinson, C. and Walker, J.R. (1985). Oxidative transformations of arachidonic acid in human dispersed lung cells, disparity between endogenous and exogenous substrate. *Br. J. Pharmacol.*, **86**, 417–426

103. Al-Ubaidi, F. and Bakhle, Y.S. (1980). Differences in biological activation of arachidonic acid in perfused lungs from guinea-pig, rat and man. *Eur. J. Pharmacol.*, **62**, 89–96

104. Payne, A.N. and Lees, I.W. (1986). Cardio-pulmonary effects of arachidonic acid aerosols in guinea-pigs and rats. Presented at the *6th International Conference on Prostaglandins and Related Compounds*, June 3–6, Florence

105. Quan, S.F., Moon, M.A. and Lemen, (1982). Effects of arachidonic acid, PGF_{2z} and a PGH_2 analogue on airway diameters in dogs. *J. Appl. Physiol. (Respir. Environ. Exercise Physiol.)*, **53**, 1005–1014

106. Frey, H.H. and Dengjel, R.J. (1976). Antagonism of arachidonic acid-induced bronchoconstriction in cats by aspirin-like analgesics. *Eur. J. Pharmacol.*, **40**, 345–348

107. Sirois, P., Chagnon, M., Borgeat, O. and Vallerand, P. (1985). Role of cyclooxygenase products in the lung action of Leukotrienes A_4, B_4, C_4, D_4 and E_4. *Pharmacology*, **31**, 225–236

108. Larsen, G.L. (1985). Hypersensitivity lung disease. *Ann. Rev. Immunol.*, **3**, 59–85

109. Brigham, K.L. (1984). Pulmonary dysfunction caused by diffuse lung inflammation. In Ferruccio, B., Hurd, S. and Johnson Hegyeli, R. (eds.) *Cyclooxygenase and Lipoxygenase Modulators in Lung Reactivity, Progress in Biochemical Pharmacology*, Vol. 20, pp. 26–27

110. Sladen, A. (1976). Methylprednisolone. Pharmacologic doses in shock lung syndrome. *J. Thorac. Cardiovasc. Surg.*, **71**, 800–806

111. Rinaldo, J.E. and Rodgers, R.M. (1982). Adult respiratory distress syndrome: changing concepts of lung injury and repair. *N. Engl. J. Med.*, **300**, 900–909

112. Fallat, R.J., Mielke, Jr., C.H. and Rodvien, R. (1980). Adult respiratory distress syndrome and Gram-negative sepsis. *Arch. Intern. Med.*, **140**, 612–613

113. Kaplan, R.L. and Sahn, S.A. (1979). Incidence and outcome of the respiratory distress syndrome in Gram-negative sepsis. *Arch. Intern. Med.*, **139**, 867–869

114. Pepe, P.E., Potkin, R.T., Reus, D.H., Hudson, L.D. and Carrico, C.J. (1982). Clinical predictors of the adult respiratory distress syndrome. *Am. J. Surg.*, **144**, 124–130

115. Hudson, L.D. (1982). Causes of the adult respiratory distress syndrome – clinical recognition. *Clin. Chest Med.*, **3**, 195–212

116. Wardle, E.N. (1984). Shock lungs; the post traumatic respiratory syndrome. *Q. J. Med.*, **211**, 317–319

117. Fine, A.M., Lippman, N., Holdzman, H., Eliarz, A. and Goldberg, S.K. (1983). The risk factors, incidences and prognosis of the adult respiratory distress syndrome following septicemia. *Chest*, **83**, 40–42

118. Bachofen, M., Bachofen, H. and Weibel, E. (1979). Lung edema in the adult respiratory distress syndrome. In Fishman, A.P. and Renkin, E.W. (eds.) *Pulmonary Edema*, pp. 241–252 (Baltimore: Williams and Wilkins)

119. Gorin, A.B., Weidner, W.J., Demling, R.M. and Staub, N.C. (1978). Non-invasive measurements of pulmonary transvascular protein flux in sheep. *J. Appl. Physiol.*, **45**, 225–233

120. Prichard, J.S., Rajagopalan, B. and Lee, G. (1980). Transvascular albumin flux and the interstitial water volume in experimental pulmonary oedema in dogs. *Clin. Sci.*, **59**, 105–113

121. Brigham, K.L. and Dukes, S.S. (1985). Prostaglandins in lung disease. *Semin. Respir. Med.*, **7**, 11–16

122. Sheller, J.R. and Brigham, K.L. (1984). Effect of leukotrienes on sheep airways smooth muscle. *Am. Rev. Respir. Dis.*, **129**, A232

123. Ogletree, M.L., Snapper, J.R. and Brigham, K.L. (1982). Immediate pulmonary vascular and airways responses after intravenous LTD$_4$ injections in awake sheep. *Physiologist*, **25**, 275

124. Ogletree, M.L. and Brigham, K.L. (1984). Pulmonary vascular and hemo-dynamic effects of prostaglandin E$_1$ in unanaesthetised sheep. *Microcirc. Endothel. Lymph.*, **1**, 307–327

125. Williams, T.J. and Piper, P.J. (1980). The action of chemically pure SRS-A on the microcirculation in vivo. *Prostaglandins*, **19**, 779–789

126. Albert, R. and Henderson, W. (1982). Leukotriene C$_4$ increases pulmonary vascular permeability in excised rat lungs. *Fed. Proc.*, **41**, 1503

127 Dahlén, S., Bjork, J., Hedqvist, P., Arfors, K.E., Hammarström, S., Lindgren, J.A. and Samuelsson, B. (1981). Leukotrienes promote plasma leakage and leukocyte adhesion in post-capillary venules. *Proc. Natl. Acad. Sci. USA*, **78**, 3887–3891

128. Fletcher, J.R. and Ramwell, P.W. (1980). Indomethacin treatment following baboon endotoxin shock improves survival. *Adv. Shock Res.*, **4**, 103–111

129. Short, B.L., Gardiner, M., Walker, R.I., Jones, R.S. and Fletcher, J.R. (1981). Indomethacin improves survival in gram-negative sepsis. *Adv. Shock Res.*, **6**, 27–36

130. Pingleton, W.W., Coalson, J.J., Hinshaw, L.B. and Guenter, C.A. (1972). Effects of steroid pretreatment on development of shock lung. *Lab. Invest.*, **27**, 445–456

131. Snapper, J.R., Hutchinson, A.A., Ogletree, M.L., Brigham, K.L. and Stahlman, M.T. (1983). Effects of cyclooxygenase inhibition on the response to group B streptococcal toxin in sheep. *Pediatr. Res.*, **17**, 107

132. Brigham, K.L., Bowers, R.E. and McKeen, C.R. (1981). Methylprednisolone prevention of increased lung vascular permeability following endotoxemia in sheep. *J. Clin. Invest.*, **67**, 1103–1110

133. James, P.M. (1975). Treatment of shock lung. *Am. Surg.*, **41**, 451–456

134. Du Toit, H.J., Erasmus, F.R., MacFarlane, C.M., Taljaard, J.J.F., King, J.B., Klerk, A.J. and Elk, E. (1984). Methylprednisolone and the adult respiratory distress syndrome. *S. Afr. Med. J.*, **65**, 1049–1053

135. Blackwell, G.J., Carnuccio, R., Di Rosa, M., Flower, R.J., Parente, L. and Persico, P. (1980). Macrocortin: a polypeptide causing the anti-phospholipase effect of glucocorticoids. *Nature (London)*, **287**, 147–149

136. Jones, R., Reid, L.M., Zapol, W.M., Tomashefski, J.F., Kirton, O.C. and Kobayashi, K. (1985). Pulmonary vascular pathology: human and experimental studies. In Lenfant, C. (ed.) *Acute Respiratory Failure*, pp. 23–160. (New York: Marcel-Dekker)

137. Marsico, S.A., Severi, B., Grillone, G. and Zanoni, A. (1980). Ultrastructural changes in the non-cardiogenic pulmonary oedema. *Bronchopneumologie*, **32**, 111–129

138. Adamson, I.Y.R., Bowden, D.H. and Wyatt, J.P. (1970). Oxygen poisoning in mice – ultrastructural and surfactant studies during exposure and recovery. *Arch. Pathol.*, **90**, 463–472

139. Kistler, G.S., Caldwell, P.R.B. and Weibel, E. (1967). Development of fine structural damage to alveolar and capillary lining cells in oxygen-poisoned rat lungs. *J. Cell Biol.*, **32**, 605–628

140. Nucci, G., de, Astbury, P., Read, N., Salmon, J.A. and Moncada, S. (1986). Release of eicosanoids from isolated lungs of guinea-pigs exposed to pure oxygen: effect of dexamethasone. *Eur. J. Pharmacol.*, **126**, 11–20

141. Blackwell, G.J., Flower, R.J., Nijkamp, F.P. and Vane, J.R. (1978). Phospholipase A$_2$ activity of guinea-pig isolated perfused lungs: stimulation and inhibition by anti-inflammatory steroids. *Br. J. Pharmacol.*, **62**, 79–89

142. Nucci, G. de and Moncada, S. (1985). Inhaled corticosteroids for respiratory distress? *Lancet*, **2**, 1061

143. Reinitz, E.R., Motoyama, E., Smith, G.J.W. and Kerstein, M.D. (1977). Pulmonary sequelae of experimental pancreatitis. *J. Surg. Res.*, **22**, 566–579

144. Kerstein, M.D. and Iannou, N. (1984). Pulmonary surface tension after nontoxic experimental pancreatitis. *Ann. Surg.*, **50**, 375−376
145. Cunningham, A.L. and Hurley, J.V. (1972). Alpha-naphthylthiourea-induced pulmonary oedema in the rat: a topographical and electron-microscope study. *J. Pathol.*, **106**, 25−35
146. Meyrick, B., Miller, J. and Reid, L. (1972). Pulmonary oedema induced by ANTU, or by high or low oxygen concentrations in rat − an electron microscopic study. *Br. J. Exp. Pathol.*, **53**, 347−358
147. Pankhania, J.J. and Bakhle, Y.S. (1985). Effect of pulmonary oedema induced by α-naphthylthiourea on synthesis of cyclo-oxygenase products in rat isolated lungs. *Prostaglandins*, **30**, 37−49
148. Weiland, J.E., Davis, W.B., Holter, J.E., Mohamed, J.H., Dorinsky, P.M. and Gadek, J.E. (1986). Lung neutrophils in the adult respiratory distress syndrome: Clinical and pathophysiological significance. *Am. Rev. Respir. Dis.*, **133**, 218−235
150. Fink, J.N. (1984). Hypersensitivity pneumonitis. *J. Allergy Clin. Immunol.*, **74**, 1−10
151. Olenchock, S.A. (1977). Animal models of hypersensitivity pneumonitis. *Ann. Allergy*, **38**, 119−126
152. Yoshizawa, Y., Nakazawa, T., Ripani, L.M. and Moore, V.L. (1982). Development of chronic pulmonary inflammation in immunised guinea-pigs by aerosol challenge with antigen: relationship of immune complex disease and cell-mediated hypersensitivity. *J. Allergy Clin. Immunol.*, **70**, 114−119
153. Calvanico, N.J. and Garancis, J.C. (1985). Specificity and duration of post inflammatory suppression in rabbit-lungs challenged with aerosolized antigen. *Clin. Exp. Immunol.*, **59**, 336−342
154. Gardner, D.L. (1972). *The Pathology of Rheumatoid Arthritis.* (London: Edward Arnold)
155. Klareskog, L., Urba, F., Scheynius, A., Kabelitz, D. and Wigzell, H. (1982). Evidence in support of a self-perpetuating HLA-DR-dependent delayed-type cell reaction in rheumatoid arthritis. *Proc. Natl. Acad. Sci. USA*, **79**, 3632−3636
156. Winchester, R.J., Kunkel, H.G. and Agnello, V. (1971). Occurrence of gamma globulin complexes in serum and joint fluid of rheumatoid arthritis patients: use of monoclonal rheumatoid factors as reagents for their demonstration. *J. Exp. Med.*, **134**, 286S−295S
157. Good, R.A., Rotstein, J. and Mazzitello, W.F. (1957). The simultaneous occurrence of rheumatoid arthritis and agammaglobulinaemia. *J. Lab. Clin. Med.*, **49**, 343−357
158. Balow, J.E., Austin, H.A. and Tsokos, G.C. (1984). Plasmapheresis therapy in immunologically mediated rheumatic and renal diseases. *Clin. Immunol. Rev.*, **3**, 235−272
159. Billingham, M.E.J. (1983). Models of arthritis and the search for anti-arthritic drugs. *Pharmacol. Ther.*, **21**, 389−428
160. Smith, M.N., Tucker, M.J. and Billingham, M.E.J. (1982). Experimental arthritis in the rat: a disease caused by periosteal cell activation? In *Proceedings of FECTS VIIIth Meeting Copenhagen*, p. 167
161. Vane, J.R. (1971). Inhibition of prostaglandin synthesis as a mechanism of action for the aspirin-like drugs. *Nature (London)*, **231**, 232−235
162. Aspinall, R.L. and Cammarata, P.S. (1969). Effect of prostaglandin E_2 on adjuvant arthritis. *Nature (London)*, **224**, 1320−1321
163. Zurier, R.B. and Quagliata, F. (1971). Effect of prostaglandin E_1 on adjuvant arthritis. *Nature (London)*, **234**, 304−305
164. Trentham, D.E., Townes, A.S. and Kang, A.H. (1977). Autoimmunity to the type II collagen: an experimental model of arthritis. *J. Exp. Med.*, **146**, 857−868
165. Courtenay, J.S., Dallman, M.J., Dayan, A.D., Martin, A. and Mosedale, B. (1980). Immunisation against heterologous type II collagen induces arthritis in mice. *Nature (London)*, **283**, 666−668
166. Andriopoulos, N.A., Mestecky, J., Miller, E.J. and Bradley, E.L. (1976). Antibodies to native and denatured collagens in sera of patients with rheumatoid arthritis. *Arthr. Rheum.*, **19**, 613−617
167. Trentham, D.E., Dynesius, R.A., Rocklin, R.E. and David, J.R. (1978). Cellular sensitivity to collagen in rheumatoid arthritis. *N. Engl. J. Med.*, **299**, 327−332
168. Sloboda, A.E., Birnbaum, J.E., Oronsky, A.L. and Kerner, S.S. (1981). Studies on type II collagen-induced polyarthritis in rats. Effect of anti-inflammatory and anti-rheumatic agents. *Arthr. Rheum.*, **24**, 616−624

215

169. Klein, D.C. and Raisz, L.G. (1970). Prostaglandins: stimulation of bone resorption in tissue culture. *Endocrinology*, **86**, 1436–1440
170. Leslie, C.A., Gonnerman, W.A., Ullman, M.D., Hayes, K.C., Franzblau, C. and Cathcart, E.S. (1985). Dietary fish oil modulates macrophage fatty acids and decreases arthritis susceptibility in mice. *J. Exp. Med.*, **162**, 1336–1349
171. Prickett, J.D., Trentham, D.E. and Robinson, D.R. (1984). Dietary fish oil augments the induction of arthritis in rats immunised with type II collagen. *J. Immunol.*, **132**, 725–729
172. Dumonde, D.C. and Glynn, L.E. (1962). The production of arthritis in rabbits by an immunological reaction to fibrin. *Br. J. Exp. Pathol.*, **43**, 373–383
173. Hunneyball, I.M. (1984). Use of experimental arthritis in the rabbit for the development of antiarthritic drugs. In Otterness, I., Capetola, R. and Wong, S. (eds.) *Advances in Inflammation Research*. Vol. 7, pp. 249–262. (New York: Raven Press)
174. Blackham, A., Farmer, J.B., Radziwonik, M. and Westwick, J. (1974). The role of prostaglandins in rabbit monoarticular arthritis. *Br. J. Pharmacol.*, **51**, 35–44
175. Henderson, B. and Higgs, G.A. Synthesis of arachidonate oxidation products by tissues of the synovial joint during the development of chronic erosive arthritis. *Arthr. Rheum.*, **30**, 1034–1042
176. Higgs, G.A., Salmon, J.A. and Spayne, J.A. (1981). The inflammatory effects of hydroperoxy and hydroxyacid products of arachidonate lipoxygenase in rabbit skin. *Br. J. Pharmacol.*, **74**, 429–433
177. Fitzgerald, M.F., Henderson, B., Higgs, G.A., Parente, L. and Pettipher, E.R. (1985). The levels of PAF and lyso-PAF in the joint fluids of rabbits with antigen-induced arthritis. *Br. J. Pharmacol.*, **86**, 422P
178. Issekutz, A.C. (1983). Comparison of the effects of glucocorticoid and indomethacin treatment on the acute inflammatory reaction in rabbits. *Immunopharmacology*, **5**, 183–195
179. Hellewell, P.G. and Williams, T.J. (1985). Suppression of inflammatory oedema in rabbit skin by two PAF antagonists, 48740RP and L-652731. *Prostaglandins*, **30**, 713
180. Glynn, L.E. (1968). The chronicity of inflammation and its significance in rheumatoid arthritis. *Ann. Rheum. Dis.*, **27**, 105–121
181. Robinson, C. and Holgate, S.T. (1985). New perspectives on the putative role of eicosanoids in airway hyperresponsiveness. *J. Allergy Clin. Immunol.*, **76**, 140–144
182. Cuss, F.M., Dixon, C.M. and Barnes, P.J. (1986). Inhaled platelet activating factor causes bronchoconstriction and increased reactivity in man. *Am. Rev. Respir. Dis.*, **132**, A212
183. Morley, J., Page, C.P. and Sanjar, S. (1985). Pharmacology of the late response to allergen and its relevance to asthma prophylaxis. *Int. Arch. Allergy Appl. Immunol.*, **77**, 73–78

Index